Recovery in Mental Health

World Psychiatric Association *Evidence and Experience in Psychiatry* Series

Series Editor: Helen Herrman (2005 -)
WPA Secretary for Publications, University of Melbourne, Australia

The *Evidence & Experience in Psychiatry* series, launched in 1999, offers unique insights into both investigation and practice in mental health. Developed and commissioned by the World Psychiatric Association, the books address controversial issues in clinical psychiatry and integrate research evidence and clinical experience to provide a stimulating overview of the field.

Focused on common psychiatric disorders, each volume follows the same format: systematic review of the available research evidence followed by multiple commentaries written by clinicians of different orientations and from different countries. Each includes coverage of diagnosis, management, pharma and psycho- therapies, and social and economic issues. The series provides insights that will prove invaluable to psychiatrists, psychologists, mental health nurses and policy makers.

Depressive Disorders, 3e
Edited by Helen Herrman, Mario Maj and Norman Sartorius
ISBN: 9780470987209

Substance Abuse
Edited by Hamid Ghodse, Helen Herrman, Mario Maj and Norman Sartorius
ISBN: 9780470745106

Schizophrenia 2e
Edited by Mario Maj, Norman Sartorius
ISBN: 9780470849644

Dementia 2e
Edited by Mario Maj, Norman Sartorius
ISBN: 9780470849637

Obsessive-Compulsive Disorders 2e
Edited by Mario Maj, Norman Sartorius, Ahmed Okasha, Joseph Zohar
ISBN: 9780470849668

Bipolar Disorders
Edited by Mario Maj, Hagop S Akiskal, Juan José López-Ibor, Norman Sartorius
ISBN: 9780471560371

Eating Disorders
Edited by Mario Maj, Kathrine Halmi, Juan José López-Ibor, Norman Sartorius
ISBN: 9780470848654

Phobias
Edited by Mario Maj, Hagop S Akiskal, Juan José López-Ibor, Ahmed Okasha
ISBN: 9780470858332

Personality Disorders
Edited by Mario Maj, Hagop S Akiskal, Juan E Mezzich
ISBN: 9780470090367

Somatoform Disorders
Edited by Mario Maj, Hagop S Akiskal, Juan E Mezzich, Ahmed Okasha
ISBN: 9780470016121

Recovery in Mental Health
Reshaping Scientific and Clinical Responsibilities

Written by

Michaela Amering and Margit Schmolke

Based on a translation by Peter Stastny

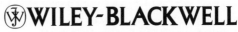

A John Wiley & Sons, Ltd., Publication

Library of Congress Cataloging-in-Publication Data

Amering, Michaela.
　　[Recovery. English]
　　Recovery in mental health : reshaping scientific and clinical responsibilities / written by Michaela Amering and Margit Schmolke ; translated by Peter Stastny.
　　　p. ; cm.
　　Includes bibliographical references and index.
　　ISBN 978-0-470-99796-3
　1. Mental health services. 2. Recovery movement. I. Schmolke, Margit. II. Title.
　　[DNLM: 1. Mental Disorders–rehabilitation. 2. Health Policy. 3. Treatment Outcome. WM 400 A5133r 2009]
　　RA790.5.A45 2009
　　616.89–dc22

　　　　　　　　　　　　　　　　　　　　　2008044599

ISBN: 978-0-470-99796-3

A catalogue record for this book is available from the British Library

Typeset in 10.25/12 Times by Laserwords Private Limited, Chennai, India
Printed in Singapore by Markono Print Media Pte Ltd

First impression   2009

Contents

Foreword

Recovery in mental health – reshaping scientific and clinical responsibilities, is not just 'another text' on mental illness. To fully understand the wisdom this book offers, the reader needs to appreciate the different perspectives these two authors provide. Michaela Amering and Margit Schmolke, both personally and professionally, honour the knowledge-base that emerges from those who have struggled and triumphed over illness and distress. Although the addition of this 'lived experience' knowledge-base to the dominant discourses of psychiatry is both challenging and paradoxical at times, its use for providing supportive environments for people experiencing mental illness/distress can ultimately transform how we think about supporting another in distress.

When I was first diagnosed with a mental illness over two decades ago, the concept that I could recover and reclaim a life beyond illness was not something ever discussed by my treating team. In fact, the opposite was discussed more vigorously: much time and effort was devoted to educating and convincing me that the illness was permanent, and most likely to prevent me living a full life. Plans were drawn up for my long-term care and treatment in environments that risked disconnecting me from my roles, opportunities, rights and responsibilities. These are not the messages of encouragement and hope that you expect from health professionals. I can remember desperately trying to find information that would contradict this prediction and provide me with hope. The bookshops and libraries that I visited had numerous books depicting the demise of a person diagnosed with a mental illness, which only served to reinforce the downward spiralling predictions given to my family and myself of what lay ahead.

What I needed was to find *this* book amongst the many bookshelves that I scoured. I often wonder how the course of overcoming a mental illness might have been different, if anyone had dared to utter anything about the possibilities of overcoming and reclaiming a life beyond illness. Sadly, my story of poor expectations, cautious outcomes, and lack of belief in the possibilities of recovery, is not mine alone, but one encountered by many.

FOREWORDFOREWORD

Overcoming the impact of a mental illness and its treatment is not easy: it is even more impressive when people recount stories of how they have triumphed in spite of negative and cynical predictions and without encouragement from others. The effort involved in reclaiming a life beyond illness belongs to the individual. It is a journey that requires great determination, self-belief and personal effort. It is also a journey that each person must ultimately decide upon, take responsibility for and be central to.

Somewhere along the way, I lost my sense of being able to 'self-right', owing to the nature of having a mental illness and the constant focus on what was wrong, what needed changing and what was still ahead to achieve. Ultimately, I was filled with a sense of failure – that being so, the experience of recovery was far beyond me. If anything changed for the positive, I named the external supports that were propping me up as the reason. I named the doctors, nurses, hospital admissions, support groups, day programme, case managers, family, friends, medications, etc., but I did not name myself. I had lost my sense of what I could do to contribute to my own well-being, and this only served to reinforce my sense of failure and impotence. This idea that they are incapable of 'self-righting' due to their illness, becomes a perpetually self-fulfilling prophecy for both the person receiving support, and for the care provider, who then feels they need to provide total support to prevent a person from succumbing. Nobody learns of other ways to be with each other unless we step outside our comfort zone and dare to try something different.

No one else, whether they are family, friends or workers, can 'recover' a person, no matter how much they long for that to be occur. What then, is the role of the 'other', if not to create recovery for them? The role of the 'other' is to be in genuine relationships with people and create environments of support in which a person can negotiate their sense of 'self-righting'. If we dare to name ourselves as a supporter of another, then we must adhere to a number of foci in our support. Firstly, we must believe that a person has the capacity to 'self- right' or recover. Secondly, we must work 'as if' recovery is always real, present and possible, even though we might never have the privilege of being a full witness to it. We have to ensure that the environments of support provided are sufficiently accessible for a person to be able to exercise their recovery-effort within them, and we have to be mindful not to stand in the way of, nor to inhibit their unique efforts to overcome.

There are numerous personal, professional and societal core beliefs that underpin the manner in which treatment and care are provided. The core belief that people will always need support and that they cannot determine and self manage their life-journey is an old story – one that is not supported by the growing evidence from those with a lived experience of being 'in recovery' from mental illness. The authors extend an invitation to us to embrace this growing and emerging evidence that people can reclaim their lives and often thrive beyond the experience of a mental illness or distress.

In this book, Michaela and Margit highlight the importance of creating alternative environments of support; they stress that peer support, peer-controlled and -operated services need to be integral to any comprehensive system of care. The value for those who have been in receipt of good peer support is repeated within many lived-experience narratives, be it natural, informal or professional peer support. How the nature of peer support provision differs from the support of non-peer providers is a question that services should reflect upon. Peer support asks the supporter to draw on their lived experience as their main informant on how to support another in distress. This is not a formally acquired knowledge and skill-base, but one that has been gathered through the triumphs and struggles over illness or distress, instilling an inherent 'knowing' that recovery is real, ongoing, full of discovery, takes effort and is ultimately transforming. With this focus, a peer is able to create a space for another, to support kindly and challenge where necessary, encouraging similar triumph over illness and distress.

This relationship has been repeatedly named as essential, when people are asked what helps and what hinders their recovery processes. The authors have rightfully challenged the beliefs, held by some, that place the role of the therapeutic relationship in health outcomes as 'soft evidence'. People with a lived experience have clearly named what is helpful and unhelpful within therapeutic encounters. It is not the technical skills provided that usually get named, but whether a person experiences relationships as either helpful or unhelpful. To remedy this, health professionals must risk bringing their full personhood to the relationship, not just their professional identity.

There is more to well-being than the absence of illness. There is much more to recovery than the absence or presence of symptoms. If the management or treatment of symptoms alone becomes the focus of a person's interaction with health professionals, then the risk of adopting an illness-saturated identity is extremely high. Being viewed through an illness-centric lens is a consistent and universal lament from many who receive services. When systems of care focus on the modification, amelioration, management, treatment or support of illness alone, the risk for many is an increasing sense of institutionalization, difference and ultimately alienation. This is the essence and root of stigma, discrimination and institutionalization and the foundation of disability.

Michaela and Margit remind us to be ever mindful of the invitation to replace our person-centric gaze with an illness-centric focus. In our relationships with others, we need to ensure that a person has opportunities to realize their capacity to influence their distress, re-establish their authorship of their own lives, connect with their sense of sameness, and be in awe and wonder at their constant efforts of 'self-righting'. This is one of the greatest gifts that we can offer another.

Michaela and Margit have provided us all with an opportunity to reflect on how our practices can be informed by those with a lived experience of overcoming, ultimately enhancing how we relate to and provide environments of support. This opportunity to learn is not just in the reading of this work, but in the invitation to continually seek out the lived-experience wisdom that constantly surrounds us.

Helen Glover

September 2008

CHAPTER 1

Introduction

Over the last few years important English-speaking countries such as the USA, the UK, Ireland, Australia, New Zealand, and Canada have embraced recovery-orientation as a guiding principle of their mental health policy. Major stakeholders and different professional groups have expressed their loyalty to the concept. Guidelines, training modules and system transformation initiatives have followed swiftly and experiences and data as well as complex and controversial discussions are emerging.

Interestingly, the rest of the world has not yet reacted in any discernible way. In 2005 we felt a strong need to bring these developments, at that time known mainly only to English speakers, to a German-speaking audience (Amering and Schmolke, 2007). Our book was greeted with great interest throughout the Swiss, German and Austrian mental health community.

Our participation in the World Psychiatric Association (WPA) and other international initiatives led to the idea of translating the book into the different languages of interested mental health professionals, users and carers. We had started to make plans for Turkish, Ukrainian, Serbian and Spanish editions when English-speaking colleagues and friends pointed out that comprehensive accounts of the background, developments and uses of the term and concept of recovery were not yet readily available in English. And indeed, while much has been written about recovery, most of it is in electronic form or in scientific articles and policy papers, no doubt reflecting the pace of change in this fast-moving field.

Wiley-Blackwell decided to venture on a translation of the book. We updated and amended the material and edited the specific references to the situation in the German-speaking countries. The book was originally written for an audience for whom the recovery-concept was new. This English language version will reach many more people who have perhaps only recently become interested in recovery. At the same time it will also be available to audiences in countries like the US and the UK, from where the main impetus of the concept came and where the mental health field has been in close contact with the concept for many years as it is government policy in those countries. The extremely fast development from a bottom-up concept into a top-down policy approach, with all the resulting implementation efforts and bureaucratic power struggles must have created challenging problems, some of which will have had aspects peculiar to their specific locations. The speed of the development of the concept and the challenges that have arisen during its implementation could well make a fresh and comprehensive look at recovery both timely and welcome.

This is a WPA book and we hope that it will help people all over the world who work locally but who also read and communicate internationally in English. Also, as in the

Recovery in Mental Health: Reshaping scientific and clinical responsibilities Michaela Amering and Margit Schmolke
Copyright © 2009 John Wiley & Sons, Ltd

original German version we did try to write in such a way that the book would be a resource not only for researchers, policy-makers and clinicians with a professional psychiatric background, but also for interested readers with other professional or experiential backgrounds and people with a lived experience of mental health problems in their own life or in the lives of their loved ones and friends. Peter Stastny's expert translation has certainly also added to this aspect of the book.

For individuals who are facing the challenge of a serious psychiatric disorder, recovery has always been a very significant path from the limitations of patienthood to a self-determined and meaningful life. Bolstering resilience is an essential element of the healing process, which involves marshalling the powers of resistance and providing a constructive adaptation to difficult circumstances, and also the mobilization of energies in order to protect the person from demoralizing resignation and self-stigmatization. Professional help is often a crucial aspect of recovery-processes. However, it often fails to respond to important opportunities, and may even be a hindrance to the efforts people make towards their own recovery.

Ever since users of mental health services have gone beyond merely telling their stories, to recording, publishing, organizing and researching them, their invaluable experiences and what they have learned have become accessible to the general public. Professional circles have been quick to respond. Recovery-concepts were adopted and their implications for research and practice are being spelled out. Recovery-oriented supports are being called for and increasingly promulgated. New research designs are being explored and put into practice. Newly defined criteria for remission and recovery are being formulated and should lead to higher expectations and to the development of new kinds of support. These new kinds of support need to be evaluated according to the extent to which they can contribute to the strengthening of the resilience and the health of individuals with serious mental health problems.

Is hope as a precondition for recovery indeed justified? We believe that you will come away from reading this book with an affirmative answer to this question. All scientific data about course and treatments for severe mental health problems are pointing in a direction where it no longer makes sense to be swayed by a diagnosis towards an unfavourable prognosis. The fact that psychiatric disorders can have highly variable courses should not lead us to assume the worst. The difficult job of overcoming the temporary strain of an illness-episode should not induce us to take refuge in prognostication for the future.

Pronouncements such as "You are too ill for talk therapy" or "You will never be able to pursue a career as a dancer" are as inappropriate as "Everything will be just like before" or "He will never be able to rely on himself". Such predictions are not just factually wrong, but also quite harmful. We know how destructive such statements can be. To destroy someone's dreams for their life is a catastrophe, especially at a time when a person is making every effort to overcome a mental health crisis. And we know very well how important it is to envision the possibility of new developments, aspirations and solutions to the current situation.

To some extent, these facts have been known for a long time. The same applies to the prejudices and misguided traditions in this area. Obviously, it can take a long time for certain facts to be recognized and certain attitudes to be transformed accordingly. On the other hand, there are times when paradigms topple rather precipitously and we may be in a period when just such a thing is occurring. The stigma of immutability and incurability can be overcome. Over time an exciting and autonomous research domain area has emerged, in which people with a lived experience of mental health problems and services develop and carry out scientific projects. There have been many important collaborations between researchers and service users. Service users are contributing their expert opinions directly to clinical work, and are working as providers, advisors and trainers, as well as working in their own autonomous services and on other projects. Governments have begun to endorse these collaborative efforts by establishing recovery-orientation in their health service policies. By doing this, they aim to enhance the effectiveness of existing services and research projects, while at the same time promoting and establishing new initiatives and concepts.

As clinicians and researchers we are impressed by the challenges and opportunities that the recovery movement presents to the field of mental health. And we recognize the new scientific and clinical responsibilities in support of people with mental health problems in their efforts towards making full use of their health and resilience in order to achieve their goals in life. In this book we address conceptual issues as well as different ways of contrasting, delineating, and combining existing strategies and concepts with the current new definitions and meanings of recovery. The implications of recovery-orientation for our scientific responsibilities include the development of novel research policies and methodologies for many urgent research questions. Consequences for mental health policy, service provision and therapeutic relationships include new strategies and tools as well as evaluative data and attempts at system transformation from different regions. All this, as well as the consideration of obstacles, misunderstandings and problems, are arranged around the core of the book, which consists of exemplary stories of people who, as pioneers, have made their own stories and their experience in self-help and advocacy – in addition to their traditional professional expertise – available, and who have created models and language for recovery, which have laid the groundwork and made their way into planning and practice. The collaboration between mental health professionals without a lived experience and users and former users of services is a key condition for the implementation of recovery-concepts and will appear as a major topic in all parts of the book.

CHAPTER 2

Recovery – Developments and Significance

Recovery is nothing new. The notion of recovery has always been part of the medical discourse in different ways. However, in mental health, the issue of recovery has taken on a rather urgent dynamic in recent years. Clinicians, policy-makers, health-care planners, politicians, advocates, managers and scientists are busy trying to make recovery into a goal and a central concept of their efforts. For an exploration of *The Roots of Recovery: What can be Learned from 300 Years of Efforts to Treat People with Mental Illnesses as People* see Larry Davidson, in press at Wiley-Blackwell. To explain the current 'rediscovery of recovery' in its 'new meaning' Ramon *et al.* (2007) suggest several factors, including long-term follow-up studies and the consequences of de-institutionalization. They highlight the recognition and the essential impact of the user movement and experiential knowledge as well as the social model of disability, with its focus on the interaction between individual and environment and the acceptance of the strength model and the focus on counteracting stigma and fostering social inclusion. Recovery in its 'new meaning' talks about outcome as well as about process, about agency as well as interdependency, broaches risk avoidance as well as risk-taking, moves away from a deficit model towards empowerment, resilience and hope and formulates transformative implications for society, health and mental health policy, services and users of services. Mental health services can be helpful for recovery if they succeed in fostering control, choice and hope, but harmful if they undermine self-determination and convey pessimism and hopelessness.

The current convergence of the interests and activities of service users and those of mental health professionals is a central element in coming to an understanding of these new developments. These would not have been possible other than as an extension and logical consequence of the achievements of the consumer movement. What is new in the role that recovery plays today is the increasing readiness and expertise of those users and mental health professionals who are engaged in collaborative efforts. The fact that empowered service users have had many successes and have been able to find ways of understanding and influencing the professional mental health system, is key for any current developments towards recovery. Most conceptual and political considerations and decisions have evolved from collaborations between people with and without a lived experience of mental health problems and the psychiatric service system. Many of the most influential publications on this subject were written by users and ex-users

Recovery in Mental Health: Reshaping scientific and clinical responsibilities Michaela Amering and Margit Schmolke
Copyright © 2009 John Wiley & Sons, Ltd

of services and work-groups that have brought together individuals with and without personal experiences as psychiatric patients.

'Recovery-based practice is the synthesis of professional and lived experience knowledge-bases, and is not simply an additional aspect to the way we already deliver services. If recovery-based practice knowledge is to be authentically developed then it will require constant attention to the synthesising of professional and lived experience knowledges, ultimately fusing into a shared knowledge-base' (Glover 2005, p 2). The positive aspects of recovery as a broad umbrella concept have been pointed out, for example, by Rachel Perkins (Turner-Crowson J, Wallcraft J 2002, p 249)–'Whether mental health problems are viewed in biological, social, psychological or spiritual terms, recovery is still a necessary process' or by Wesley Sowers (2007, p 5) 'Recovery creates a community that all can take part in as it erases the distinctions of position, age, skin colour, religion, language, and education and joins us in our common humanity. If we fail to recognize this capacity for recovery to unite us, we will have squandered a great opportunity to integrate our highly fragmented and siloed service systems. If we fail to understand that we are all engaged in a similar struggle, we will miss the opportunity to empathically engage those who seek comfort and hope'.

Recovery reflects 'common sense' (Amering 2008). But is it a 'common purpose' (Roberts and Hollins, 2007)? Concerns by mental health professionals are often expressed in terms of fear of misunderstandings and illusionary hopes and expectations, lack of clear definition and lack of scientific evidence (Roberts and Hollins, 2007). The idea that for recovery-orientation to survive and gain impact research evidence is essential is quite prevalent among professionals thinking about policy change and system transformation (for example, Slade and Hayward 2007; Liberman and Kopelowicz, 2005). Other specific obstacles have been highlighted, for example a funding system that is aiming at programmes for user populations and does not allow individualized packages, services' pessimism and avoidance of even calculated risks (Ramon *et al.* 2007) and the need for professionals to share power. Worries also concern the possible misuse of the concept in order to cut services (Roberts and Hollins, 2007), which would be a cynical further aggravation of an already deplorable situation of 'scarcity, inequity, and inefficiency' of resources for mental health care and the protection of the human rights of people with mental health problems all over the world (Saxena *et al.* 2007). Users, user advocates and researchers with a lived experience have voiced concerns along the lines of the 'risk of professional colonization of this very special and very different knowledge-base' (Glover 2005) and co-option of the recovery movement and dilution of its challenges by the mental health system.

The essential element of what started out as the recovery movement in the 1980s is the voice of the user movement. Through successful co-operation between different stakeholders the essential expertise through lived experience and the results of user-led and user-controlled research should provide the mental health field with a multi-perspective evidence-base for policy and development (Rose *et al.* 2006). This should in turn strengthen the growth and impact of 'a civil rights movement dedicated to the liberation of people with mental illness from being marginalized, from being excluded, and from being shunned' (Thornicroft, 2006).

We do not know yet, whether languages other than English will have a term they want to use to describe the possible meanings and definitions of recovery or whether they will want to adopt the English term into their language. However, important aspects of the 'vision of recovery today' with its values of 'person orientation, person involvement, self-determination, choice and growth potential' (Farkas, 2007) are expressed, for example, in the 2005 Action Plan endorsed in the Mental Health Declaration for Europe by ministers of health of the member states in the WHO European Region (WHO, 2005a, p 1). This Action Plan identifies as one of five priorities for the next ten years the need to 'design and implement comprehensive, integrated and efficient mental health systems that cover promotion, prevention, treatment and rehabilitation, care and recovery'. It also prominently includes a call to 'recognize the experience and knowledge of service users and carers as an important basis for planning and developing services' and collectively 'tackle stigma, discrimination and inequality, and empower and support people with mental health problems and their families to be actively engaged in this process'.

CHAPTER 3

Recovery – Basics and Concepts

DEFINITION

'... a deeply personal, unique process of changing one's attitudes, values, feelings, goals, skills and roles. It is a way of living a satisfying, hopeful, and contributing life even with limitations caused by the illness. Recovery involves the development of new meaning and purpose in one's life as one grows beyond the catastrophic effects of mental illness' (Anthony, 1993, p 13).

William Anthony's statement has become one of the most frequently quoted to define what recovery – 'as a guiding vision' – is or can be (Slade *et al.* 2008).

'Recovery does not refer to an end product or result. It does not mean that one is "cured" nor does it mean that one is simply stabilized or maintained in the community. Recovery often involves a transformation of the self wherein one both accepts one's limitation and discovers a new world of possibility. This is the paradox of recovery i.e., that in accepting what we cannot do or be, we begin to discover who we can be and what we can do. Thus, recovery is a process. It is a way of life' (Deegan, 1996, p 13).

Pat Deegan was one of the first people who eloquently described how she and other people with the experience of psychosis and a diagnosis of schizophrenia have moved beyond a patient role and have lived in recovery, building meaningful lives and enjoying success and a great deal of health instead of a life 'in the sometimes desolate wastelands of mental health programmes and institutions' (Deegan 1996, p 3). Recovery in these definitions is not a return to a 'premorbid' state. It is rather a development of personal growth and overcoming the often negative personal and societal implications of receiving a diagnosis, especially the traditionally attached prognosis, that can hinder this process and the full use of coping strategies and resilience.

While the term 'recovery' has a long history in the medical discourse the above definitions speak a completely new language of life, aspiration and opportunity and try to capture a process of many facets, phases and forms:

'Recovery is a process, a way of life, an attitude, and a way of approaching the day's challenges. It is not a perfectly linear process. At times our course is erratic and we falter, slide back, regroup and start again... The need is to meet the challenge of the disability and to re-establish a new and valued sense of integrity and purpose within and beyond the limits of the disability; the aspiration is to live, work, and love in a community in which one makes a significant contribution.' (Deegan 1988, p 15)

Davidson *et al.* (2005a) conducted a Webster-dictionary search and came up with four different definitions of recovery:

- a return to a normal condition;
- an act, instance, process, or period of recovering;
- something gained or restored in recovering;
- the act of obtaining usable substances from unusable sources, as with waste material.

When considering these four definitions it becomes obvious that they can all be relevant in the context of illness and health. Trying to find possible demarcations between these four definitions makes sense but only within the understanding that various types of recovery-efforts coexist and complement each other in the actual lives of individuals, and that they lead to success in various combinations.

A return to a normal condition

Acute physical illnesses, such as a cold or a fracture sustained in a skiing accident are most relevant to this definition. The goal is a return to a normal state of affairs, to the way things were before. This is the classical use of the term and a widespread definition of recovery. It could also be called reconstitution. Nevertheless, even such obvious examples might go along with changes in the immune status or an altered bone structure in the area of the fracture, which should not be overlooked. Such changes might not impair the normal state of affairs, but could manifest themselves in the future as enhanced resistance or a source of resilience, and they could become useful as warning signs in connection with individual risk factors. This applies especially to illnesses with a risk of relapse – and there are few which do not carry such a risk. But with all conditions that are ongoing over a period of time, or illnesses that don't develop acutely, a reconstitution of the previous, in other words the purported 'normal state', is not necessarily the primary aim. Therefore, it does not make sense to hold on rigidly to this definition of recovery when it comes to such long-term conditions.

A procedure, a period of time, a process

The second definition which emphasizes recovery as a process has its origins in trauma theory. Following traumatic events, a return to the preceding situation is not desirable, instead we aim for the integration of an experience which frequently and often dramatically changes how a person sees the world and his or her situation in the world. According to this definition, recovery becomes an active process which should bring about a situation by life is thwarted neither by denial nor by a continuous experience of victimization. Recovery following a trauma can be a lengthy process. It essentially aims at understanding the experience and regaining control over safety and life as a whole. The pathways from a damaged person to a survivor, from victim to victor, are essential elements in accounts of experiences with life-threatening illnesses such as certain cancers and AIDS.

Reconstitution and gain

Becoming whole again and thereby gaining something has long been a central element in the self-help activities of individuals with addiction problems. Usually, abstinence is a central goal. To achieve a healthy life, given the risk of relapse, it is essential to confront one's tendency towards addictive behaviour. The causes and effects of these problems which are not directly linked to substance abuse must be dealt with. It is not sufficient to gain control over the drugs, a person needs to find a way to become in charge of their life as a whole. This usually has nothing to do with returning to a pre-existing state of being, but rather, has to do with creating a situation – often for the first time – where a meaningful life with maximum control becomes possible. Consequently, the gain from confronting and surmounting an addiction problem can be quite substantial, affecting many aspects of life and identity.

Because psychiatric conditions have a rather variable course, the potential meaning of recovery must also differ. While many people might find themselves back in the previous 'normal' situation after experiencing an episode of depression or psychosis, corresponding to the first definition of recovery, such an acute and extraordinary experience can have its own traumatic aspects. We know that psychotic experiences and certain elements of acute treatment can be traumatizing. Such situations require that these experiences are worked through and integrated. Naturally, beyond returning to the pre-existing condition, additional gains of experience, insight and raised consciousness can be achieved.

A process, whereby something useful can be gained from basically useless sources

The recovery movement of users and mental health advocates is primarily concerned with ways to develop new approaches to long-term psychiatric problems with uncertain outcomes. This represents on the one hand an analogy to the self-help movement of alcohol users, where abstinence is considered a precondition for a healthy lifestyle, but which also requires that a person's vulnerability and proneness to addiction should not be cast aside, but rather become a part of the person's identity: 'reshaping of one's personal identity through a holistic sense of self that includes the psychiatric disability but does not center on the psychiatric disability as a defining aspect of life' (Onken *et al.* 2007). All symptoms of an illness do not need to disappear for a person to have control over his/her life, deal constructively with individual propensities and idiosyncrasies and enjoy self-reliance and freedom of choice. Some of the most prominent representatives of the recovery movement are especially keen to point out that a successful and meaningful life can unfold even with persistent symptoms and disabilities. This might happen by employing a disability concept or, in the case of hearing voices, by stripping the phenomenon of its meaning as pathology and coming to a place where it can be experienced as an individual and relatively common idiosyncrasy which may even be enriching. We are frequently impressed by individuals who report that a psychiatric condition they had experienced as unhelpful, senseless and causing unjustified suffering, did lead to a life changed for the better, beyond merely coping with an illness. Symptoms can be understood within the framework of an illness and can be brought under control, to a point where they no longer interfere with life. This in turn can then catalyze helpful insights beyond any distressing experiences. The same applies to the recognition and acceptance of limitations tied to an illness or disability. Concepts of illness or disability can be determined by psychological, biological and social factors, or a combination of these.

The large variety of mental health problems and the course of defined disorders, as well as the emphasis on individual choices and paths towards recovery should make it obvious, why a clear-cut and generalizable definition of recovery would be hard to come by. What needs to be underlined is that change in the direction of health and reconstitution is actually – and frequently as a surprise to all participants – possible at any time, even all of a sudden in the midst of a crisis when a person starts to feel much better than before, or more gradually after a prolonged illness. Of equal importance is the realization that in any life situation or phase of illness, health is lived and experienced at the same time, a fact that is often overlooked.

However, putting any kind of pressure on people to conform to some general commandment of health is certainly wrong and should be completely avoided. We are rather inclined to agree with Albert Camus who has Abbe Galiani say to Madame d'Epinay in *The Myth of Sysiphus*: 'The important thing is not to be cured but to live with one's ailments' (Camus 1983, p 38) and to thank Helen Glover for her warning against exchanging the 'entrapment of chronicity' for the 'entrapment of recovery': 'My gift and your gift are our brokenness and woundedness. No one is perfect. Accepting our woundedness and our brokenness and imperfections builds our resilience and our immune system against the desire to reach the "pure" recovery whiteness' (Glover 2003).

Two and more meanings

Many efforts to conceptualize recovery distinguish between internal and external factors. Nora Jacobson and Dianne Greenley (2001) consider hope and health internal factors – both in the sense of an identity and self-worth beyond any illness and with regard to having control over one's life. Relationships to others also play an important role. External factors are shaped by the situation of human- and patient-rights, and the opportunities for vocational and social integration. A positive culture, which promotes participation and empowerment among its citizens is essential, as is a mental health system that works in a recovery-oriented fashion.

The idea of two meanings of recovery is a recurring one and often corresponds to a focus on internal and external factors. A classical discussion concerns 'clinical' and 'social recovery', with the traditional clinical outcome definitions such as symptom reduction and functioning and quality of life, corresponding to the former and economic and social independence to the latter. 'Recovering from' an illness in the clinical sense is defined as an outcome and thus is quite differently defined from the process of being 'in recovery' (Davidson and Roe, 2007), which is usually defined around self-determination and a life in the community, despite symptoms or illness or disability. Bellack's suggestion of 'scientific' versus consumer models (Silverstein and Bellack 2008) also deals with the measurability of recovery as an outcome – usually in the form of symptoms, severity and functioning scales versus an ongoing process of overcoming adversity and striving towards what is important in an individual's life, a notion that has also been defined as 'personal recovery' (Slade *et al*. 2008). The distinction between outcome and process is often viewed as critical (Meehan *et al*. 2008) and sparks the essential discussion on how to develop new assessments and methodologies in order to measure outcome in a valid form in a recovery-oriented clinical and scientific context (Slade and Hayward 2007).

Onken *et al*. (2007) also describe a juncture between two perspectives. Interestingly, they highlight it with regard to the process of 'contextualizing recovery in the light of symptomatology' (p 14). The distinction they discuss here concerns 'those who believe recovery is the absence of symptoms' and those 'who view recovery as a positive sense of self achieved in spite of continuing symptoms or in recognition of one's surmounting the social impact of illness' while discussing the importance of symptom self-management without necessarily 'calling for the absence of symptoms'. This is probably one of the most important points when discussing possibly fundamental differences between clinical and personal recovery, clinical and social or clinical and rehabilitative models, and service-based and user-based recovery. It might actually be key to the question whether and how best to communicate between the two different meanings.

Onken *et al*. (2007) do link the lack of consensus with regard to the definition of recovery to the lack of consensus regarding the definition of mental illness. To this the problems of definition of psychiatric disability and those of defining and assessing mental health can be added. Notably, the Substance Abuse and Mental Health Services Administration of the US Department of Health and Human Services' (SAMSHA) national consensus statement does not include the term 'mental illness': 'Mental health recovery is a journey of healing and transformation enabling a person with a mental health problem to live a meaningful life in a community of his or her choice while striving to achieve his or her full potential.' (del Vecchio and Fricks, 2007). A comprehensive expert panel arrived at 10 fundamental components of recovery for SAMHSA (www.mentalhealth.samhsa.gov; 13.5.08):

- self-direction
- individualized and person-centred
- empowerment
- holistic
- non-linear
- strengths-based
- peer support
- respect
- responsibility
- hope

which is rather centred around the individual and accompanied by the following comment on society's interest in the recovery endeavour: 'Mental health recovery not only benefits individuals with mental health disabilities by focusing on their abilities to live, work, learn, and fully participate in our society, but also enriches the texture of American community life. America reaps the benefits of the contributions individuals with mental disabilities can make, ultimately becoming a stronger and healthier nation.'

Onken *et al*. (2007) in their overview on definitions come up with elements of recovery grouped into *person-centred* ones such as: hope, sense of agency, self-determination, meaning and purpose, awareness and potentiality; *re-authoring* elements of recovery such as coping, healing, wellness and thriving; *exchange-centred* elements such as social functioning and social roles, power, choice among meaningful options, and *community-centred* elements such as social connectedness/relationships, social circumstances/opportunities and integration. This list and grouping correspond to their suggestion of an ecological framework that considers an interactional dimension between different parts of a system in need of change. This ecological perspective takes full account of the complexities and the 'dynamic interplay of forces that are complex, synergistic, and linked' that can facilitate or hinder recovery as well as 'the dynamic interaction among characteristics of the individual (such as hope), characteristics of the environment (such as opportunities), and characteristics of the exchange between the individual and the environment (such as choice)'. Also, Onken *et al.* (2007) suggest – with Watzlawick – distinguishing between first order change, which 'occurs within a given unit of a system but the system itself remains unchanged', second order change within the system itself, and interactions between changes in different parts of the system and the system itself.

In 'hazarding' a 'provisional consensus' from the literature – 'recovery is difficult, idiosyncratic, and requires faith – but it is possible' – Hopper (2007) arrives at four themes that approximate recovery's 'meaning in use':

- renewing a sense of possibility
- regaining competencies
- reconnecting and finding a place in society
- reconciliation work.

In examining the efforts to implement recovery-orientation at a service system level he concludes that 'what was true of recovery narratives' – namely 'avoidance of rude quotidian realities' – 'is no less true of state plans'. He addresses material deprivation as well as justice disparities and brings up the requirements of social demands and system-level reforms. The resulting tensions and major challenges lead him to introduce Amartya Sen's capabilities approach to recovery (Hopper, 2007), an approach providing a framework to constructively address some of the major confusions and serious conflicts of the recovery debate, especially around the issues of political-economic and social implications for real change and system transformation.

In conclusion, the joy about the diverse and constructive approaches to such a complex topic should override any disappointment about the absence of strict rules, definitions and regulations. What can be clearly stated is that the rights to participation, self-determination and to be protected from discrimination are central preconditions for recovery. In summary, recovery can be defined as a development that describes a movement from the limitations of the patient role to a self-determined life in the community. For the most part, at an individual level, such developments are ongoing, determined by the values and aims that each person deems essential.

The supports which people need when they are advancing along a recovery pathway are manifold and informed by individual priorities. If supports are meant to enable people to gain control over their life in terms of empowerment and recovery, a move away from a traditional model which describes mental conditions basically as deficits must strive towards a resource-oriented approach. In planning a modern mental health service, a flexible, mobile, and person-centred approach is fundamental, because it is guided by individual requirements for support and the needs and resources of each person in their living environment, instead of demanding an adjustment to existing services. Within therapeutic relationships, participatory models that allow shared decision-making and joint crisis plans and advance directives for acute crises are replacing paternalistic compliance models. The relationships between service users and providers are being considerably transformed through these innovations as new roles and expertises emerge. However, these kinds of changes can only be sustained if the policy-makers show they are behind them by creating the necessary conditions for their implementation.

POLITICAL STRATEGIES

Many English-speaking countries such as the UK, Canada, Australia and New Zealand have redirected their health planning in terms of a recovery-orientation. The US Government has expressed this most pointedly in the 'New Freedom Commission on Mental Health' (US Department of Health and Human Services 2003):

'We envision a future when everyone with a mental illness will recover, a future when mental illnesses can be prevented or cured, a future when mental illnesses are detected early, and a future when everyone with a mental illness at any stage of life has access to effective treatment and supports – essentials for living, working, learning, and participating fully in the community.'

The commission emphasizes three obstacles which currently stand in the way of these innovations:

- stigma that surrounds mental illnesses;
- unfair treatment limitations and financial requirements placed on mental health benefits in private health insurance;
- the fragmented mental health service delivery system.

These three issues clearly demonstrate that in spite of all the differences between Europe and the USA, the basic problems are identical and difficult to overcome. Many Western countries have similar strategic plans to address these problems. The future will show where the overall situation is most likely to be successfully transformed.

The National Health Service in the UK is currently placing recovery front and centre of its strategy and its guidelines. (There is more about this in the section on system transformation in chapter 7). Many essential elements are not just applicable to mental health care, but to health care in general. The central role of service users and family members remains a key aspect. Many demands articulated by these constituencies are being reflected in mental health plans, and it is clearly provided that they are to play an active role in all steps towards implementation. Users and family members are already represented on many councils and advisory bodies. In the UK health care system, no council that aims for political relevance can afford to function without user and family participation. Dan Fisher is a member of the US Commission on Mental Health. He will be introduced more fully further down, in the section on the 'Empowerment Model of Recovery' in chapter 4. In addition to his credentials as a psychiatrist, he brings his experiences as someone diagnosed with schizophrenia and as the director of the National Empowerment Center in Washington, DC. Similarly, the Action Plan for Mental

Health endorsed in the Mental Health Declaration for Europe which was approved by the EU-ministerial conference in Helsinki in 2005 proposes an active role for users and collaboration on all levels as a key element of its plans and recommendations.

The following noteworthy example of the Scottish Recovery Network as an example of a regional initiative to implement recovery-orientation illustrates essential collaborations on different levels.

The Scottish Recovery Network

The Scottish Recovery Network (SRN) was founded in 2004 in Glasgow as one of four official initiatives within the National Programme for Improving Mental Health and Well-Being (www.scottishrecovery.net).

Since the beginning of the network, a number of events and workshops have been held, with the aim of promoting and examining recovery from long-term mental health problems in Scotland. As a result, a diverse group of organizations came up with a detailed proposal to formally put together the Scottish Recovery Network as a learning forum for the exchange of ideas around the topic of recovery.

Members of the network are convinced that recovery is a subject for everyone. Therefore, the SRN wants to work with local communities and various stakeholder-groups, including users with long-term mental health problems, their friends, relatives, mental health professionals, with a variety of services inside and outside the mental health system and with citizens in general.

They use the internet for dialogue among users and other interested parties, and offer discussion forums that include lectures and articles about recovery. Furthermore, they are disseminating information about their collaboration with other centres, for example, in New Zealand. Individuals with psychiatric symptoms are invited to present their personal stories and to publish them anonymously on their website.

Members of the network are convinced that recovery is not about a new 'model' or concept within psychiatry. Neither should recovery be considered a new ideology. They attempt to find out what helps people to stay or become healthy and are eager to share this information with other individuals and centres.

Their basic idea is that people can recover even from the most severe types of mental disorders. Recovery implies that a person has a chance of a satisfying and fulfilled life, with or without psychiatric symptoms. The path and the experience of recovery cannot be the same for two separate individuals. Attitudes and values have a profound impact on the further course of recovery for each person. Recovery is more than the absence of symptoms. Recovery is a profound personal process. The expectation of recovery and the understanding about the kinds of things that help people regain control over their life, is a key aspect.

Simon Bradstreet summarizes the collected insights about recovery from the international literature in his survey article, 'Elements of recovery: international learning and the Scottish context', which can be accessed on-line (www.scottishrecovery.net). He understands recovery in the broadest sense of the term, offering the definition of William Anthony's (1993) that outlines a satisfying, active and hopeful life even within the limitations of the illness. Developing a new sense and meaning of life is essential while growing beyond the catastrophic outcomes of a psychiatric condition.

Bradstreet summarizes the following shared elements of recovery from the international literature:

- *Hope:* Without hope recovery is not possible. There can be no change without the belief that a better life is both possible and attainable.
- *Meaning and purpose:* People find meaning in very different ways, for example, some people may find spirituality important while others may find meaning through the development of stronger interpersonal or community links.
- *Potential for change:* A recovery approach requires a fundamental belief that everyone has the potential for change. It challenges the traditionally pessimistic outlook of mental health professionals, which is influenced by a historical belief in the chronic nature of some mental health problems. It also proposes that episodes of illness, while clearly distressing, can in fact be developmental and educative experiences.
- *Control:* It is central for recovery to have the subjective experience of having regained control over one's life. People who use mental health services are sometimes denied an adequate level of involvement in their own care and treatment.
- *Active participation:* In contrast with being a passive recipient of services, recovery aims at active individuals who take personal responsibility for their care, often in collaboration with friends, family, supporters and professionals.
- *Holistic and inclusive approach:* Recovery considers all elements of a person's quality of life. It recognizes that the extent to which someone enjoys good health and well-being is influenced by a wide range of social, environmental and individual factors and is much more than the management of symptoms.
- *Environment:* External factors such as stigma and discrimination, employment and training opportunities, housing and social exclusion have a strong influence on recovery.
- *Optimistic and realistic approach:* Recovery is rarely a linear process, people will have periods where their recovery is slowed by a bout of illness.
- *Creative risk-taking:* Services are rightly concerned about managing risk but the danger is that it becomes the overriding concern. For someone to overcome a disabling illness and become actively involved in their community requires an element of creative risk-taking.

Narrative research in Scotland

Members of the Scottish Recovery Network (SRN) are insisting that recovery should not be understood as an adjunct to other mental health services, but rather that it should be promoted and supported by the entire health system, starting with the first diagnosis. Officials within the Scottish mental health system are especially supportive of recovery approaches and positively inclined towards the SRN. Therefore, the SRN sees as one of its central missions the need to examine the many factors that promote or interfere with recovery.

The SRN also aims to establish an evidence-base of all important characteristics within Scottish recovery experiences by using a qualitative methodology. The value of individual experiences as evidence is essential for this undertaking.

This research project has several goals which will mark all future work of the SRN. Members are hoping that the collected stories will yield common factors of recovery in Scotland, while at the same time providing information about the uniqueness of each person's experience. Such 'anecdotal evidence' gleaned from individual stories can help to improve health care policies and practices in all areas of Scotland, while gaining a better understanding of the elements that bolster the well-being of each individual. The project works on the assumption that the stories told will include references to a variety of services and programmes (medical care, housing, social work, volunteerism), as well as to the ways that the broader society influences recovery as studies from other countries have shown that job development and supported employment, or meaningful activities, education, art, sports and physical exercise have a significant impact on promoting recovery.

During 2005 members of the SRN collected the first personal accounts of recovery from 67 individuals with psychiatric problems at six different locations in Scotland. Participants for the project were recruited primarily through the national and local press, although web-based support groups, the email list of the SRN, user-organizations and public events were also used. The stories were collected in semi-structured interviews. Participants were asked to share their stories anonymously with two interviewers, who also prepared an audio-recording for purposes of transcription. The results of the study are now available to participants and other interested parties on the SRN website.

The members of the SRN realize that while this project can only be a snapshot of the lives of the people who were interviewed it can, nevertheless, serve as a reflection of their recovery-processes. To introduce more dynamic elements and a longitudinal perspective, the participants could be followed for a period of three to five years along their recovery processes, for instance by seeking feedback at various points in time. Alternatively, those who had already been interviewed could be invited for another interview within three to five yeas, in order to reflect the recovery process they had already gone through. Additional information could also be provided by using the same qualitative methodology with individuals who provide support, such as friends, relatives and mental health workers, or by obtaining views from the community at large.

The ethical guidelines with respect to study participants, employees and network members have been taken very seriously. Participants received assurances that they would not be left to their own resources after a potentially stressful interview. Qualified individuals, who could be called on for support, were available. The participants had the opportunity to review the transcripts of their interviews and make changes, for example, by clarifying the meaning of certain statements, or by eliminating others. The participants were also asked to provide informed consent for all aspects of the study (questionnaire, interview, etc.). The researchers and interviewers in this project participated in a specific training programme to make sure they were capable of addressing all emotional aspects that might come up during an interview. In addition, a therapeutic consultant was available throughout the project if needed, for study participants as well as for research staff.

The Scottish Recovery Network is an example of a courageous initiative that attempts to apply international experiences concretely to the situation in Scotland and to create, right from the start, a transparent system of evidence at all levels. It will be exciting to watch the further developments of this project.

Below we summarize the main results of the narrative research project, which searched for factors that helped and factors that hindered the participants' recovery from long-term mental health problems. It highlights several common elements which were found to be helpful for recovery. These included:

- developing a positive view of yourself and having hope for the future;
- having meaningful activities and purpose in life, and having contributions and choices in life validated and valued;
- having supportive relationships;
- having the right mix of treatments and support.

Building a good base for recovery

The authors conclude that getting some of the practical aspects of life sorted out can create a safe space from which a person can start their recovery journey. For some of the people they spoke to, this was linked to finding secure housing. For others it was linked to getting access to benefits or managing debts, taking time off work or confronting the past.

Example: 'When I got the flat that I am in now, for the first time it was my house and it was my space and I could fill it with my memories and, you know, there wasn't any baggage there... and it was a place where nobody knew me, nobody knew that I had mental health problems, nobody knew who I was. I was just a person who had moved into this flat...'

Believing recovery is possible

Many people the authors spoke to talked about the importance of believing in the possibility of recovery. They described how taking a more hopeful and optimistic approach to their illness created hope, a feeling of self-worth and confidence. It helped them create a new identity as a person who was in recovery.

Example: 'I think sometimes, certainly myself, the thing that prevented recovery was that I didn't know anything else. I'd got a mental illness. There's some safety in being ill. Although I hated every minute of it, there was still some security in that.'

Being in control of your own recovery

Some people talked about a realization that they were letting symptoms control their lives and affect people around them.

Example: 'Me..., that's what's changed. Me..., it was a control thing... There was an unconscious release of control on my part. (For twenty years) I let other people control what I was doing and what I wasn't doing. I let the symptoms of my illness become the centre of my universe, and the symptoms of my illness aren't the centre of my universe.'

Looking for the positives in life

People often tend to be more aware of their weaknesses and problems than they are of their strengths and abilities. Everyone has strengths and being aware of what they are can help maintain well-being. Some people told the authors about the strength they had gained through living with mental health problems.

Example: 'I do feel I'm a stronger person for having the experiences that I've had. I do think I've benefited as an individual, from the entire, what would you call it? Experience.'

Finding the right support and treatment

Recovery is a unique and individual process. The things that help or support one person may not work for another. This means that getting good quality advice and information is very important. Many participants said that finding the right mix of support and treatment helped them in their recovery.

Example: 'Talking therapies are no good without my medication, I need both. Helping people understand that what might suit one person might not suit another...'

Keeping busy and finding meaning and purpose

Everybody needs meaning and purpose in their life. Many of the participants found this by doing things with their time. Some people talked about the need to 'give back'. Many of the people the authors spoke to were very creative. Arts and creativity gave them a voice at different stages in their recovery.

Example: 'I get a lot out of creating and actually being able to give, to give to people something that I've actually spent time on, and that's something that I can do when I'm well.'

It's a personal thing

This project provides a summary of some of the things the researchers learnt during the Narrative Research Project. Of course it is not possible to report all findings and reflect the experience of all readers. The authors' personal hope is that it helps people on their own Route to Recovery.

Example: 'It is – it's a personal thing. You can't say to someone do this, do that, and do the next thing and you'll be fine... you have to take ownership – you have to want to move on.'

The results of this project were published in 2007 in an on-line booklet with the title *Routes to Recovery. Collected wisdom from the SRN Narrative Research Project* (www.scottishreceovery.net) and can be translated into other languages and converted to large print and audio on request. It is supported by the Scottish Government as part of the National Programme for Improving Mental Health and Well-Being. The full research report is available on request from the Scottish Recovery Network. The booklet called *Journeys of Recovery* includes twelve of the recovery stories gathered as part of the project. These stories are also available in audio formats.

COLLABORATION WITH USERS OF PSYCHIATRIC SERVICES

The situation in the UK is conducive to the evaluation and the use of recent experiences of changed roles and collaborative working conditions between services users and providers. Collaborations have concerned planning, implementation and evaluation of psychiatric services. Many participants in collaborations have recorded their observations. Some of these are anecdotal, some ideological, and some are described in scientific language. Reviewing this material quickly reveals that the call for change and equal standing has not always been greeted with joy among mental health professionals. At times this takes the form of distrustful statements implying that user-involvement might be a ruse, broadly speaking, to justify unpleasant and unfavourable changes, especially cost-saving measures. The argument about costs is not to be taken lightly and the consideration that demands urging self-reliance could lead, in a worst case scenario, to a curtailment of services, is certainly justified. On the other hand, it is equally reasonable to assume that a system which propagates freedom of choice and individual service-planning might turn out to be rather expensive. Overall, it is becoming clear that the critique and the demands of the user movement might indeed reveal that certain budget items cannot be justified, and new ways of distributing funds might be called for. In some instances this might indeed mean cuts in certain areas that are dear to the heart of mental health professionals.

Another decisive question would be whether the involvement of users should be seen within a broader development of participatory democracy, or whether the involvement of users has been conceived as an element of a specific intervention designed to advance the empowerment of individuals who are suffering from a lack of self-confidence and self-efficacy. Most likely, both of these aspects need to be kept in mind. Needless to say, psychiatry is part of societal developments – such as the strengthening of patient rights – and also shares more general developments in health policy, which might, for example, imply a reduction in relevance and thereby a cut in the funding of inpatient services.

Key aspects of the general argument for involving users are the benefits that can be derived from their expertise in order to enhance the quality of services and interventions. Beyond this, a better understanding of psychiatric problems and how they are overcome can be expected, as well as impulses for new and alternative developments. No one would deny such benefits, but what desired and untoward outcomes might occur beyond this is cause for much concern. And finally, there is the issue as to how this should be happening in practice. The questions and problems listed below make this rather obvious: In the UK, the political climate is such, that users are being involved at all levels. This means that an oversight agency might confront a programme manager with a decision-making body which included a person whom he/she had known earlier only in a therapeutic context. Even the immediate administrative structures might now include users of the very same service. Does this mean that service users have to be consulted before any decisions are made? Might these users, who are essentially lay people, thwart decisions that are perfectly well justified? What about a potential veto? Or must all plans and discussions inevitably be complicated a priori by involving users in every conversation at all levels?

The answers to these questions are intimately tied to other questions, such as: Who are these users, after all, who desire and who are supposed to be sitting on boards and committees? What entitles them to do so? How are they paid? Or are these honorary tasks? Are they doing this for personal gain? And how will this affect them therapeutically? Are they now our colleagues? Are they less qualified, since they never worked here, or more qualified, because they are familiar with the other side? Are patient representatives something like a new kind of labour union? Tait and Lester (2005) summarize the obstacles for user involvement based on reports about the difficulties with this new policy:

- lack of information
- financial and time costs
- concerns over representativeness
- resistance to the idea of users as experts.

The first three items illustrate matters that are hard to ignore. If we want to transform and improve psychiatry by involving service users at all levels equitably, then this would constitute a major adjustment. Even those mental health workers who see this as a fabulous chance have to realize how much experience, expertise and good advice is still lacking. No one knows as yet, how to deal with such an opportunity. In order to obtain the necessary knowledge to approach this task responsibly, time and money is needed. Opportunities for training and supervision are already being offered by consumer experts such as *How to successfully include people with psychiatric disabilities on boards and committees: overcoming the barriers and providing support* by Patricia E Deegan PhD and Deborah Anderson MSW, a primer booklet that can be obtained for US$ 20 via Pat Deegan's website (www.patdeegan.com).

Good intentions are not sufficient. We know that the process of such a reconfiguration would be exciting and instructive, but it is also quite obvious that setbacks will need to be tolerated and disappointments worked through, including problems that no one had expected.

One of these problems is frequently expressed by the following question: to what extent are those users who are suddenly appearing on boards and work groups, and participating in discussions and votes, actually representative. 'Representative for whom and for what?' would be the next question, and while thinking about this it is easy to slip into a very basic discussion. In practice, this can take the following form: Those who are sitting on boards are usually people with considerable dedication and the talent to use such situations to deliver critiques and proposals for change. Mental health professionals are sometimes concerned that those patients who generally appear calm and content are not represented in these forums. They might be of the opinion that those 'other patients' – known to them from therapeutic contacts – are quite different, even needier, but not as demanding or self-determined.

User representatives might counter that mental health workers and doctors would also not like to be represented by those colleagues who are the least eloquent and assertive. They know about the concerns and desires of their peers, who confide in them a great deal that they would not share with providers in one-to-one contacts. Many of these activists have considerable experience in self-help, which they are now able to apply. Rutter *et al.* (2004) go further by asking: are we talking about representative users or rather about representative perspectives? How does a person become representative? By being democratically elected? Or by a statistical procedure? Who would be entitled to vote? Is there to be a requirement that a person be moderately ill or moderately healthy in order to represent other patients? Or is this basically about the notion that user-representatives should conform to our image of a 'typical patient'?

It makes sense to consider these questions within the context of all new social movements. When a group becomes empowered to participate in discussions, the problems that arise are generally quite similar. It is comparable to organized labour, the women's movement and the appearance of green parties in parliaments. And it is far from clear whether over time there will be a sufficient amount of activists to sustain these type of organizations.

My (M.A.) personal experience of collaborating with people with a lived experience in clinical work and the self-help movement makes me feel quite optimistic about the future. In Birmingham, where Ron Coleman worked as a member and advisor of the Assertive Outreach Team that I also worked on (cf. the first section in chapter 4), I was impressed by the ways in which Ron could engage with individuals whose experience in general and with psychiatry in particular was marked by coercion and violence, and thereby contribute much to de-escalating certain situations. His expertise, based on personal experiences with comparable situations, opened up new opportunities for non-coercive interventions that would not have been imaginable without his special contribution.

Also, the availability of a user-run crisis house which offered spaces as an alternative to hospitalization meant considerable relief and considerable enrichment of the team's opportunities for intervention and support. These experiences, as well as the contact with user-run organizations in New York in the course of a research project, clearly demonstrate to us that a substantial enlargement of the panoply of supports and interactions through the involvement of users as service providers or leaders of psychosocial agencies offers considerable opportunities for recovery-oriented clinical work.

Colleagues and leaders who have their own experience of recovery inspire just those kind of interventions that aim to enhance the motivitation and self-reliance of users, and to disrupt the tendencies towards chronification of traditions that are stultified by an emphasis on 'stabilization'. But it is certainly not only their personal example that is effective here. They are also demonstrating techniques and methods and new types of relational work. These can often be formulated rather concisely and taught to others, even to those without personal experiences of recovery, and would make their work more effective. When enough funds, time and opportunities for training and supervision are available, as mentioned earlier, then we should not underestimate the potential of these transformations to assist in the struggle against burnout of mental health workers in general.

Needless to say, this new professional group, whose expertise derives to a considerable extent from their own experiences, will need regulation, training requirements and career ladders. Successful models for involving peers as members and leaders of therapeutic teams in the area of addiction treatment might serve as guidelines here. On the website of the US American National Empowerment Center (www.power2u.org) there is up-to-date information about research projects that assess the effectiveness of consumer-operated service programmes and consumer-driven initiatives for system transformation (see also

Chapter 7). In the UK there is some experience with such services, but no clear-cut studies that might elucidate the pro and cons of teams with peer members for the users of such services. Conceptually speaking, it is obvious that additional benefits and greater effectiveness can be expected. Graham Thornicroft and Michele Tansella (2005), the authors of today's most important European textbook of community psychiatry, are asserting that current and former service users can make essential contributions to all nine core principles of community mental health work:

1. autonomy
2. continuity
3. effectiveness
4. accessibility
5. comprehensiveness
6. equity
7. accountability
8. co-ordination
9. efficiency

Also, Thornicroft and Tansella declare their high expectations towards what is to be gained from user-involvement in mental health research (cf. Chapter 6).

At another level, I (Michaela) also experienced the relevance of user-involvement with regard to recovery-orientation. In Birmingham, users were also involved in the hiring committees for job applicants. A user-colleague who participated in the hiring process of a senior psychiatrist addressed an applicant thus: 'When I was 18 I was first admitted to a mental health service and learned later from the records that my diagnosis had been paranoid schizophrenia. Say you are on call at night and I ask you: "They told me I had a psychotic break. What is that and what is likely to happen in the future?" He wanted to find out whether the answer would be honest and communicate hope and strength, or would lead to despair and resignation. In preparation for such a job interview, an applicant might learn to think in this fashion and to handle such questions successfully.

There is plenty of evidence that involving persons with a lived experience of health problems and treatments improves the quality of what is being taught. The problems and obstacles we have described are similar to those in the areas of clinical work and planning. How are they being paid? How to prevent burnout and overextension? What about differences in status? The first studies on involving consumers in the teaching curriculum come from rheumatology, diabetology, cardiology and oncology. In the meantime, psychiatry has been catching up.

In our opinion, psychiatry, with its expertise in therapeutic contacts and communication in difficult circumstances, could and should be in the vanguard of implementing new forms of co-operation between users and clinicians. It is gratifying to see that psychiatry is indeed gaining ground in these areas and we hope that this will be followed by further developments.

The European Union project, EX-IN (experience involvement, www. ex-in.info), is an important European initiative with participants from six countries (Germany, Sweden, Norway, The Netherlands, UK, and Slovenia) taking part in 14 projects. It is being funded as part of the EU-employment initiative, Leonardo da Vinci, and co-ordinated by

Jörg Utschakowski from Bremen, Germany (www.initiative-zur-sozialen-rehabilitation.de 12.8.2008). This project goes a long way towards a practice of user involvement:

1. The pilot-project will compile the different experiences of experts and organizations with user involvement in different countries and different contexts in Europe;
2. Existing studies about methods and outcomes of user involvement will be compared and new studies carried out within and through the partnership;
3. The qualification systems and attainable qualifications in the different countries will be compared;
4. The training needs of people with lived experience will be described in order for them to be able to take part in teaching and delivery of services;
5. Description and development of useful, innovative training methods;
6. Development of modules (especially those modules which ensure the transfer of the knowledge of people with lived experience in the training and caretaking process);
7. Development of a curriculum which gives people with lived experience and with different backgrounds, useful training to enable them to gain the ability and the acknowledgement to participate in the mentioned fields;
8. The conditions for an official registration will be checked with the aim to achieve such conditions.

www.ex-in.info (16.2.08)

Participating countries have committed themselves to take responsibility for implementing the results of the project, at least partially. This could be a decisive step towards improving the chances for future developments in this area. The experiences and insights of users are entering the curricula and study materials, which could qualify them as teachers and colleagues.

In many countries local groups and projects are springing up and developing ideas, structures, teaching and research programmes as well as innovations and alternatives to traditional services. That users and ex-users as well as carers are bringing their immense experience to the field represents a formidable opportunity for psychiatry. When we consider the involvement of users in the planning, implementation and evaluation of mental health services carefully, as we are doing here, it appears to be eminently necessary, self-evident, and quite 'do-able'. However, due to the fact that such involvement requires a fundamental rethinking within the mental health field and a real readiness to share power, it is clear that the successes of user-run projects and initiatives will also bring about power struggles with the established system, and therefore 'we are likely to be facing a divided health system for some time to come: on the one hand, the medically prescribed order, and on the other side, the "disorder" of personal healing that is being propagated by user/survivors' (Stastny 2004, p 275).

RESILIENCE–A DYNAMIC RECOVERY-FACTOR

In the 1970s, the resilience paradigm emerged from a) the findings within a research agenda of investigating risk for psychopathology, and b) a political agenda of discontent with the prevailing deficit models in psychology in general and in clinical psychology particularly. Therapists had begun to note that the exclusive focus on psychopathology, deficits and problems was neglecting the positive and adaptive aspects of functioning that are inherent to human nature (Coatsworth and Duncan 2003). In the USA, a group of researchers were charting a programme of study on risk for schizophrenia. While studying the development of children identified to be at risk for the disorder, the investigators observed that many of the participants did not show signs of deficits and poor development; rather they showed signs of manifest competence, well-being and positive adaptation (Garmezy, 1974, 1985). Since then, programmes of 'resilience' have contributed a lot to the understanding of the natural phenomena of resilience.

Resilience as the mental capacity to resist adversities is directly linked to the recovery process. Resilience can be seen as a driving force for recovery. In the course of the recovery process, forces of resilience are increasingly developed. Helen Glover (2003) situates this relationship in an important context: 'Being diagnosed with mental illness/distress does not preclude someone from the ability to build resilience. Identifying too fully with mental illness and its implicit limitations may prevent someone developing their personal meaning and responses to negative emotions and experiences.' At their Institute for the Study of Human Resilience at Boston University, founded in 2001, Courtenay Harding (2005) and Pat Deegan (2005a) have investigated, over the last few years, specific processes of resilience and restitution following a psychiatric condition. Interest in and publications about resilience have increased tremendously in recent years, a welcome development in comparison to the numerous publications of studies about traditional risk factors. In 2002, the data-base PsycINFO yielded a total of 1600 scientific studies on the subject of resilience, while in 2004 a total of 2400 scientific papers were found.

Some researchers are, however, warning that the term 'resilience' might become a fancy word, and as such could be promulgated in popular science without much actual knowledge to back it up. Another risk is that resilience might be seen as a 'mystical power' that can bestow limitless invulnerability on a person. Scientific findings so far are keeping this myth within bounds by promoting more realistic expectations.

Fortunately, resilience has been afforded a central role in international psychiatry as one of the factors connoting positive health. Juan Mezzich, President of the World Psychiatric Association from 2005–2008 (Mezzich 2005a), emphasizes that pathology has occupied a monopoly in the discussion of health and clinical care and positive aspects of health have been largely ignored in research and clinical psychiatry. He includes the following elements among the central aspects of positive health: a) functioning and resilience, b) resources and support and c) quality of life.

The concept of resilience emphasizes the complexity of psychopathology, helps elucidate the possibilities of prevention, and gives cause for hope in clinical practice. Wolff (1995) advocates greater efforts in science to spread the insights about resilience. The public and politicians need to be informed to what extent decisions about housing, employment, social benefits, education and justice can impact child development and what kind of changes in the macro-sphere can safeguard and enhance the resilience of children.

Health promotion – an increasingly important field for prevention and clinical treatment – considers resilience an important factor in the healing process. Other positively formulated approaches to processes of healing are hope, newly learned optimism, self-help activities and supportive social networks, to mention but a few (Schmolke and Lecic-Tosevski 2003a; Seligman and Peterson 2003). Resilience is not reduced to mental resistance. Recent studies have shown that promoting mental health can avert the development of physical illnesses (Raphael *et al.* 2005; Herrman 2005) – in line with the adage 'There is no health without mental health' (New York City Department of Health and Mental Hygiene, 2003).

What do we mean by 'resilience'?

The term 'resilience' comes originally from engineering and connotes the impact-strength, resistance, stability or durability of a material vis-a-vis the forces of weight, physical assault, pressure, friction, centrifugal power and other potentially disturbing or destructive forces – according to various dictionaries. 'Resilience' also means elasticity, malleability, tension, bounce, flexibility, and pliancy (bending rather than breaking) – all terms used in technical fields.

In clinical psychology and psychotherapy, the term 'resilience' has come into use only in recent years. Here it implies the power to resist, mental elasticity and regaining the former mental stability following a stressful period or event.

Resilience is understood by resilience researchers as follows:

- Psychic resistance or the process of adapting well in the face of adversity, tragedy, or high levels of stress (Rutter 1995);
- Elastic capability of resistance (Bender and Lösel 1997);
- Motivational power (Richardson 2002);
- The process by which children, youth and adults withstand sources of challenge and also the patterns of bouncing back or recovering from such conditions (Coatsworth and Duncan 2003);
- A class of phenomena that is characterized by good outcomes despite serious threats to adaptation or development (Masten 2001);
- The capability to come out of the most adverse conditions in a more resistant way and equipped with more resources than would have been the case without these difficult conditions (Walsh 1998).

Experts on resilience emphasize that resilience does not refer to fixed powers of an individual which might be directed against noxious influences from the outside, but rather suggest a flexible dynamic energy commensurate to the situation, in other words a 'bio-psycho-social competency' (Gunkel and Kruse 2004). In analogy to biological processes, mental resilience is being understood by Lösel (2005) in terms of:

- Processes of protection (for example, the immune system);
- Processes of repair (for example, the healing of wounds);
- Processes of regeneration (for example, sleep).

The concept of resilience and its study

There are many stories of people who succeeded in functioning well socially in spite of having been challenged by the symptoms of a physical or mental condition, or who bounced back after a period of extreme stress. The study of resilience involves a scientific analysis of such biographical accounts. This implies an attempt to understand the biographies of such individuals and to retrace how they were able to overcome their difficulties and to live a productive and fulfilled life. Learning from these experiences and applying this knowledge to an improvement of prevention- and treatment programmes, is an essential goal of such efforts (Coatsworth and Duncan 2003).

The conceptual development and empirical understanding of resilience has occurred since the 1980s, primarily within the fields of developmental psychology, psychopathology and pedagogy. Its prominent exponents are, for example, Sir Michael Rutter (1985) in England, Emmy Werner (1993) and Norman Garmezy (1991) in the USA, and Friedrich Lösel (1994) and Günther Opp (1999) in Germany.

Research has shown that resilience is more than an adaptation to adverse conditions and also more than simply enduring or surviving. An individual does not demonstrate resilient behaviour in spite of adverse circumstances, but rather *because* of them. Experiences of extreme stress can elicit strengths in a person that he or she may have never thought possible before. 'In the midst of winter I realized that there was an invincible summer within me' wrote Albert Camus – a sentence that Rosemarie Welter-Enderlin has chosen as a motto for her conference on resilience in Zurich 2005 (Welter-Enderlin and Hildenbrand 2006).

In general, there is a consensus that resilience cannot simply be equated with social competence or mental health. Resilience is not determined by static, but rather by dynamic protective factors that can moderate multiple and cumulative risks (Rutter 1985).

Child psychologists and child psychiatrists have recognized the following factors, among others, that contribute to protection and resilience in situations when a developing individual is facing massive mental, physical and psychosocial stressors (for example, Werner and Smith 2001; Bender and Lösel 1997):

- positive sense of self (self-efficacy);
- positive social behaviour;
- active coping;
- an intact home;
- positive relationships with other competent and caring adults;
- good intellectual capabilities;
- attractiveness;
- confidence in the meaningfulness of life;
- religious belief/spirituality;
- good education;
- socio-economic advantages.

Resilience is closely linked to other concepts, such as 'emotional intelligence' (Edward and Warelow 2005), 'self-regulation' (Buckner *et al.* 2003) and 'self-organization' (Cicchetti and Rogosch 1997). The Israeli medical sociologist Aaron Antonovsky (1987) with his concept of 'salutogenesis' wanted to find out more about the reasons why certain people enjoy a rather intact development in spite of considerable risk factors and why they are able to deal with traumatic experiences faster and better than others. The resilience-construct has also become increasingly important in gerontology. In that context, resilience is not merely considered a counterbalance to vulnerability, but also as a 'factor of well-being for elderly persons'. Resilience here means the ability to make an active and constructive effort of adaptation, which allows a person of advanced age to successfully master challenges, reconstitute a normal functional capacity after a traumatic event and pursue a satisfactory management of losses and privations (Foster 1997).

Protective factors within the individual and the environment

Scientific results are in remarkable agreement about the characteristics of a child and its environment with respect to resilient outcomes. Such characteristics are often referred to as 'protective factors' since they are capable of diminishing and attenuating the effects of major stressors, traumatic events and cumulative risks on a person (Rutter 1995).

Nearly all environments harbour some risks, but when there are sufficient protective factors available to a young person and their family, resilience can develop. Such protective factors can safeguard the child from diseases that loom when he/she is subject to risks or stressors.

Masten and Reed (2002) describe the effects of protective factors at various levels:

Individual attributes, such as good intellectual capacities, an attractive and friendly personality, a high degree of self-confidence and trust in others, spirituality/belief, as well as talents that are recognized by their bearer and by others.

Families are important sources of protective factors. When family members convey positive and optimistic opinions and values, when they communicate meaningfulness to the entire family, then they are able to protect the children and promote their resilience (Walsh 1998). Other protective factors include a high level of organization and stability, solidarity among family members, and clear, open communication.

Communal factors, such as the availability of resources that support the family and its growing members by giving them the opportunity to become engaged in meaningful activities, as well as social cohesion among the members within a community.

Resilience is not an extraordinary capacity

Ann Masten at the University of Minnesota has emphasized in her article 'Ordinary Magic' (2001) that the most surprising result of resilience research is that resilience is not born from rare, extraordinary, or unique qualities, but rather anchored in the magic of common human resources, in other words, rooted in the mind, brain and body of every young person, in their families, and in their relationships and the communities of which they are a part.

The results of her studies of children who grew up under stressful and disadvantageous circumstances led the author to conclude that resilience should be considered as the successful functioning of basic human systems of adaptation. Some of these systems are aspects of an individual person, while others are elements of the relationships between an individual and his/her immediate social and ecological environment. Examples of these basic systems are: 1) attachment systems that provide social connections between people; 2) the central nervous system that provides for cognitive development and learning; 3) family systems, and 4) community organizations.

Coatsworth and Duncan (2003) developed these ideas further by suggesting that resilience as an effective system of adaptation encompasses a multitude of possible interventions. For instance, promoting resilience does not necessarily imply an intervention on an individual level. The most effective and long-lasting interventions are generally those that affect multiple systems and their interactions. Such interventions might generate protective families and communities, which in turn could strengthen the resilience of its younger members.

Capturing the 'resilience' construct

Freitas and Downey (1998) provide an overview of the scientific results regarding resilience, which suggest that:

- particular characteristics rarely serve exclusively risk or protective functions;
- individuals who seem resilient on one index often do not seem so on other indices, and;
- individuals often are not equally resilient across contexts.

These findings support a 'dynamic conceptualisation of resilience', which might help us understand why the ways children cope with stressors vary across domain, development and context. The authors are pursuing the question why certain children respond with resilience to certain stressors, while others have difficulties. This requires clarification of the following elements: a) the content of and relational structure among relevant psychological mediators such as competencies, expectancies, values and goals; and b) the relation between these psychological mediators and relevant features of the environment. The authors illustrate the application of their approach by investigating the relationship between IQ and behavioural problems among adolescents.

Luthar, Cicchetti and Becker (2000) have reviewed critical studies about the conceptual and methodological definition of resilience. The main critical points are the following:

- ambiguities in definitions and central terminology;
- heterogeneity in risks experienced and competence achieved by individuals viewed as resilient;
- instability of the phenomenon of resilience and;
- concerns regarding the usefulness of resilience as a theoretical construct.

The authors conclude that the study of resilience offers an important opportunity to find out more about the processes that influence individuals in situations of high risk and stress. They are encouraging continuing scientific attention to the conceptual and methodological difficulties, which are outlined by sceptics as well as supporters of the resilience concept.

Today, instruments that measure resilience as a personality variable have been developed and are in the process of being validated (Wagnild and Young 1993; Friborg *et al.* 2003; Leppert 2002; Connor and Davidson 2003; Oshio *et al.* 2003).

Some results from studies of resilience

The Kauai longitudinal study: resilience among high-risk families

Emmy Werner, a psychologist and pioneer of research on resilience at the University of California, made her name with the famous Kauai-Study (Werner 1993; Werner and Smith 2001).

Her group of collaborators followed 698 children born in 1955 on the Hawaiian island of Kauai over four decades. Psychologists, paediatricians, nurses and social workers examined their development at the ages of 1, 2, 10, 18, 32 and 40. Two hundred and ten study participants (ca. 30%) grew up under exceedingly difficult circumstances, plagued by poverty, parental illness, neglect, divorce and abuse. Emmy Werner was especially interested in these children-at-risk and wondered what kind of a development they might have experienced throughout the years, and whether they had the chance of a relatively problem-free life. At first, this question received a negative answer for about two thirds of the children so burdened. Between the ages of 10 and 18 they had notable learning and behavioural problems, ran into trouble with the law, and suffered from emotional problems.

However, one third of these 210 high-risk children developed rather positively. At none of the follow-up points could the researchers identify any kind of behavioural problems among these children. They were successful in school, founded a family, were embedded in social life and set realistic goals for themselves. At the age of 40 nobody in this group was unemployed nor had any of them run into trouble with the law and nobody was dependent on the support of social welfare institutions.

This resilient third, which showed a favourable long-term outcome, had grown up with some degree of protection, since they did not have to go through a significant separation from their primary caretaker in the first year of age, nor had they had to share parental attention with a sibling before the age of two and they had also been able to develop a sufficiently close relationship to a primary attachment figure. Kauai inhabitants who experienced neurological trauma during childbirth developed no problems as adults as long as they grew up in a stable and economically comfortable home. However, even quite a few of those children who had several risk factors (birth trauma, economical problems, broken home) turned out to be rather successful later, especially those who were able to develop an attachment to one adult person.

Further results of the study are that resilient children were endowed with protective factors which could attenuate the negative effects of adverse circumstances: they found support in a stable emotional relationship to adult parental figures outside of the disrupted family. Grandparents, a neighbour, a favourite teacher, a priest and even siblings provided a refuge for such neglected or abused children and affirmed that they were worthwhile individuals. When Werner and her co-workers assessed them at the age of 18, many of the adolescents named a favourite teacher who had become a role model, a friend or a confidant and who showed them how problems could be solved constructively and supported them particularly in times when their own family was in conflict or threatened by disintegration.

It is also important that a child who has experienced neglect and violence in the parental home is challenged early to develop some responsibility. For example, they might be asked to look out for younger siblings, or assume a function in school. Individual attributes also play a role: resilient children usually seem to have a 'calm' temperament and are less excitable. They have the capacity to approach others openly and thereby activate sources of support for themselves. And they frequently have a special talent which enables them to receive recognition from their peers.

Emmy Werner comes to an optimistic conclusion: the assumption that a child from a high-risk family necessarily turns into a failure, is contradicted by the research on resilience.

Bielefeld study on invulnerability

Doris Bender and Friedrich Lösel (1997) of the University of Erlangen in Germany examined 144 foster children who came from environments with multiple problems. A sub-group of 66 adolescents (the 'resilient' ones) developed considerably better than the remaining 78 study participants.

The resilient youth were much less impulsive, dealt with problems actively and assertively, had access to reliable attachment figures outside the family, were able to find support in school and experienced the situation in the foster home as positive. In sum – not unlike Emmy Werner's findings – the 'resilient' ones more frequently had the following protective factors:

- a stable emotional relationship to an adult during childhood, ideally one of their parents;
- the availability of social support and role models for constructive problem-solving (for example, older siblings, teachers);
- early challenges to achievement and assumption of responsibility;
- an intellectual prowess to overcome traumata;
- favourable requisites based on temperament.

Western Sydney Study: living with schizophrenia and developing a resilient self

Rene Geanellos (2005), a researcher in the nursing sciences at the University of Western Sydney, has conducted a qualitative study to investigate the subjective experiences of individuals living with the diagnosis of schizophrenia. He examined the personal accounts of 19 individuals which had been published in the renowned US journal *Schizophrenia Bulletin* in its section on First Person Accounts between the years 1990 and 2003. Some of these accounts had been published anonymously. The author subjected these biographical accounts to the hermeneutic method proposed by Hans-Georg Gadamer, which opens itself up vis-a-vis the text in an attempt to understand how the experience of schizophrenia is 'felt' without filtering it through an overarching concept (such as the notion of recovery).

A central finding of this study was that resilience moves along a continuum: according to circumstances, time and space, resilience exists to a greater or lesser degree in the biographical accounts that were examined. Individuals living with the diagnosis of schizophrenia experience cycles of resilience, i.e. their selves and their resilience are in a state of transformation.

These results seem to support the idea that living with schizophrenia might provide opportunities to develop resilience, due to the fact that the self adapts to this condition in unexpected and unplanned ways. The illness transforms life and the self in a profound and encompassing fashion. In the context of this study, adapting to the burden of schizophrenia means, according to the author, living a) wisely, i.e. understanding the nature of self-with-schizophrenia and of life-with-schizophrenia; b) mindfully, i.e. keeping understandings in conscious thought; and c) purposefully, i.e. acting deliberately.

In order to achieve this, people gather together their energy, develop willpower, seek out effective resources, establish supportive relationships and generate a stable, meaningful life along with a transformed, more resilient self.

Four principal themes and 18 sub-themes emerged from the biographical accounts of the study. The meta-theme which enveloped all the themes was entitled 'Adversity as opportunity: living with schizophrenia and developing a resilient self'.

The four principal themes were:

Fragmentation – compromised resilience and the vulnerable self:
This includes a desperate attempt to maintain the semblance of normality, considerable fear and urgent suffering that each individual must bear by him/herself and without help from others. Stigmatization by others and by oneself took place. The predominant feeling was one of being hopelessly mentally ill.

Disintegration – broken resilience and the submerged self:
Subjects were feeling overwhelmed by everyday life, isolated due to fractured relationships, and their general health was deteriorating. Fear, confusion, an 'inner storm' took over, madness escalated and the person felt disconnected from him/herself, from others and from reality.

Re-integration – recovered resilience and the re-established self:
The people experienced a desire to seek help and to strive for a turning point in their life. They struggled against destabilizing forces and yearned to resume control. They discovered many helpful activities that could enhance their well-being and they aimed to find the appropriate supports at the right time.

Reconstruction – renewed resilience and the recast self:
The people began to accept that the condition was likely to last and learned to recognize and accumulate the strengths which could help bring about stability once again. They were ready to resume contact with others and to deal constructively with their lives, realizing also that they could be useful to others even with their illness.

The author concludes that reaching the phase of reconstruction is an arduous and painful path for people diagnosed with schizophrenia. They have to deal with the distinction between their current life and the way their life might have turned out without this illness. This includes feelings of disappointment and mourning. They have to learn how to live within the restrictions and consequences of this condition, which was uncalled for and for which they were unprepared. Understanding how to live with a diagnosis of schizophrenia does, however, enable a capacity to transform and rearrange one's self. Reconnecting with life results from a fundamentally reoriented perspective of the person's self and his/her own life. Resuming a connection with life is an active process, promoted by many activities and relationships to others. Some persons who live with schizophrenia succeeded in looking beyond their own lives, feeling the need to help others with similar experiences and to tell them about their lives and give them advice. For instance, one person created a personal internet website and wrote up his own experiences of the diagnosis of schizophrenia in order to help and educate other people with the same diagnosis.

The author of this study considers stressors and difficulties as a potential opportunity to adapt to the challenges of life and to bolster one's own resilience. Resilience counts, since it enables adaptation and makes it possible to build on the person's inner strength to make use of helpful relationships and to foster talents and creativity in dealing with life's demands. In this way, resilience and adaptation become mutually dependent: resilience fosters adaptation and the other way around. This study suggests that people living with schizophrenia are actually dealing with their burdens in this fashion. The characteristics of their resilience are: vigilance, purposeful actions, persistence, courage, the ability to confront the unexpected and the ability to move along in spite of the difficulties.

In practice, these results imply that seeing resilience along a continuum spells opportunities for intervention. A nurse might, for instance, help a person to strengthen her/his resilience at a time when it has reached quite a low level during the phase of disintegration. Such an intervention requires, however, that clinicians become aware that individuals can adapt to the challenges of life and understand the process. 'Resilience along a continuum' also means that clinicians need to know the extent to which the resilience of service users can be compromised, and how it can be regained along the path towards reconstruction.

Scandinavia and Los Angeles a secure attachment and an efficient right brain hemisphere as early factors of resilience

Per Svanberg (1998) provides an overview of results coming from attachment research and developmental psychopathology that sets up a scientific framework for primary prevention and early interventions with respect to mental health. There is some evidence for successful interventions taking place as early as during pregnancy. The author concludes: A secure attachment relationship to primary parental figures, which has been established during the very early years of a child's life, is conducive to equipping the child with the necessary resilience to cope with many adverse life events as an adult, without developing psychiatric symptoms.

The review includes practical suggestions and interventions for a comprehensive primary prevention strategy with the principal aim of facilitating resilience and social competence from earliest childhood on.

Allan Schore (2001) from the University of California at Los Angeles School of Medicine includes the following data from various disciplines in his research endeavours in order to arrive at a deeper understanding of the psycho-neuro-biological mechanisms that may be the foundation for mental health throughout childhood: a) data from attachment studies on dyadic affective communications; b) data from neuroscience on the early developing right brain; c) data from psychophysiology on stress systems; and d) data from psychiatry on psycho-pathogenesis. According to the author, the infant's early developing right hemisphere has deep connections into the limbic and autonomic nervous systems and is dominant for the human stress response, and in this manner the attachment relationship facilitates the expansion of the child's coping capacities. This model suggests that adaptive infant mental health can be fundamentally defined as the earliest expression of flexible strategies for coping with the novelty and stress that is inherent in human interactions. Allan Shore describes this efficient right brain function as a resilience factor for optimal development over the later stages of the life-cycle.

Study of accident victims in Kiel, Germany

In this study the researchers Dieter Frey *et al.* (1985) were able to confirm the hypothesis that resilient individuals show less of a tendency to internalize the causes of negative events, personal failures or disasters. In other words they tend not to attribute the causes of such events to themselves, but are rather inclined to favour external attributions of causality, i.e. assigning guilt to others. They interviewed victims of accidents soon after their admission to hospital, regarding the causes and the possible inevitability of the accidents. Furthermore, the researchers asked them about their perception of the extent to which they themselves might have had an impact on their recovery. Subjects who were able to see a positive side to their situation and who did not consider themselves responsible for the accident, which they took as a given, recovered more rapidly from their injuries than those who believed the accident could have been prevented and who therefore reproached themselves and quarrelled with their fate. The latter group took an average of 140 days to be ready to resume working, while the duration of convalescence for the more optimistic group was only an average of 80 days.

Belfast review on risks and resilience in situations of emotional abuse

The psychologist Dorota Iwaniec and colleagues (Iwaniec *et al.* 2006) at the Belfast Institute of Child Care Research have surveyed studies that identify factors which can predict the psychosocial functioning of children following experiences of emotional abuse. Special attention was paid to factors that could determine risks and resilience in children. These factors include:

- predisposing factors such as early care-giving experiences;
- precipitating factors such as the frequency, intensity and duration of the abuse;
- factors intrinsic to the child, such as working models of the self and others, internal or external attributions, behavioural and coping strategies, self-esteem, and disposition;
- external factors such as school and availability of supportive relationships.

The researchers recommend that attention be given to the particular vulnerabilities and protective factors belonging to each child who experienced emotional abuse, in order to effectively reinforce their inherent resilience.

A study on resilience among women who experienced sexual abuse (Michigan, USA)

Judy Lam and Frances Grossman (2006) examined the relationship between protective factors and adult adaptation in a non-clinical sample of 264 undergraduate women. They found two groups without childhood sexual abuse, again one high (n = 109) and the other low (n = 99) on protective factors. In the two other groups with childhood sexual abuse, again one was high (n = 17) and the other group low (n = 27) on protective factors. The first hypothesis that higher levels of protective factors would be significantly associated with higher levels of functioning for all individuals was supported by the study data. The second hypothesis that the women with childhood sexual abuse and higher levels of protective factors would appear similar in adaptation to those without childhood sexual abuse was also supported. The findings further suggested that though the protective factors were beneficial for most individuals, they were significantly more helpful for those women with childhood sexual abuse.

Protective factors of Tibetan refugees in India who survived torture

A retrospective study from India (Holtz 1998) examined 35 refugee Tibetan nuns and lay students who had been taken prisoner and were tortured. The study group was matched with 35 controls who were not arrested or tortured. All participants in this study had fled from Tibet to India. The subjects were tested with the Hopkins Checklist-25, evaluating anxiety symptoms, affective disorders, somatic complaints and social impairment. The prevalence of symptoms scores in the clinical range for both cohorts was 41.4% for anxiety symptoms and 14.3% for depressive symptoms. The torture victims had a significantly higher proportion of elevated anxiety scores than the non-tortured control group (54.3% vs. 28.6%), but not of depressive symptoms. Results suggest that the experience of torture had negative long-term effects on mental health over and above the effects of being uprooted, fleeing one's country and living in exile as a refugee, though the additional effects were small. The following factors served to foster the resilience among the group of torture victims and prisoners and protected them against negative psychological sequelae: political commitment, social support in exile and prior knowledge of and preparedness for confinement and torture. Furthermore, the contribution of Buddhist spirituality plays an active role in the development of protective coping mechanisms among Tibetan refugees.

Implications of resilience research for practical interventions and research

Researchers who study resilience do not believe in resilience as an attribute that is distributed to individuals by chance. They do not consider emotional hardiness as a matter of luck. Some individuals are able to use their capacities under their own steam, while others require specific and tailor-made support. The results of resilience research have motivated mental health professionals to enhance and broaden their clinical and preventive interventions. The results of this research have changed the way that service providers conceptualize their interventions, from solely deficit-oriented to strengths-based models and frameworks. The results not only brought badly needed hope to the fields of prevention and treatment but also the messages of possibilities and optimism. In order to have an effect, 'resilience research must influence the attitudes and beliefs of human service personnel, as well as the way that service systems operate' (Coatsworth and Duncan 2003, p 6).

Educational implications

The American Psychological Association (APA 2008; Newmann 2005; Kersting 2003) assigns specially trained psychologists to elementary schools to teach children how to best cope with the unavoidable adversities of life. They are rehearsing resilient behaviours with their students. This programme aims to help children cope constructively with everyday stressors (for example, harassment, low grades), and not capitulate in the face of more serious situations, such as parental neglect, divorce and experiences of violence. Similar approaches to promoting resilience are being implemented in German day-care centres. Every educator can contribute to a child's well-being by how they behave in everyday situations. By observing such behaviour the child may well gain confidence in his/her own strength and capabilities and experience him/herself as valuable and capable of effecting changes in their own behaviours (Wustmann 2004).

Implications for prevention and health promotion

In summary, we can say that the scientific findings about resilience so far have broad and important consequences for prevention and health promotion. Preventive interventions are a natural extension of resilience research. It is much better to increase capacities to do well despite adversity than it is to treat individuals after maladjustment has crystallized (Albee and Gullotta 1997). Although the historical task of prevention focused exclusively on reducing risk factors for disorder, more recent studies have shown that the most powerful effects tend to come from both reducing risks and increasing protection (Pollard, Hawkins and Arthur 1999).

The foundation of resilience can be situated rather early in human development by looking at the security of the dyadic relationship between the infant and its primary attachment figure. When such an attachment is promoted early on, this leads to success-ful affect regulation and an expansion of the coping abilities of the child. For example, programmes for first-time mothers living in poverty and adolescent mothers, are helpful. These preventive interventions help to nurture and build the natural attachment relation-ship between the mother and the infant, help the mothers to build their own beliefs in their capacity to change the course of their lives, and also help to build the mother's sense of efficacy. An example of such an intervention is the Nurse Family Partnership, which is a programme for first-time mothers living in poverty (Olds *et al.* 1998).

Resilience is not a static or given dimension, but rather the result of active processes of adaptation and coping, which may be painful and difficult but which can transform each individual life to a greater or lesser degree. Empathic support and attendance throughout these subtle and complex processes, also later in life, is indicated.

Resilience is an exciting and young area of research, which is likely to yield results that can benefit many disciplines in both clinical and non-clinical areas. At the conference of the World Psychiatric Association (WPA) in Cairo (2005) a special symposium took place on the subject of 'Resilience in Mental Health Promotion: Interdisciplinary Perspectives'. The symposium included psychologists, psychoneuroimmunologists and oncology and public health specialists (Schmolke 2005, Ray 2005, Riba 2005, Herrman 2005). We are especially keen on seeing the future contributions to resilience from interdisciplinary research in neuro-endocrino-immunology, a field that examines the complex interactions between the various systems within a person and the material and social environments.

Implications for treatment

Resilience research does not translate directly into a specific kind of therapy, nor does it suggest that one kind of therapeutic approach will be superior to another. Instead, it suggests more general practices that are useful across different therapeutic approaches.

One treatment approach that directly reflects resilience research is called 'reframing'. It aims at helping clients to cognitively and affectively process life events in a way that builds on the positive, does not deny the negative, and allows them to incorporate the reality of these experiences into their own self concept. Reframing is a common technique in family therapy and is comparable in some respects to the technique of positive cognitive restructuring used in cognitive behavioural therapy (Rutter 1999). According to Rutter's recommendation to family therapists, the reduction of negative 'chain reactions' and the promotion of positive ones can determine the extent to which the consequences of stressors are likely to become permanent. New experiences or changes within family life can bring about a positive turning point. Even if positive experiences per se do not have a particularly protective effect, they can still be useful when they are able to help neutralize some of the risk factors.

In more general terms, resilience is connected to the mind, brain and body of individuals, to their families and to the communities in which they live. Consequently, practical interventions can be directed to these areas. That means that resilience can develop a priori or later on, that is to say, it can be learned whenever a person confronting a seriously stressful situation is enabled to activate the necessary protective factors which function:

- within a person (for example, hope);
- in a social or treatment context (for example, professionals who are knowledgeable about resilience; peers with similar experiences and therefore with an expert knowledge that has developed accordingly, along with a heightened sensibility); and/or
- in a macro-social context (for example, outpatient services that are not only oriented towards psychopathology; positive encounters with peers or colleagues in school or work place, etc.).

Resilience can also be seen as a counterforce to stigmatization. Many stigmatized individuals report that they gained strength and learned important lessons for their life whenever they were confronted with the negative consequences of stigmatization (see also Chapter 5).

Implications for research

Michael Rutter (2006) provides conceptual clarification of resilience, proposes various ways of assessing resilience methodologically and outlines what we can learn from resilience research. The author draws a distinction between the traditional concepts of risk and protection on the one hand and resilience on the other. Risk and protection both start with a focus on variables and then move to outcomes. There is an implicit assumption that the impact of risk and protective factors will be broadly similar in everyone, and that outcomes will depend on the mix and balance between risk and protective influences. By contrast, resilience starts with a recognition of the huge individual variation in people's responses to the same experiences. There is evidence that much of the variation in psychopathological outcomes can be accounted for by the combined effects of risk and protective factors. More importantly, resilience as understood as an interactive concept can only be studied if there is a thorough measurement of risk and protective factors. 'In short, resilience requires the prior study of risk and protection but adds a different, new dimension' (Rutter 2006, p 3).

Rutter (2006) proposes three broad research implications that derive from resilience findings:

1. Since resilience is not a general quality that represents a trait of the individual, research needs to focus on the processes underlying individual differences in response to environmental hazards, rather than resilience as an abstract entity.
2. Because resilience in relation to adverse childhood experiences may stem from positive adult experiences, it is necessary to adopt a life-span trajectory approach that can investigate later turning point effects.
3. Due to the importance of gene-environment interaction, it will be necessary to combine psychosocial and biological research approaches and to use a diverse range of research strategies (such as functional imaging of cognitive processing, neuroendocrine studies, investigation of mental sets and models, and the use of animal studies of various kinds).

Resilience findings – according to the author – provide five key implications for scientific understanding of substantive effects:

a) Resistance to hazards may derive from controlled exposure to risk rather than its avoidance (for example, exposure to feared object in behavioural therapy as opposed to its avoidance; the latter may lead to persistence of fear);
b) Resistance may derive from traits or circumstances that are either risky or neutral in the absence of the relevant environmental hazard (for example, for children who have been exposed in early life to parental abuse or neglect, adoption can be highly advantageous, according to a study by Duyme et al. 1999);
c) Resistance may derive from physiological or psychological coping processes, rather than external risk or protective factors. That means it requires a move from a focus on external risks to a focus on how these external risks are dealt with by the individual. (for example, young people who had a prolonged psychiatric hospitalisation, showed three features which were strongly characteristic of resilience: personal agency and a concern to overcome adversity; a self-reflective style; and a commitment to relationships – according to a study by Hauser et al. 2006);
d) Delayed recovery may derive from 'turning point' effects in adult life (for example, by marrying a non-deviant, supportive spouse in adulthood and thereby entering a new protective circle of family and friends; see Laub and Sampson 2003); and
e) Resilience may be constrained by biological programming or by the damaging effects of stress/adversity on neural structures.

Rutter (2006) points out that the study of dynamic processes, including a person's cognitive/emotional mechanisms, to discover how external risks are dealt with by the individual, may require qualitative methods to generate hypotheses (although quantitative measures will still be required to test the hypothesis so generated). Michael Rutter (2005) gave his assessment of the current research on resilience: 'We are just beginning to understand how to use research results on resilience for prevention and psychosocial intervention'.

RECOVERY, PREVENTION AND HEALTH PROMOTION

Throughout the past twenty years, growing interest and active promulgation of a new conceptualization of health and innovative research efforts in the areas of prevention and health promotion have been notable. We can observe a clear shift from the concept of pathogenesis that has been dominant so far towards salutogenesis. These developments have come about primarily as a result of the work of health- and social scientists. One of the reasons for this growing interest is the fact that the high rates of morbidity and chronicity have not abated in spite of considerable progress in the knowledge about aetiologies and treatment approaches. Therefore it has become imperative to emphasize perspectives of prevention and health promotion in general discussions, even though these fields still carry much less weight than acute interventions, within overall health care. The reasons for this development are convincing. Health promotion and focused preventive measures can lead to the avoidance of certain illnesses; they may have a positive impact on risk factors and facilitate the timely recognition and treatment of early symptoms and they may also allow stabilization and improvement of long-term illness courses.

There are conceptual and historical differences between prevention and health promotion. Traditional prevention aims to contain and avert the initial breeding grounds and risks for illnesses. Preventing the spread of infectious diseases is a classic domain of prevention. This requires knowledge of pathogenic factors, i.e. knowledge about the development and the course of an illness at individual and communal levels. The traditional concept of prevention which relies on a model based on risk-factors runs into difficulties whenever the promotion and maintenance of health is concerned.

Health policies in the 21st century will need to be constructed from the key question 'What makes people healthy?' (Kickbusch 2003, p 386). Health is achievable not merely by prevention and treatment of illnesses, including mental conditions (Orley 1998). Consequently, the rather young field of health promotion aims to implement salutogenic knowledge in practice, in relation to the individual as well as social, cultural and economic conditions. Compared to prevention, health promotion has a larger and potentially more varied field of intervention, addressing a greater number of target groups. The various types of interventions in the fields of prevention and health promotion are no longer strictly separate, but are rather seen as complementary, depending on the situation and the target group, which may call for one or the other measure to achieve its goals. Ultimately, both areas are aiming for gains in health status, but by different means. While prevention tries to achieve this through relieving the burden of illness and consequently pays most attention to illness-related risk-factors, health promotion spends more energy on the harnessing of resources and health-supporting protective factors (Herrman, Saxena and Moodie 2005; Malterud and Hollnagel 2004).

Bengel, Strittmatter and Willmann (1999) understand health promotion as a social-ecological model. Preventive measures are targeted at active and responsible participation of the layperson in the establishment of health-promoting conditions and at the collaboration between laypersons and professionals. The authors regard the concept of health promotion as being similar to the empowerment approach which grew out of North-American communal psychology (Rappaport 1981). Empowerment refers to the strengthening of competence, responsibility and resourcefulness of persons or groups.

The scientific section, 'Preventive Psychiatry', of the World Psychiatric Association (WPA) has broadened its view on prevention by including perspectives on positive health and health promotion. The section starts its consensus-paper on psychiatric prevention with the following words, which give cause for optimism:

'Mental illnesses are among the leading causes of disability worldwide. Therefore, psychiatrists and other mental health professionals should put all their efforts to decrease the mental health "epidemic" in the society, by preventive and health promotion programmes. Conventional, illness based treatment should be broadened to a comprehensive, multidimensional approach to mental health and mental disorders. This includes the enhancement of positive attitudes and reduction of prevailing scepticism regarding the possibility of prevention and cure. Combining illness-focused treatment with health promotion interventions and strengthening positive mental health such as life skills, would decrease psychological distress, enhance quality of life, i.e. self-esteem, mastery of one's life, life satisfaction, competence and psychological adjustment. It would break the spiral of stress, increase psychobiological immunity, and reduce inpatient treatment and stigmatization of people with mental illnesses.' (Lecic-Tosevski *et al.* 2003, p. 307)

The aims of promoting general and mental health

The main ideas of health promotion were developed by the WHO in the 1986 Ottawa Charter. An explicitly strong position was assigned to positive capacities for health and to a strengthening of the multiple resources that are available to the individual as well as to the community as a whole. According to the Ottawa Charter, health is no longer understood as a primary goal of life, but rather as an essential element of daily life that can be actively shaped. Health is more than mere absence of illness, and correspondingly must be formulated in positive terms. Accordingly, health is created and lived by people in their everyday environments, i.e. where they are playing, learning, working and loving (WHO 1986).

Today there is a special branch of health promotion that addresses mental health in particular (mental health promotion). Many experts agree that interventions that occur only once a mental disturbance has taken hold are coming too late. Furthermore, when interventions are limited to treatment, they can only address certain aspects of the disturbance. A fundamental rethinking seems necessary in the direction of a more integrative view, which reflects the entirety of life circumstances. Berger (1999) refers to the biopsychosocial model of Engel (1976) and Antonovsky's concept of salutogenesis (1979), which has been incorporated into the WHO Ottawa Charter.

According to the broad definition of WHO (2001), promoting mental health encompasses all strategies that aim to have beneficial effects on mental health. This includes rediscovering and promoting personal resources, capacities and abilities, as well as enhancing the socio-economic environment. Mental health is defined as '. . . a state of well-being in which the individual realizes his or her own abilities, can cope with the normal stress of life, can work productively and fruitfully, and is able to make a contribution to his or her community' (WHO 2001, p. 1). In this positive sense, mental health is the foundation of well-being and effective functioning for an individual and for a community.

There are proponents of the view that 'mental health promotion' should not be separated from health promotion in general, since the 'emotional' aspects cannot be isolated from all other social and physical domains, as they are interlocking and complement each other (Seedhouse 2002).

Anderson and Jenkins (2003, p 241) consider the following aspects of the Ottawa Charter of WHO to be its most revolutionary elements:

• It left the medical domain outside the concept of health promotion. Instead, the idea of 'returning power to people' can be understood as taking the power from medicine to be returned to people;
• Health promotion is characterized by positive approaches and messages rather than paternalistic or restrictive educational strategies.

Some experts emphasize that health promotion should not simply be a top-down intervention, and that NGO-type initiatives are just as promising as those coming from communities and individuals themselves. The most successful programmes have been developed in collaboration with community members at large, instead of those based on a top-down approach – according to Helen Herrman (2001), the renowned Australian health promotion researcher. The 'silent voices and signs', changes in society and culture, that can have a long-term impact on mental health, must be carefully noted and taken into consideration (Anderson and Jenkins 2003, p 241).

Since the core values of health promotion are very much tied to seeing individuals as subjects of their own lives, empowerment and real participation are being seen as basic elements of any health-promoting activities (Raeburn and Rootman 1998; Tones and Tilford 2003). Several innovative WHO programmes started in the early 90s, such as Healthy Cities, Healthy Islands and Health-promoting Schools and Hospitals. For example, the programme on health-promoting schools emphasizes the strengthening of communicative and emotional competencies, the advance of conflict resolution strategies and the development of a culture of non-violent dispute (WHO, UNESCO and UNICEF 1992; Berger 1999). The Declaration of Ottawa formed the cornerstone for a host of activities that range from health-promoting policies, environments and communal actions to the development of personal competencies (life-skills), as well as calling for a re-orientation of health services (WHO 1986).

European principles of mental health promotion

Of late, a network of general hospitals has been founded that is committed to the implementation of health-promotion projects as part of their clinical services. Hartmut Berger (1999, 2008) from the Walter-Picard Hospital in Riedstadt, Germany, is the co-ordinator of this network, which brings together the various components of this exciting project. Its central strategies follow the empowerment-concept, i.e. the transmission of knowledge and capacities that aim to enhance personal resources and to enable active coping-strategies (Berger 1999). So far, 600 hospitals have joined this network, which is supported by the WHO (Lobnig *et al.* 1999). In 1998, the Task Force on Health Promoting Psychiatric Services emerged from this network and now includes over 100 member institutions. Based on this co-operative enterprise, basic principles of health-promoting psychiatric services, along with several best practice models for health promotion in psychiatric services, have been developed (Berger *et al.* 2005; www.hpps.net). Accordingly, health-promoting mental health services need to:

- orient themselves to a holistic concept of health and disease;
- orientate their activities to human dignity, equality and solidarity, always in respect of the varying needs of the different cultural groups within the community;
- orientate themselves to the well-being of the patients, families and staff and obligate themselves to the protection of the environment;
- use their resources wisely in accordance with the measure of their contribution to health;
- apply their efforts to active co-operation and networking with other health services.

These principles have already been applied to 137 projects which have been presented since 1998 at annual conferences of 'Health Promoting Hospitals' in Europe. The Task Force of Health Promoting Psychiatric Services is funded by the European Community and is dedicated to the implementation of health promotion and prevention of psychiatric conditions in Europe. These projects have led to the development of guidelines for mental health promotion and prevention of mental illnesses (www.imhpa.net) as well as to the so-called Green Book (European Commission 2005) and the mental health action plan (WHO Ministerial Conference on Mental Health 2005; internet: www.euro.who.int 30.08.08) which include strategies for the promotion of mental health in the European Union.

'There is no health without mental health'

Any amelioration of mental health is closely tied to improvements in physical health and behavioural changes. Empirical studies from several countries affirm the complex inter-actions between mental health and education, work productivity, supportive relationships within families and the community at large, as well as lower crime rates – according to Australian experts in health promotion (Herrman *et al.* 2003; Walker and Rowling 2002).

Health policy-makers from Anglo-American countries have pointed out clear relation-ships at the political, economic and public health levels between the physical and the mental health of citizens. The federal US Government has noted that 'mental health is fundamental for health in general' (US Department of Health and Human Services 1999). And according to the UK health system, promoting mental health brings a broad spec-trum of health-related and social advantages, such as improved physical health, greater emotional resilience, stronger social integration and participation, and greater economic productivity (Department of Health, UK 2001).

The resulting document, which has the title 'There is No Health without Mental Health', summarized the results of a health survey among 10,000 inhabitants of New York City. People who had experienced high levels of emotional stress were found to have three times greater rates of poor general health. Significant emotional stress (associated with depression, anxiety, nervousness, sadness, hopelessness, low self-worth) is highly correlated with physical illnesses such as diabetes, obesity, asthma, hypertension and health-compromising behaviours, which include a lack of exercise, excessive alcohol and nicotine use and poor nutrition (New York City Department of Health and Mental Hygiene 2003).

A study of the health of older people in Thailand illustrated the interplay between physical and mental health. Among the daily health-promoting activities of these subjects are good nutrition and regular physical exercise. They increased their knowledge about health and pursued religious activities, had good relationships with others and managed their finances and expenses carefully – all this leading to high satisfaction with life (Othaganont et al. 2002).

The influence of social and environmental factors on poor health are manifold and include behavioural mechanisms as well as physiological parameters, which are related to neuro-endocrine and immunological functions. Interpersonal relations, environmental influences and individual experiences can have a positive impact on biological processes, and especially on brain regions that might even have an impact on the regulation of genes (Bauer 2004). The strong health-promoting effect of 'social energy', equally involving physical as well as mental processes, has also been pointed out by Ammon (1983). This refers to intensive emotional and social exchange among individuals at large, as well as within therapeutic and non-therapeutic groups.

Social support is part of the key resources that have been the subject of study in the field of health promotion for many years. The consensus is that people who live in isolation are facing a higher mortality and morbidity risk. Studies were able to show a connection between social support and the survival rates from myocardial infarction (Mookadam and Arthur 2004). Social support is considered to be a health-promoting factor when it generates a feeling of belonging and intimacy and when it leads to people experiencing themselves as more competent and self-efficient (Berkman 1995; House 2001). Supportive social networks in the community can exert a protective effect for individuals when they experience a high degree of trust within a tight-knit group (Fisher et al. 1999).

A qualitative study by King et al. (2006) investigated the relationship between social support and adaptation of people with chronic conditions such as cerebral palsy, spina bifida and attention deficit disorder. They experienced three different types of social support, which are related to self-perception and positive convictions:

- emotional support (positive affirmation and acceptance lead to the perception that they are trustworthy and also to greater self-esteem);
- instrumental support (instruction and making strategies available that lead to greater self-efficacy);
- cognitive support (encouragement, esteem and new perspectives lead to a coherent self-concept and worldview).

The mutual influences of mental and physical health are also addressed in a chapter by Raphael et al. (2005) which is part of the substantial volume by the WHO on mental health promotion.

Connections between health promotion and recovery

A broader understanding of health as an 'essential component of daily life' and the philosophy that individuals are subjects and agents of their own lives, illustrate the conceptual connections and the overlap of certain areas in health promotion and recovery. These shared connections relate to the following positively formulated elements: subjective variation in healing and convalescence; hope; re-learnt optimism; resilience; manifold self-help activities; coping mechanisms; supportive social relations and networks. And that is just to mention a few. Health and recovery-processes are viewed rather subjectively and at the same time situated within the context of social networks in the community and everyday life. In this sense, health promotion can be seen as a meta-concept for all these processes. Whenever we are thinking beyond a partial task of health promotion, i.e. the 'stabilization and amelioration in the course of an illness', then the recovery-process can assume a meaningful role in the broad innovative vision of health.

It could be said that the 'hard' definition of recovery comes from clinical outcome research and asserts the following conditions for recovery: a person should no longer display any clinical symptoms or any limitations that may be related to such symptoms, and should be in a position to function independently of the help of others. As presented in detail above a more comprehensive definition of recovery, stemming from the user movement and the Independent Living Movement in the USA, has assumed an increasingly important role in more recent literature on rehabilitation. It suggests that recovery does not necessarily imply an improvement or elimination of symptoms and deficits, but rather relates to a learning process that enables people to live with long-term limitations and teaches them how to cope or compensate for them and to participate in community life as actively and satisfactorily as possible. Such an understanding of recovery also applies to people who have not yet managed to overcome their symptoms or other illness-related limitations and who are in the midst of their recovery-processes (Davidson *et al.* 2005b).

Another connection between health promotion and recovery involves the consideration of factors that can have an impact on individual illness- and convalescence-related processes. There are many examples of individuals with serious psychiatric and physical illnesses that provide evidence of the multiple paths and developments that may include temporary or ongoing stability, set-backs, increase of frequently painful insights, a growth in creative powers and a life with a stronger and more mature identity. These documented experiences in the biography of individuals, who have often had a rather long and tortuous path to recovery, have given rise to the comprehensive definition of recovery.

The concept of health promotion also emerged from the realization that objective parameters are no longer sufficient and need to be augmented by subjective views, if health is to be understood in all its complexity and within its very specific social and cultural context. The investigation of the great variety of personal, social and material resources is just one of the many approaches to individual and communal health.

Co-existence of health and illness

The commonalities of health promotion and recovery also include a relative and process-oriented understanding of illness and health. It is not possible to clearly delineate these from each other and to consider them in neatly separated categories, such as those used by medical science, according to defined parameters. As the Swedish social scientist Alain Topor (2001) has shown in his differentiated empirical study, successful recovery implies living with contradictions. It is not about being 'either sick or well' but rather about being 'both at the same time', in other words, being ill and healthy concurrently (see pp 168 in this book).

This corresponds to the continuum of health proposed by the Israeli medical sociologist Antonovsky (1987), according to whom, a person at any point on the continuum can move towards more or less pronounced health. This means that a person is never totally ill or completely healthy. In the field of mental health promotion, the allocation of health and illness occurs similarly. Mental disorders and positive mental health are not seen as the opposite poles in a linear scale, but rather as two overlapping and interrelated components of one whole concept of mental health (Detels *et al.* 2002).

In her own study of protective factors among people diagnosed with schizophrenia in their everyday life, Schmolke (2001) found similar results. At that time she had no awareness of the recovery-concept, but her study took place simultaneously with several of the studies that later on provided her with important insights about recovery. One result of her study was that the participants experienced themselves as healthy most of the time, and as sick only when they were in the midst of an acute psychotic episode and needed more intensive support. The participants made use of many personal resources while having to deal with extremely stressful demands and illness-related limitations. Paradoxically, many factors that were usually considered as highly problematic and risky (such as an alcoholic partner, whose demands pulled his friend out of a very withdrawn and isolated state), had an enormously supportive and health-sustaining effect for certain individuals. The study was embedded in the conceptual framework of health promotion.

Thomas Bock, the founder of the first psychosis seminar in Hamburg, Germany (a seminar, also called a trialogue, with service users, relatives and professionals as participants in a non-hierarchical manner, see pp 189–190), believes that health and illness have become erroneously and unnecessarily polarized in the sense that 'health is desirable and illness a must to avoid at all costs'. Accordingly, a successful concept of life would be equated with physical and mental health and illness would deserve nothing but pity. The idea of 'absolute health' would put people who are chronically ill or disabled in complete isolation (Bock 1992). An interdisciplinary conference was held in Germany in the early nineties that was dedicated to this dialectical subject and carried the title 'How healthy are the sick?' (Lutz and Mark 1995).

Protective, health-promoting resources and positive health can sometimes co-exist with severe psychopathological symptoms – as documented in several recovery-narratives. This implies that in clinical services (i.e. in assessment, treatment and rehabilitation), psychopathological symptoms and functional limitations on the one hand and strengths, capacities and personal efforts towards recovery on the other, must be captured and related to each other. Interventions and health promotion programmes should not be implemented separately from clinical practice. In other words, a person who is sick also needs the kind of things that make him feel good and strengthen him, just like anyone else. This integrated approach culminated in a special issue with the title 'Health-promotion – an essential component of effective clinical care' (Schmolke and Lecic-Tosevski 2003a).

Practical examples of health promotion activities

Diagnosis

Juan Mezzich has developed a conceptual connection between health promotion and diagnosis. According to the author, diagnosis as part of an integrative understanding must go beyond the standardized assessment of psychopathology and include positive aspects of health, as well as recommendations for specific health promotion strategies, in addition to standard treatment planning (Mezzich 2003, Mezzich 2005a). In a separate section, this book also includes further details about the International Guidelines for Diagnostic Assessment (IGDA) of WPA (2003) (see pp 206 in this book).

Self-help groups

In a special issue of a Swiss mental health journal (*Pro Mente Sana Aktuell*, 1999), several projects are described under the rubric of 'Health Promotion and Prevention: Stepchild Psychiatry', which aim to bolster individual health. In one of the articles, Vogelsanger (1999) presents self-help groups as an essential element of health promotion. They are said to generate the following positive effects. They:

- counteract social isolation;
- provide orientation;
- encourage brain storming and discussions;
- generate information and knowledge;
- dispense new meaning to life.

For example, self-help groups on the subjects of anxiety and panic attacks, obsessions and addiction, or for survivors of incest and other traumas, are making an important contribution which might prevent an emotional disturbance from turning into a chronic illness.

Individuals with emotional problems can also have physical and social difficulties, which might be the focus of the self-help group they have chosen. Conversely, there are probably many members of self-help groups for physical disorders who also suffer from psychiatric conditions. In a self-help group for individuals with depression, one woman expressed the difference between somatic and emotional illness as follows:

'I spent several weeks in hospital after a heart attack, which was an entirely new experience for me. I could not believe how many letters, flowers, and visits I received. There was so much empathy. Before, when I was hospitalized for depression, this was quite different. Hardly anyone got in touch with me and any contact was so tense, that I soon rather avoided them. In the end it is much simpler to have something "real".' (ibid. p 14).

'What does health mean to you?'

The same journal also includes two articles with several interviews that ask what health meant personally to the participants and what they would do for their own health. The following two examples show clearly that people with and without psychiatric problems do not display great differences in their health-promoting activities and their subjective meaning of health. To the question 'What does health mean to you?' they answered as follows:

Example 1: 'Health is a broad concept for me, which includes quality of life, satisfaction, living-in-the-centre, engagement with my environment and joyful encounters with people. I always look for physical recreation, be that by taking a walk, a yoga-type exercise, going to the gym, or taking my god-child to Disney Land. Even reading a book that has nothing to do with my work, or getting enough sleep, are good for me. I find it important to critically evaluate the demands placed on me and on my co-workers. How much can be expected realistically? Is there a risk of burnout? And I give myself permission to be sick, which for me is also part of health.' (Quotation from a leading health administrator in Switzerland, *pro mente sana* 1999, p 24).

Example 2: 'When I like to get up in the morning and tackle my work; when I feel vibrant and no pain, no nasty thoughts and no arguing. I feel healthy when I like to move myself, use my senses consciously, find myself interested in the environment, and when I pay attention. Giving and receiving love is also part of it. When I am able to make plans for the future, still find room in my heart, when I am able to help someone, or don't have financial worries, then I feel at my best. Also when sleeping and dreaming instils no fear, when I have no bad feelings or anxieties, and when I'm able to laugh. Constant rage is bad for my health, it even makes me feel angry in my muscles.' (Quotation from a participant with a psychiatric diagnosis, *pro mente sana* 1999, p 4).

Knowing – Enjoying – Better Living

This is the title of a new psycho-educational group seminar for individuals with psychotic experiences, developed by Michaela Amering, Ingrid Sibitz and colleagues from the Department of Psychiatriy and Psychotherapy at the Medical University of Vienna (Amering *et al.* 2002; Sibitz *et al.* 2006). This seminar goes beyond the traditional psycho-educational themes by focusing on increasing quality of life, i.e. on factors that strengthen well-being beyond the illness. Four units are devoted to each of two thematic sections. The seminar addresses individuals who have been diagnosed with a psychosis from the group of schizophrenias and who have expressed an interest in the content of the seminars. Participants gather for nine weekly meetings.

The first thematic section gives participants the opportunity to inquire about the following illness-related subjects:

- How can I reduce my vulnerability?
- How can I cope with symptoms?
- What are the effects of medication?
- How can I deal with prejudice and discrimination?

The second thematic section encourages people to discover activities and needs that might help improve their quality of life. This includes the following questions:

- How do I enhance my well-being?
- How do I stay in shape?
- How can I feel good around others?
- How can I plan and actively fashion my life?

In this manner, the facilitators continue to learn about new aspects of the illness by hearing a great variety of touching and authentic accounts from the participants, who are speaking about their experiences of psychosis. The facilitators gain insight through these narratives and learn to recognize which ways of dealing with service recipients might be helpful and which not. Another advantage is that all participants, including the facilitators, learn how to live better through participating in discussions about improving quality of life. 'Knowing – Enjoying – Better living' becomes a motto for everyone. Many participants say in their feedback that they find the mutual exchange, the style of the seminar and the possibility of learning something new and of making new contacts as quite positive. The realization that they are not alone with their illness is a great relief for everyone, as is hearing from others how they are coping. After attending the seminar, the participants describe themselves as 'stronger, more courageous, more active and more motivated'. One participant gave the following feedback: 'and then you get the feeling that you are not as overwhelmed. You can do something about it – which is also a huge mental strength' (Sibitz and Amering 2003 p 31).

Health promotion services for people with psychiatric disabilities

In 2004 at Boston University's Centre for Psychiatric Rehabilitation, a colloquium was organized on the topic of 'Health and promotion of health of people with psychiatric disabilities'. The papers arising from the colloquium were published in 2006 in a special issue of the *Psychiatric Rehabilitation Journal*. The authors aimed not only to stimulate a dialogue about the critical health issues of people with psychiatric disabilities, but also to encourage the translation of caring actions into caring policies, programmes and practices that promote the health – not the illness – of people who live with psychiatric disabilities. They argued that people who live with psychiatric disabilities have a 'right to a healthy life', a right to thrive and not just survive, and that clinicians have a responsibility to address these issues (Hutchinson and Henry 2006). The authors point out that the issue of health promotion is particularly critical because the life expectancy for individuals with serious mental illnesses is significantly lower than that of the general population. According to Hutchinson *et al.* (2006), physical illnesses frequently accompany mental illnesses, thereby compounding the disease burden. People with serious mental illness often live below the poverty line, lead sedentary lives, consume poor diets, are heavy tobacco users and have much lower rates of recommended health behaviours than the general population.

Hutchinson *et al.* (2006) aim to include concepts of wellness into health promotion programmes for persons with psychiatric disabilities. They point out that the wellness concept has advanced the idea of the importance of engaging in certain health-promoting behaviours within healthy environments, not simply for the purpose of preventing or better managing a disease, but also to enhance one's well-being and quality of life. While primary prevention emphasizes 'forestalling dysfunction, particularly in those situations of high risk', wellness enhancement emphasizes 'promoting psychological health and physical well-being in all people, not just those at high risk' (p 241).

The authors point out that people with serious mental illnesses have a right to optimal health and that they can be well even if their psychiatric diagnoses suggest that they are ill. Furthermore, various health promotion practices could increase their health and well-being. According to Mullen (1986), experiencing psychiatric symptoms or disability does not preclude experiencing wellness. Results from a survey document that people with mental illnesses strongly agree and use a variety of integrative and complementary health practices and treatments as they pursue improved well-being and increased community integration (Ridgeway et al. 2002). For example, Copeland (1997), a US recovery activist, has developed wellness education materials and tools which offer empowering opportunities to achieve health and wellness despite the general lack of attention to health promotion services within the mental health system (see pp 83 in this book).

Hutchinson et al. (2006) have developed a conceptual framework for integrating health promotion services into the mental health system. They define wellness as 'people's growth toward healthy physical, mental and spiritual lifestyles expressed in healthy environments, and the reduction of co-morbid health conditions and disorders' (p 245). In their framework, the wellness concept should be consistent with a public health approach (i.e. an integrated method of functioning oriented toward maximizing the potential of which the individual is capable). The authors plead that the concept of wellness must be integrated into the already existing system of other mental health services that are desired by people with severe mental illnesses. 'Health promotion services for people with severe mental illnesses must be compatible with the fact that other services exist (for example, crisis intervention, treatment, rehabilitation), yet expansive enough to insure that wellness thinking is brought into the field as a full partner in the pursuit of recovery from severe mental illnesses.' (Hutchinson et al. 2006, p 244).

The following principles of health promotion for people with serious psychiatric disabilities have been formulated (Hutchinson et al. 2006, p 247):

- Health and access to health care are universal rights of all people.
- Health promotion recognizes the potential for health and wellness for people with psychiatric disabilities.
- Active participation of people with serious psychiatric disabilities in health promotion activities is the ideal.
- Health education is the cornerstone of health promotion for people with psychiatric disabilities.
- Health promotion for people with psychiatric disabilities addresses the health characteristics of environments where people live, learn and work.
- Health promotion is holistic and eclectic in its use of many strategies and pathways.
- Health promotion addresses each individual's resource needs.
- Health promotion interventions must address differences in people's readiness for change.

The authors give examples of health promotion activities and interventions for persons with psychiatric disability which have already been put into practice (ibid., p 247f.):

- Stationing a nurse practitioner in a community mental health centre to engage people in order to ensure that each receives optimal primary health care and screenings. This way, this professional could offer health education, individualized encouragement and health advocacy within the larger health system;
- A person teaching people positive self-care behaviours and health promotion strategies in day treatment programmes, clubhouses and outpatient services rather than many 'services as usual';
- Introducing medical identification cards that people carry, indicating their health issues, their providers and choice of care to help reduce the tendency to treat medical conditions as psychiatric symptoms;
- Implementing physical activity interventions in mental health settings (for example, Richardson *et al.* 2005);
- Enhancing communication between mental health and medical providers in order to help inform, co-ordinate and provide better treatment and reduce costly poly-pharmacy.

In conclusion, the authors state that while there are promising evaluation studies of health promotion interventions for people with serious mental illnesses, many are lacking in the methodological rigour that is required for a service to be labelled 'evidence-based'. They believe that it is essential to study the effect of 'services as usual' in combination with health promotion services, on recovery outcomes. The effects of health promotion interventions must be assessed in terms of both human and financial benefits. 'Only in this way can health promotion services be funded to take their rightful place in the repertoire of essential services for people with severe mental illnesses.' (*Hutchinson et al.* 2006, p 248).

Joint dimensions of health promotion, prevention and recovery

In concluding we want to offer a few thoughts about the shared dimensions of health promotion, prevention and recovery, which have originated from different positions, historical concepts and specialty fields. They do have in common a comprehensive, holistic understanding of health, which considers health not merely as the absence of illness. All domains can influence and cross-stimulate each other. Once we know more precisely what leads to healing and convalescence from serious mental problems, as outlined in the recovery-concept, health promotion and prevention can build on this. And vice-versa, once we have assembled more details about the factors that promote and maintain the general health of individuals, in the interplay with social, cultural, material and environmental factors, then recovery-experts can benefit from this. Finally, more refined modern prevention programmes can consider the salient points in their intervention, such as the risks of relapse on the way to recovery. Successful health promotion can play an essential role in preventive success at various levels.

We hope that the available knowledge and the rich trove of experiences about recovery, and about the promotion of positive health, will enter day-to-day clinical practice, and that clinicians will become more open to these new perspectives. The 'therapist as a person' and the sometimes life-saving relationships between clinicians and help-seekers are key resources in the recovery process.

One potential risk needs to be pointed out here: The many autobiographical narratives of (ex-) users reveal a profound understanding of the experience of mental health problems, which would otherwise not be accessible to clinicians. However, there is the risk that autobiographical reports could be quickly transposed by clinicians and researchers into the medical or therapeutic 'lingo', which they have acquired in the course of their professional socialization. Should such a transformation take place, much valuable and authentic material would be lost again. Hatfield and Lefley clearly pointed out this risk in their 1993 book, which provided an important platform for many people with mental problems and their personal recovery-narratives.

RECOVERY AND QUALITY OF LIFE

In medicine as well as psychiatry, assessing quality of life (QOL) offers important insights about the subjective experiences of individuals with certain conditions. Therefore, many clinicians and researchers are interested in determining the patient's quality of life levels. Unlike merely illness-related parameters, QOL-assessments provide feedback about general life-satisfaction, well-being and functioning in social roles. Such feedback has become widely established in assessing treatment effects beyond symptom reduction or fewer hospital days. In many psychosocial and medical domains, QOL-assessments that aim to capture the perspectives and subjective experiences of patients, have become indispensable (Katschnig *et al.* 2006).

In a parallel development, research- and evaluation-projects conducted by users have also focused on subjective assessments and on definitions of process- and outcome-variables, which should include recovery, satisfaction with services, QOL and empowerment (cf. Campbell 1997; Faulkner 2000; Rose 2001). The main emphasis in these studies is placed on capturing subjective views of the participants, i.e. by using empowerment- and recovery-instruments and qualitative statements, based on semi-structured interviews and methods of observation which provide access to subjective experiences. Stastny and Amering (2006), in their chapter on quality of life, have noted with surprise that the dimension Quality of Life has been afforded relatively little attention in the course of user-run studies. It seemed to these authors that the findings of QOL experts and user-run studies have barely influenced or cross-fertilized each other.

This seems especially surprising, since users as researchers explicitly aim to improve the life of users of mental health services. Therefore, it could be assumed that the QOL concept might be of interest to them, in that it might help them to assess the impact of self-help and other user-driven interventions. On the other hand, it is equally astonishing that QOL researchers who are interested in subjective experiences, have not found a bridge to enable a dialogue with user researchers. It is lamentable that this shared area of interest has not led to more significant changes in attitudes or more collaborative projects over recent years. Integration of user-values and QOL has not taken place and these two areas seem to be moving forward as 'parallel universes'.

To determine the possible cause of these parallel processes, it is necessary to take a closer look at the developments in research, from a user perspective that has already redefined the parameters for therapeutic goals and outcomes. Such a user perspective was sought in a large-scale California study about user-satisfaction with mental health services, which involved its subjects in all phases of the research (Campbell and Schraiber, 1989). It turned out that users favoured different priorities and outcome variables than the professional researchers. Only one of eight thematic areas concerned the subject of 'Wellbeing and quality of life'. Users responded to the question: 'What would make your life better right now?' by emphasizing socio-economic factors such as 'a decent home, a job, independence, a reasonable income and good friends', topics that have been considered as subjective and 'objective' components of QOL by the research community. A similar research project in the UK came up with similar results. In addition, users emphasize the significance of nature and the extent and quality of their relationships with others, including to their peers (Faulkner and Thomas 2002).

Other studies (Dumont and Campbell 1994) cited the following domains as most important to users: legal issues; the impact of users on services and on the mental health system as a whole; oppression and racism; coercive measures and control; preserving the integrity of individuals; harmful effects of treatment; alternatives to traditional services; civil rights; quality of life; work, and the validity of research. Here too, quality of life was only one variable among many. In the late 90s, recovery began to occupy a central role in research, and has possibly taken the place of the earlier interest that users had in quality of life concepts. Among an extensive listing of recovery-oriented instruments there was no mention of a specific QOL measure (Ralph *et al.* 1999). Instead, a parallel development ensued, with the new concepts of recovery and resilience on the one side and quality of life on the other. The idea that even people with prolonged and complex mental health problems could develop resilience by learning about, and living in, recovery has taken centre stage in studies that are run or influenced by consumers. Differences in research design also became apparent. While the tradition of recovery emphasizes a person-centred and process-oriented approach along with qualitative methods, QOL research still favours studying cohorts of subjects, using measures that are either cross-sectional or administered pre- and post-intervention. Following the precepts of action research, the empowerment-concept has also found resonance in user-directed studies that aim to effect a change in the roles of participating individuals and organizations by moving them from passive research subjects to active participants. A greater exchange between the scientific field of QOL research and the concepts of recovery and resilience seems highly desirable and is likely to yield promising results. Quite apart from the important role that the experiences and perspectives of users of professional services have played with regard to recovery, and could also potentially play in regard to quality of life, the empowerment concept could be an important bridge which would bring these unfortunately divided domains into greater contact.

One of the reasons for the lack of endorsement of the quality of life construct by people with lived experience of mental health problems and disabilities might well be the serious problem of the relationship between objective and subjective assessments of quality of life. This problem is further aggravated when one looks at the research findings of small and fragile associations between objective and subjective assessments. There is ongoing debate about which one should take precedence and there are arguments that they are two different kinds of data altogether (Warner 1999). The sad story of many people living under dire circumstances due to serious mental health problems, discrimination and social exclusion who rate their subjective quality of life rather highly – probably by 'cutting their coat to suit their cloth' – and other problems that Warner captured in his suggestion as to the understanding of the 'emics and etics of quality of life assessments' (Warner, 1999) illustrates what might discourage people from this field of research.

Recently, the introduction of the capabilities approach, with a focus on agency and opportunities, connectedness and citizenship (Hopper 2007; Ware *et al.* 2007), which has led 'to a framing of quality of life following psychiatric disability that prioritizes capacity for reflective action over satisfaction and functioning' introduced a truly new dimension to this discussion and might prove to be better at fostering research which deals with 'what really matters' (Ware *et al.* 2008). Such a development might well bring experts with a lived experience on board.

RECOVERY AND EMPOWERMENT

Like recovery, empowerment is a complex construct. Empowerment, self-determination and self-efficacy are essential elements of recovery-processes (Corrigan 2006). This leads to the assumption that empowerment can have a measurable impact on recovery. A study conducted at Yale by Resnick *et al.* (2005) addressed the problem of an empirical basis for recovery. The researchers decided to consider recovery as an attitudinal variable. This reflects an orientation based on a process-model of recovery, but also means that such an attitude – like all attitudes – can be measured and, in the right context, used as an outcome variable.

This study included more than 1000 participants with a diagnosis of schizophrenia. Several available measurements that might be applicable to recovery – such as hope and optimism; quality of life and empowerment; knowledge of dealing with support systems; social networks; satisfaction and autonomy – were analyzed in a complex statistical operation. The goal was to identify the salient dimensions of recovery and to render them measurable with a newly designed instrument.

Four central areas were identified:

- the capacity to feel empowered in one's life;
- self-perceptions of knowledge about mental illness and available treatments;
- satisfaction with quality of life;
- hope and optimism for the future.

The authors consider that the instruments they developed to measure recovery-attitudes to be a contribution to scientific development in the direction of evidence-based treatment. They derive recommendations from their results as to which interventions are more likely to contribute to a recovery-attitude; these can then be assessed accordingly. Empowerment was the strongest factor. This also means that interventions which enhance self-esteem might have a particularly strong impact here. Treatment must aim at teaching service users to make autonomous decisions and to trust them. But it goes further than taking responsibility for your own decisions by virtue of being able to act in ways that correspond with the service system. Services must be capable of supporting the goals of their clients but must also be capable of helping them first to define and clarify these goals. Empowerment certainly relates to quality of life and to the knowledge of how to deal with the mental health system. Also, the relationship between empowerment, social support and social inclusion is an essential one. It is not surprising that the promotion of empowerment seems to be an important part of recovery-oriented work.

Another study on the relationship between recovery and service empowerment (Crane-Ross *et al.* 2006) has also shown that the subjective assessment of empowerment in a treatment setting exerts the greatest influence on measures that are associated with recovery (level of functioning, quality of life, symptomatology and the proportion of met needs). Notably, this applies to a larger degree to the level of empowerment of the users' views as compared to the views of service providers. Considerable difference was noted between users' and providers' estimation with respect to empowerment levels within services. Therefore, it is essential that users and providers engage in thoroughgoing exchanges about the ways in which services can actually contribute to recovery. The motivation for such exchanges should be high, given that the important contribution of empowerment to recovery is now widely accepted.

Laugharne and Priebe (2006) conclude that empowerment seems to have impacted more at an organisational level than on individual care and suggest that this might reflect the fact that the power differential between service users and providers is an extremely stubborn phenomenon, with a tendency to persist even in 'person centred' and consumer-led services. Along the same lines, Laugharne and Priebe (2006) warn that the ethical and the economic arguments for patient choice should not be confused, the latter possibly granting a person choice between different institutions offering the same paternalistic approach to treatment decision-making.

With empowerment and recovery-orientation promoting new roles and responsibilities for patients in their treatment and a focus on shared decision-making and individual choice, the prospect of real change regarding power confronts mental health professionals with areas of conflict. The 'top ten concerns about recovery encountered in mental health system transformation' (Davidson *et al.* 2006a) not only prominently address the issue of resources, but also focus on issues of risk. Client choice appears as a possible source of 'neglect under the banner of recovery' (Meehan *et al.* 2008) as well as a source of provider risk: 'If recovery is the person's responsibility, then how come I get the blame when things go wrong?'. Advances in the science and practice of risk assessment are seen as sources of improvement (Davidson *et al.* 2006b; Meehan *et al.* 2008) of this difficult situation and advance directives are viewed as promoters of change (Onken *et al.* 2007) and protection for mental health professionals, who, however, 'will continue to err on the side of caution until they are assured that the system will support them in times of crisis' (Meehan *et al.* 2008). It would be advantageous – especially from the point of view of avoiding stigmatization and discrimination – if psychiatry could move closer to the medical health field, which is in no way connected to such problems. In order to succeed in such a move 'we must be careful to distinguish between a person making (from our perspective) a dumb or self-defeating choice, and a person who is truly at risk' in order to embrace the all important concept of the 'dignity of risk' and the 'right to failure' (Deegan, 1996). This is an essential step towards parity and equality in terms of patients' and of human rights including the option of a capacity law that covers all medicine instead of a special legal situation for mental health as distinct from health (Dawson and Szmukler 2006; see also page 22).

RECOVERY AND EVIDENCE-BASED MEDICINE

Currently there is an ongoing debate in all of medicine as well as in psychiatry about 'evidence-based medicine'. Evidence-based means that the only kinds of medical interventions which should be offered are those which have been scientifically shown to be helpful and effective for a large group of individuals. Most likely everybody is by now familiar with this discussion through the media. Frequently, newspapers report about whether third-party payers should cover so-called complementary treatments, and if so, which ones. A recent study of homeopathic treatments, which many people experience as helpful, could not demonstrate their effectiveness. Consequently, in 2005 Switzerland issued a restriction on reimbursement for certain alternative treatments; similar discussions and decisions are taking place in many countries. Those who offer homeopathic treatments have argued that the kind of scientific methods which are likely to generate results that would be considered adequate evidence, are not appropriate for the evaluation of this type of treatment. Even within established medical practice, such instances have occurred. A simple example of the difficulties of trying to apply evidence-based research methods to certain treatments is the demand for random assignment to comparison groups and for placebo control groups. Scientific studies that use random assignment to comparison groups in double-blind designs (i.e. neither the subjects nor the investigators know who is getting the active treatment and who is not) – for instance a certain drug and a placebo that looks just like it – are considered to be generating the highest quality of evidence. While such studies can be done fairly easily with drugs, they demand very complex designs to test, for example, different models of residential rehabilitation. Subjective decisions and preferences play a decisive role here, and it is not to be expected that a simple random assignment to one form of housing or another could be judged according to the same criteria. It is also difficult, in many situations, to offer a placebo-intervention in the same way as a placebo-pill. Therefore, there is currently a lively discussion about the kind of scientific evidence that should be regarded as meeting the criteria of evidence-based medicine.

To this day we still have a clear hierarchy of evidence: at the top there are meta-analyses – which are also methodologically quite problematic – in other words, analyses that are a composite of several randomized clinical studies. Not unlike therapeutic guidelines and consensus-statements, which are generally based on the opinions of academic researchers, such meta-analyses have only limited impact on service provision and planning.

There are practical, political, and scientific reasons to support the admission of other kinds of evidence, and to foster new ways of obtaining scientific knowledge and consensus. Most of these considerations concern quantitative methods that are used to investigate effects on large samples through the use of statistical analyses. These yield information that can be applied to large groups of people. The evidence consists of probabilities that apply to certain groups of individuals, usually defined by diagnoses, and certain – more or less well defined – treatment situations. The significance of such results for individual patients or particular treatment situations is not always easy to discern. For many service providers this discrepancy leads to a general mistrust towards guidelines and 'evidence-based' rules, which frequently seem like a poor match for everyday situations and divergent contexts. Ideographic and qualitative methods, which place individual and contextual factors at the centre of attention, are generally viewed as part of the humanities rather than the natural sciences, and traditionally, are less valued.

However, there is a clear transformation in process. Qualitative research methods are gaining coinage, because they are steadily improving (see also pp 187). At the same time, much of the research stimulated or conducted by user researchers is of a qualitative nature, or at least a mixture of qualitative and quantitative methods. This leads to the next level of development in evidence-based research and planning. No longer is expertise derived solely from medical professionals, but also from people with a lived experience as users of services or family members. Furthermore, administrators, economists and social scientists have also begun to provide their perspectives to a multi-stakeholder evidence-base in medical care and policy (Rose *et al*. 2006).

To continue in a practical vein, we proceed with Fred Frese, a psychologist and user activist with a diagnosis of schizophrenia. He and his co-authors (Frese *et al*. 2001) have suggested that two different intentions must be considered in recovery-oriented services. On the one hand, relatives and mental health experts argue for interventions that are 'evidence-based'. They are particularly keen on promoting such treatments for people who are deemed incapable of speaking for themselves and who therefore must be especially protected from unproven or risky interventions. In the spirit of consumer-protection, such individuals must have access to services whose usefulness has been adequately proven and whose desired and untoward effects have been evaluated using large samples. These demands are far from being realized. We know that only a small fraction of people with a severe psychiatric disorder are being treated in a manner that is comprehensive and commensurate with the current state of the art. For example, specific psychotherapeutic interventions, which exist today for virtually all psychiatric conditions, are known to be effective. Nevertheless, they are not offered routinely. The same can be said for specific types of vocational rehabilitation and other support services. Such a lack is obviously frustrating and gives cause for political advocacy, with the aim of making such knowledge widely available in practice.

On the other hand there are many former patients who advocate for a recovery-approach that builds on subjectivity, autonomy and freedom of choice. Many people who have recovered from psychiatric conditions know that they were helped by things other than evidence-based services. Many times they benefited from individualized, unique and idiosyncratic approaches. The only proof of the effectiveness of such approaches consists in the fact that they had indeed been essential to the recovery of certain individuals. Mental health experts often tend to discourage such inventive methods because of a lack of scientific data about their effectiveness. However, for consumers such personal support may be of the essence. Frese *et al*. (2001) make it quite clear that most service users need both: evidence-based interventions as well as individual, unusual solutions. Therefore their demand is: Let's struggle together! Research must be done in both directions!

RECOVERY AND REMISSION

In 2005, the scientific debate about how the long-term course of schizophrenia should be measured, took on a new dimension. Leading US schizophrenia-researchers came together in a working group on 'Remission in Schizophrenia'. In other words, what they were concerned with was remission as it is usually understood in the traditional medical sense (Andreasen *et al.* 2005). Depending on the type of illness, remission can mean that no further symptoms of the illness are detectable or that symptoms are so minimal that they do not lead to any significant impairment in day-to-day life. For depression, anxiety and bipolar disorder, such criteria for remission had already existed for many years, and various interventions, especially psychopharmacological ones, can be assessed accordingly. According to the authors, the impetus for this new initiative was the increasing interest among not only patients, families and advocates, but also amongst professional experts, in the subject of recovery.

In their introduction the authors argue that a great variety of criteria had been used previously, that new therapies in the psychosocial and pharmacological fields had been established, and that there was scientific evidence for the fact that negative prognostic estimations for the course of schizophrenia had been overstated. They also refer to more recent data which show that certain types of symptoms, which could be associated with schizophrenia (such as hallucinations and delusions, but also a reduction in drive) occur not infrequently among the general population without leading to a diagnosis or treatment, and in fact can exist alongside a biography free of objective or subjective impairments. Therefore they propose as a criterion for remission that symptoms should be mild and not disabling. As a time criterion they suggest six months.

The European response to this proposal expresses support for the US working group's (Van Os *et al.* 2006) aim of defining clear-cut criteria for the assessment of course and outcome. The·Europeans are similarly indignant about the widespread ignorance and misjudgments concerning the course and outcome of schizophrenia. And they support the efforts of the highest calibre researchers to establish that remission of symptoms in schizophrenia has to be an important goal and should serve as a marker for treatment success.

Van Os *et al.* (2006) point out that the definition of remission by the exclusive use of symptoms has nothing in common with recovery. They see the abatement of symptoms as a necessary step in the direction of recovery. However, in both papers, recovery is defined as considerably more than this. Functioning in social roles, work, social relations and quality of life are mentioned as important criteria, even though their measurement still poses a challenge. The European authors describe recovery as 'moving forward' and 'rebuilding lives'. They express the hope that operational criteria for recovery will become available in the future, and will include constructs such as functioning in several psychosocial domains, quality of life and empowerment.

A reductionist concept of remission based on symptom-abatement has certainly given rise to criticism, since such a limited view stands to some extent in contradiction to a more differentiated recovery-concept. Nevertheless, the unanimous condemnation by the American and European authors of negative prognostic generalizations is quite powerful. Both initiatives are in agreement that information directed at service users and families should be changed to reflect higher expectations of treatment outcomes, the promulgation of hope and strong support for efforts in the direction of recovery.

There is one important difference between the American and the European publications that should be noted. The Europeans make a special point of emphasizing that the application of criteria for remission should not be connected with assumptions about the origins of the condition. They further stress that the criteria should be applied independently of the provision of treatment or lack thereof, i.e. whether recovery occurred with or without treatment. And this should also apply to the proposed criteria for a definition of recovery (Corrigan 2006). The following measurable dimensions have been proposed for recovery as an outcome that can be objectified: 'relief from psychotic symptoms; independence in matters related to housing; at least part-time work or school; regular social and recreational activities' (Corrigan 2006). Recovery as a process implies a hopeful outlook for the future, subjective well-being, goal orientation, agency and empowerment. These criteria are not only more substantial than symptoms or quantitative assessments of functioning alone, but also much more difficult to assess and to evaluate with current scientific methods. We must hope – and have some good reasons for so doing as will be shown later – that we can rise to the challenge and become engaged in savvy research into the processes of recovery.

CHAPTER 4

Personal Experience as Evidence and as a Basis for Model Development

'RECOVERY – AN ALIEN CONCEPT' - RON COLEMAN/UK

Where and when?

Ron Coleman's book, *Recovery – an Alien Concept*, first appeared in the UK in the year 1999 and is currently available in its 2nd edition (2006) from P & P Press Ltd. Like many of his other publications, such as *Working towards Recovery* (Ron Coleman, Paul Baker, Karen Taylor 2006) and the training manual, *Understanding Recovery*, it can be acquired through his website www.workingtorecovery.co.uk.

Who?

Between 1982 and 1991 Ron was a patient with a diagnosis of schizophrenia. He spent six of those years in hospitals. In 1991 he made contact with the voice-hearer movement, became their co-ordinator for the UK, and has since become a very successful international consultant and educator in the mental health field. Several of his books and training manuals have appeared in English and have been translated into other languages. He lives in Scotland with his wife and business partner, Karen Taylor, and their children.

For whom?

Ron Coleman wrote *'Recovery- an Alien Concept'* for people with mental health problems and those who have been diagnosed with mental illness, as well as for mental health professionals and other helpers. As well as his own story, the book offers a conceptualization of recovery and a personal recovery-plan that provides a stepwise plan to help users and their supporters work towards achieving the desired changes in life.

Recovery in Mental Health: Reshaping scientific and clinical responsibilities Michaela Amering and Margit Schmolke
Copyright © 2009 John Wiley & Sons, Ltd

Basic idea

The idea of recovery had become lost to people with a diagnosis of mental illness and their families and friends, as well as to mental health professionals. The idea that a person could regain his/her health had been forgotten to the point that it had become 'alien' to all. He does not mean mere stabilization, but rather the achievement of health. Ron's own story is no exception. Recovery is possible for many.

'The making of a schizophrenic'

Ron's story is about a boy who had been inspired at the age of eleven to become a priest. The sexual abuse he was suffering was both shocking and traumatic. Ron believes that he might have been able to withstand this kind of trauma without too much harm. But soon thereafter he experienced another huge tragedy. His first serious girlfriend unexpectedly took her own life. A short while later, following a sporting accident, Ron started to hear voices. He sought professional help, refused to admit himself to hospital, but was forcibly admitted a few days later. The diagnosis was 'paranoid schizophrenia'. For ten years, Ron lived as a mental patient and spent a large chunk of time in psychiatric hospitals. Drugs were of little help, the empathy and support of the staff were comforting, but contributed little towards recovery.

A recovery journey: stepping stones

It was not Ron's conviction that he could be helped which pulled him out of this situation. One of the support workers believed he might benefit from joining a voice-hearer group, and she accompanied him to one of their meetings. Other voice-hearers, new friends and mental health professionals enabled him to deal with his own voices, while pursuing his earlier interests again. This rekindled a belief in the possibility of a positive change of his situation: If you could see certain individuals as building-blocks for the edifice of recovery, you could become its cornerstone.

From victim to victor

The biggest hurdle for recovery is the person her/himself. Being a patient tends to lead you to think that help must come from others. For the purpose of recovery, you have to abandon the notion of being primarily sick and instead make space for the idea that you can step out of the patient role. To do this, you have to accept your own worth in society and begin to inhabit the role of community member and citizen. Self-worth and a high self-esteem are essential. Self-realization helps in understanding your own strengths and limitations. Learned behaviour that stands in the way needs to be recognized and transformed. It is important to assume responsibility for yourself. When Ron refers to himself as 'psychotic and proud', he is quite serious about this. A crucial prerequisite for the move 'from victim to victor' is an understanding about who you are and how you could be. The decision you make is whether you want to keep wallowing in self-pity as a poor sick person and rely constantly on the help of others, or whether you want to take the reins into your own hands. You can make the decision to set out on a recovery-journey.

Making autonomous decisions also means making mistakes. As long as you keep defining yourself through the illness, you can keep running back to psychiatry for a remedy for any mistake you have made. You can hand the responsibility over to a biological illness, instead of confronting your own humanity. Making decisions necessarily means making mistakes. You need to assume responsibility for good *and* bad choices. There is a difference between making a mistake and simply having a relapse. Taking responsibility for your decisions also means allowing yourself to have new experiences, to learn about your limitations and to make it possible to change and improve.

Freedom of choice is the cement of recovery-building. The freedom of citizens to make their own choices about life-styles and relationships is one of the foundations of democratic societies. The basic tenets of psychiatric services emphasize the need to be responsive to the decisions of clients. This is considered to be a major element in assessing the quality of psychiatric services. The reality is often quite different. Psychiatrists make decisions for their patients. Service providers are in the dark about alternatives to conventional treatment. For the most part, patients are not sufficiently well-informed to develop a solid basis for decision-making. Following hospital stays, patients are often released into environments that enhance their vulnerability. Freedom of choice must not simply mean choosing between one medication and another, for example, but rather being able to bring your own ideas to the table and having the chance to implement them. Mental health workers should not be restricting what they offer in accordance with their own ideas about patient needs, but should try to appreciate the wishes of the patients without presuppositions. As a client, you need to find out what your needs actually are and to express them clearly. Ron needed the help of a patient advocate to prepare his questions for the psychiatrists and to write them down. This enabled him to find his voice, whereas previously he had kept forgetting what he wanted to ask, in the tense circumstances of the consultation with the doctor.

'Ownership of the experience' – recognition and use of your own experiences

When Ron started to hear voices, he considered them a sign of going mad. Not only did they isolate him from others but also from himself. He talks about an alienated and fearful self, and later still about a fearful and angry self. He did not trust his own perceptions. And he could not find a meaningful context for his experiences in our society. Handing over these experiences to the psychiatric experts, he was given a diagnosis of 'schizophrenia' and was offered the corresponding treatment. But the diagnosis, the medication and the shock treatments didn't help him. Only when he started to take his own experiences seriously, after making contact with other voice-hearers, and once he had connected these experiences with his biography, did something start to change. Ron considers the time when he traded being 'Ron, the schizophrenic' for 'Ron, the voice-hearer' as the actual beginning of his recovery. He criticizes the power of psychiatry to define experiences not only because it is based on a lack of scientific validation for the diagnosis of 'schizophrenia'. It is his belief that self-worth and acceptance is diminished by reducing personal experiences to the expression of an illness and that such a reduction results in the impression of a defective self in need of repair. You have to decide to take hold of the experience and to make use of it. Only when you 'own' the experience of madness, can you take ownership of recovery.

To take ownership of your experiences once again is an act of liberation. This is not just about empowerment, but also about regaining the power that had been turned over to, or taken over by, the psychiatrists. This does not mean that professional service providers cannot make a considerable contribution to the recovery of their clients. An important chapter of Ron's book is dedicated to the role of providers who are effectively supporting the recovery of their clients. The descriptions of Ron's work with clients according to his 'choice, ownership, people, self' (COPS) recovery plan are impressive examples of recovery-work and facilitation.

The COPS Recovery Programme

Making plans is of great importance. Planning for 'person-centred help' is the relevant term, even though Coleman makes sure to emphasize that his proposal for a recovery-plan is more about development than about help. Developments can be planned and built on from a knowledge you have gained about past successes but they also need to take account of the obstacles and difficulties that must be reckoned with. Aims that can be accomplished under your own steam must be distinguished from those that require assistance from others. The person who is a designated supporter within a scheme of person-centred assistance, must be chosen very carefully. It is very problematic that users and providers cannot choose each other within mental health settings. When clients and providers cannot work with each other, this creates unhelpful and even dangerous situations. Services in which you can choose a provider, or where it is at least possible to switch in case of incompatibility, report positive experiences. Many problems and tensions can be resolved in this fashion and trusting relationships then develop more rapidly. These trusting relationships are an important foundation for a recovery-plan.

The personal recovery-plan based on the COPS programme speaks directly to the person who wants to take charge of planning their own recovery and explains briefly by whom, and why, this guide has been developed. Right from the start it is explained that each person has to decide when and with whom such a plan should be drafted, how long it will take, where they will keep their notes, and who should be allowed access to them. Certain parts may be skipped and their sequence altered. 'You are in control', states the plan and 'you make the decisions'. But there are also certain requirements, right from the start, for instance the three categorical preconditions:

• Be honest with yourself;
• Take responsibility for yourself;
• Be committed to your own recovery.

There is no point in starting without these three preconditions being in place. Correspondingly, the plan begins with phase I: 'What recovery means to me' and then moves onto your biography, important memories, experiences, predilections and important facts from various phases and domains of your life. The following sections instruct people how to describe their difficulties and coping strategies, as well as their earlier experiences with mental health services. Finally, each person can define any changes they might desire, each change being accompanied by an outline of its own paths and obstacles. All successes must be carefully documented.

The book ends on an optimistic note: the recovery concept is being put into practice. The idea lives on and the movement prevails. It is time to enjoy your own recovery.

'EMPOWERMENT MODEL OF RECOVERY' – DAN FISHER AND LAURIE AHERN/USA

Where and when?

The National Empowerment Center (NEC) in Lawrence/Massachusetts has been successful over many years in spreading the message of recovery and empowerment. This user-run organization, which is federally funded, has been distributing a wealth of information through its website and other means (www.power2u.org). The organization has become prominent in the US through media appearances, conferences and publications relevant to the discussion of mental health planning. Dan Fisher, one of the executive directors of the NEC was a member of the President's New Freedom Commission, which was charged with providing a report about the state of mental health care. Fisher was able to ensure that the report to the President contained the vision of a future where everyone diagnosed with a mental illness could recover. The NEC carries out large-scale research projects and develops training programmes on empowerment and recovery for mental health professionals, service users and planners. Its goal is a transformation from traditional psychiatry, with its dependence on institutions, towards recovery-oriented support systems.

Who?

Laurie Ahern is Associate Director of Mental Disability Rights International (www.mdri.org), an organization that protects the human rights of individuals with psychiatric diagnoses and developmental disabilities around the world. In her biography she describes herself as a survivor of sexual abuse and as a woman who recovered after being hospitalized at the age of 19 with a diagnosis of 'schizophrenia'. Today she is an impressively successful woman who travels widely in the course of her human rights work and inspects mental institutions, orphanages and other residential facilities in Latin America, Eastern Europe and the Near East. She provides training on implementing peer support and recovery all over the world.

For ten years, Laurie was one of the two executives in charge of the NEC, and the editor of their award-winning newsletter. In collaboration with Dan Fisher she developed the Empowerment Model of Recovery and PACE (Personal Assistance in Community Existence), a programme of recovery-oriented help for individuals in serious emotional distress. Their work on recovery has been very successful, while their journalistic and other writing has been translated into several languages, and has won numerous awards. Laurie spreads the word on the recovery-concept through frequent lectures, workshops and conferences for consumers, ex-consumers, relatives and clinicians.

Dan Fisher describes himself as a person who recovered from schizophrenia. He also works as a psychiatrist and has a doctorate in biochemistry. Before he decided to become a psychiatrist, he was hospitalized several times with a diagnosis of 'schizophrenia' As well as being one of the directors of the NEC, Dr Fisher works as a psychiatrist in a public mental health clinic in Massachusetts. He is the recipient of Mental Health America's Clifford Beers Award and the Bazelon Center for Mental Health Law's advocacy award.

For whom?

Ahern and Fisher are doing public relations work on a large scale. They represent national and international organizations. The PACE recovery-guide described below is aimed not only at individuals who are confronted with psychiatric conditions as consumers, family members and professionals, but also at policy-makers and service planners. PACE offers an alternative model to the PACT Programme for Assertive Community Treatment, which is currently offered as a mainstay in US mental health care. The differences between these models are clearly indicated in the recovery-guide.

Basic idea

The Empowerment Model of Recovery and PACE represent a recovery-oriented and non-coercive alternative to traditional psychiatric services. PACE is based on the assumption that people can recover even from the most difficult psychiatric problems. Laurie Ahern, Dan Fisher, Judi Chamberlain, Pat Deegan and other NEC staff offer themselves as examples. They tell their stories to encourage others, because recovery requires hope. Never give up!

Mental health services, be they hospital- or community-based, operate on the belief that mental illnesses are lifelong afflictions and that patients can never fully recover. The aims of medical and rehabilitative precepts are maintenance treatment and stabilization. While people remain ill, optimizing their functioning is the main goal. Based on recovery-research, which shows that people can recover completely as long as they get the right combination of attitude and support, Laurie Ahern and Dan Fisher present an empowerment model of recovery which they have turned into a new, practical treatment model which aims at facilitating recovery: PACE.

The principles of PACE

- People do fully recovery from even the most severe forms of 'mental illness';
- 'Mental illness' is a label for severe emotional distress, which interrupts a person's role in society;
- People can and do yearn to connect emotionally with others, especially when they are experiencing severe emotional distress;
- Trust is the cornerstone of recovery;
- People who believe in you help you to recover;
- People have to be able to follow their own dreams to recover;

- Mistrust leads to increased control and coercion, which interfere with recovery;
- Self-determination is essential for recovery;
- People recovering and those around them must believe they will recover;
- Human dignity and respect are vital to recovery;
- Everything we have learned about the importance of human connections applies equally to people labelled with 'mental illness';
- Feeling emotionally safe in relationships is vital to expressing feelings, which aids recovery;
- Understanding the meaning within severe emotional distress helps with recovery.

These principles are derived from NEC research findings. The NEC has collected data over many years about people who have completely recovered from serious psychiatric conditions. Their statements are summarized in five principal categories:

- recovery beliefs
- recovery relationships
- recovery skills
- recovery identity
- recovery community.

Recovery beliefs

It is very important to believe that at a certain point you are no longer 'mentally ill'. You cannot give up. You need people around you who trust that you are capable of starting to live your life again, to have your own dreams, friends, a job and a decent place to live. This is in opposition to the conviction that people will stay ill forever. Hope is essential. 'None of us would strive if we felt it was a futile effort'. You have to believe in yourself! You have to focus on creating a new future, not simply returning to the place where you were before you were labelled 'mentally ill' or 'schizophrenic'.

Recovery relationships

People who have recovered say that it was essential for them to have someone who believed in them, someone who trusted that they could put their life together again, take on responsibility and change things in their lives. This means that such individuals have to keep going for a long time without losing faith. In order to get into recovery, you need people whom you can trust, people you feel safe with, and also people who can give you practical advice. People who have had similar experiences with emotional crises and illnesses are particularly suited for such a role. That is why peers and peer-run projects are so important within the array of services. Mental health workers who show less professional distance and get humanly close, at times using humour to help, are experienced as more helpful. Mental health providers need to support people at their own pace and to allow them to pursue their own goals and dreams, rather than imposing or enforcing their own professional goals. Friendship and concern are expected from professional helpers as well.

Recovery skills

First of all it is important to be able to show your feelings in relationships. Anger, sadness, love and apprehension towards others need to be expressed. This is the way to make friends and to learn how to take care of yourself. It helps a lot when you learn about the things that feel good to you; this is the way you learn to take care of yourself. It may be taking a walk, meditating, writing, or many other things. You have to find out for yourself what the things are that feel good to you. Taking responsibility for yourself is an important step. You have to stop blaming an illness for all the problems you have in life, and you have to stop using some kind of chemical instability in the brain as an excuse. Nor is the opposite advisable: it makes no sense to ascribe all the guilt to yourself, or to believe that you need to be punished for something. And you have to learn to forgive yourself, to understand that certain developments and events cannot be controlled. Forgiving yourself is easier when you have friends who can forgive you. A list of personal priorities can also be helpful; it will give you a way to record your successes.

Recovery identity

It is essential not to identify yourself entirely as a patient, but rather as a full person. Remembering your achievements from before you fell ill might be helpful here. To overcome stigma and discrimination, it might be useful to become involved in the user/survivor movement. Labels like 'the mentally ill' should not be tolerated. 'Person first' language means that we are always talking about a 'person with...' a diagnosis, an illness, etc., making it clear that the person should always be seen as a whole human being. This means that we cannot be talking about ourselves or each other as 'schizophrenics', but rather we should talk about 'people with schizophrenia', and also we shouldn't use 'manic-depressive' as an adjective. To experience and refer to yourself as a whole, complete human being makes recovery possible.

Recovery community

Identity and a meaningful life are achieved within the community in which you live. The international user/survivor movement has made it possible for many to find a positive meaning in life by becoming involved, and by helping themselves and others to become empowered. Work and regular, meaningful activities were the principal therapy for many. The possibility of helping others often gives meaning to a person's own life. The way the society as a whole thinks about the potential for recovery, determines what individuals consider possible and what they might be able to achieve. A paradigm shift in the thinking about the course of mental conditions would give many people a new chance for recovery. First of all, psychiatry should transform its concepts and practices to a point where hope can prevail over resignation among service users. An appreciation of the role of losses and traumas, which contribute to the onset of mental conditions, is clearly called for from professionals in their diagnostic and therapeutic practice.

Concepts and language of PACE

The importance of language also becomes clear when reading one of the central chapters of the PACE programme brochure, which covers statements with which people are confronted when they are seeking psychiatric help. These statements, which come from the medical and rehabilitation models, are contrasted with the empowerment model of recovery.

'You are experiencing severe emotional distress which interferes with your life in the community' is closer to the truth than the assertion 'you are mentally ill'. The message of most psycho-educational initiatives: 'your mental illness is caused by a genetically or biochemically based brain disorder' falls far too short. PACE phrases it this way: 'Your distress is due to a combination of losses, traumas and lack of supports'. One of the more important differences that PACE conveys to its clients is: 'You can completely recover'. PACE never makes statements indicating that a disturbance might be permanent. Also, the idea that you can go back to work again only when your symptoms are gone, is replaced in PACE by the suggestion that you begin meaningful work as soon as you can as work helps with recovery.

Medication can be helpful in a context of self-determination: 'You may find medication helpful while you are learning self-management skills and alternative ways of recovering from severe emotional distress'. But PACE would never want to spread messages that come from 'traditional' psychiatric culture such as, for example, 'You must take your medication for the rest of your life'.

The same goes for statements such as: 'You must remain under the care of professionals forever'. On the contrary, PACE recommends that other forms of support take centre stage: 'You will be able to gain your main support from peers and friends rather than professionals'.

While traditional professional advice insists on the importance of avoiding stress, PACE wants to convey that 'you can again have dreams, meet challenges, and have a full life', that it makes no sense to assume that 'you are your illness', but that instead you should always remember that 'you are still fully human'.

Even during the acute state of an illness you should not settle for statements like 'As a result of your illness you are unable to express feelings or form relationships', but you should rather try to understand what can disturb relationships temporarily: 'You are experiencing such extreme feelings that you feel it is unsafe to show them. Eventually you will feel safe enough to understand your feelings and those of others and form close relationships'. This also means: 'You can have a significant other and have children once you have progressed in your recovery'. Finally, PACE asserts that: 'You are not more dangerous than the rest of the community' and 'You are entitled to full human rights'.

PACE promulgates the belief that everyone can become mentally ill. Therefore, we are all equal in our humanity. When your life is thwarted by serious emotional distress, and you have been given a diagnosis, this does not mean that you are suffering from an ongoing brain disease. Users always stay in control and are not subjected to force or coercion by the mental health system. The pace of recovery is up to the user and not the mental health workers. Relationships are encounters between equals and are not hampered by professional distance. Individuals who believe in you, rather than medication, are the pillars of support. Service organizations are led by peers, not by a professional mental health team. Human and patient rights are being honoured, not violated. The goal is self-determination and responsibility, instead of dependency and a lack of autonomy. Service users have a choice of the kinds of help they prefer, while traditional mental health settings are described as offering few choices and being highly focused on medication. There are no case managers to co-ordinate services, but rather 'personal assistants'. You don't have to first demonstrate compliance and agreement with all other services before becoming eligible for financial help and housing support. Such supports are independent of other kinds of help. Medication is seen as an instrument to promote self-determined coping rather than a life-long insurance policy.

The PACE Recovery Plan

Next to the above mentioned content areas, the PACE recovery-guide also includes reports about psychiatric research that support an optimistic attitude towards recovery, and stories by and about people who have lived recovery. The guide concludes with frequently asked questions about the recovery-concept:

- What causes mental illness?
- Do people still have symptoms after their recovery from mental illness?
- Is it possible to have recovered and still be taking medication?

The answers to these questions once again illustrate convincingly what this is all about, namely that human beings are complex creatures. Health and illness occur on different levels – influenced by social, emotional and cultural factors. An exclusive concentration on biological factors falls short and deprives people of hope, energy and responsibility, and makes them dependent on experts, who are expected to 'fix them'.

This does not mean that life in recovery is without problems or suffering. Here again the example of hearing voices is brought to bear, a phenomenon that can drive a person crazy, but which can also be part of a healthy life, as long as you know enough about yourself and life in general in order to integrate such experiences. Many people take psychiatric medication without being considered mentally ill. The fact that someone takes medication, does not mean they have to live a life of sickness. Everything hinges on keeping control, and seeing these drugs as one of many supports that are being used voluntarily and in a fully informed way.

Other publications about PACE and recovery by Laurie Ahern and Dan Fisher

In addition to the website www.power2u.org, there is a textbook by Laurie Ahern and Dan Fisher with videos about the principles of PACE, *Personal Assistance in Community Existence*.

Recovery through Peer Support, by Dan Fisher and Judi Chamberlain, is a training course with video materials, which is tailored for peers who work as mental health professionals in assisting the recovery of others. Judi Chamberlain is an iconic figure of the user/survivor movement and her book, *On Our Own* (1978), is a classic in the literature about user-run alternatives to psychiatry.

In the self-help manual, *A New Vision of Recovery – You Too Can Recover from Your Mental Illness*, Dan Fisher once again addresses everyone who wants to achieve recovery for themselves. He describes the values that he follows and that are keeping him well, and provides many suggestions about self-determined ways in which to deal with offers of support and support systems and about how to fashion relationships that are conducive to recovery.

Besides the freely accessible recovery-guide described earlier, there is a great deal of useful information available and there are other publications which are free of charge, for instance *The Bazelon Center for Mental Health Law* and The UPENN Collaborative on Consumer Integration's guide to self-directed mental health care, *In the Driver's Seat*. And Pat Deegan's *Re-claiming your Power during Medication Appointments with your Psychiatrist*, is a constructive guide for a self-determined approach to medication and psychiatrists.

'CONSPIRACY OF HOPE' – PAT DEEGAN/USA

Where and when?

Patricia E. Deegan, PhD, is Adjunct Professor at the Boston University Sargent College of Health and Rehabilitation Sciences and Director of Pat Deegan PhD and Associates, LLC (www.patdeegan.com, 23.08.08).

Who?

Pat Deegan was diagnosed with schizophrenia when she was a teenager. Today she is one of the most active and renowned representatives of the recovery-movements in the USA. After obtaining a doctorate in clinical psychology at Duquesne University (1984), she became programme director at the Northeast Independent Living Programme in Lawrence/Massachusetts, where she implemented a model to help people with psychiatric disabilities live in independent housing in spite of their limitations. From 1992 to 2001 she was Director of Training at the National Empowerment Center (NEC) and developed numerous self-help strategies to support people in their recovery-process.

Pat knows from her own experiences (Deegan 2005a) that before people became active representatives of the recovery-movement, they languished in states of profound apathy and indifference. Their hearts had hardened and everything seemed futile to them. They felt alone, abandoned, aimless, outside of time. Pat experienced this herself in exactly the same fashion. At the age of 17 she became psychotic for the first time. Treated with Haldol, she sat around stiffly in a chair all day long smoking cigarettes and staring into the void. Over a long period of time, her daily routine consisted of getting up (which was hard enough), smoking cigarettes, having meals, and going back to bed.

At that time, people tried to motivate her to do something. They tried, for example, to convince her to bake bread and sell it, or to join up for a boat-ride. But nothing interested her, everything seemed irrelevant. She had given up. Giving up was a solution for her, it protected her from wanting anything, from continuing to fail, from being hurt again. Time passed and nothing mattered to her. Her friends went to college and started new lives, but she didn't care about that either. She remembers that a friend of hers, who had once been very important to her, came by for a visit. Pat was sitting there, smoking, and barely said a thing. As soon as 8 o'clock struck, she cut across her friend, who was speaking, and asked her to leave, since she wanted to go to bed. Without saying goodbye she laid down. Her heart was tough, nothing mattered.

At the age of 18 she was admitted to a psychiatric hospital for the third time. When she asked the psychiatrist what was wrong with her, he answered that she had an illness called 'chronic schizophrenia'. She was told this was an illness like diabetes. If she were to take medication for the rest of her life and avoid stress, she might be able to get on with it all right. As soon as the psychiatrist had uttered these words, Pat felt their weight, and her already tenuous hopes, dreams and goals were shattered. Even 22 years later, the memory of these words still causes her pain.

Today Pat understands why this experience was so harmful for her. The psychiatrist basically gave her to understand that her fate with the label of 'schizophrenia' was already sealed. This devastating prognosis turned all her dreams and aspirations into pure fantasy, she lost all orientation to her present and kept going in a sequence of disjointed moments.

Today she knows that the psychiatrist back then had little basic knowledge. He labelled her as 'a schizophrenic', just as had been done for generations since Bleuler and Krae-pelin. He did not see her as a person, rather as an illness. Pat Deegan writes that she, along with many other people with mental health problems, had entered a dehumanizing transformation 'from being a person to being an illness', a schizophrenic, a multiple, a manic-depressive (Deegan 1992). Her personhood and her sense of self collapsed, and 'the disease' gained strength as a mighty 'It', a totally separate entity over which she no longer had any influence, just as it had been communicated to her by professional helpers.

For these reasons, Deegan demands forcefully that today's students should acquire fundamental knowledge and understanding rather than simply be taught how to recog-nize and diagnose an illness. They should encounter a person seeking help with their whole heart. The most important thing that students should learn is that human rela-tionships are the most powerful tools in working with people. That is why Pat calls the recovery-process a 'journey of the heart'. She challenges us to start at the point wherever people may be at that moment, at the place where their hearts have become hard, and where they no longer care about anything. 'It is a time when we feel ourselves to be among the living dead: alone, abandoned, and adrift on a dead and silent sea without course or bearing' (Deegan 2005a, p 60).

Pat Deegan cannot remember the specific moment when she turned from surviving to becoming an active participant in her own recovery-process. One thing she can recall, is that the people around her did not give up on her. They kept inviting her to do things. She describes one turning point: 'I remember one day, for no particular reason, saying yes to helping with food shopping. All I would do was push the cart. But it was a beginning. And truly, it was through small steps like these that I slowly began to discover that I could take a stand toward what was distressing to me' (Deegan 2005a, p 65).

For whom?

Pat Deegan speaks to and for people who have experienced major traumas in their lives (such as serious illness, physical trauma, disability or discrimination). She approaches them with the conviction that they are basically resilient and tough individuals, who could improve their healing process considerably if they had access to knowledge, self-help skills, well-trained professionals, a supportive environment and social justice.

Today, Deegan offers innovative seminars and training programmes. These include, for example, an audiotape with recordings of simulated voice-hearing. Her programme on 'voice-hearing' has been recognized internationally and is being used in the training of police, psychiatrists, mental health workers and relatives, with the goal of promoting a more empathic approach to people with psychiatric problems. She is also involved with film projects, such as *Inside Outside: Building a Meaningful Life After the Hospital*.

Pat is routinely invited to give lectures and workshops in the USA, Canada, Europe and Australia. She talks about her own recovery-story and her ideas about recovery – about the vital importance of hope and the necessity of transforming the mental health system. She has published many articles, which have appeared in books, journals and newsletters and has work available on videotapes and websites. She also writes her own online *Recovery Journal*. Her contributions have been translated so far into Spanish, Hebrew, French, Portuguese, Dutch, Norwegian, Swedish and German.

Basic idea

The New Freedom Commission in the USA has called for a restructuring of the mental health system towards recovery. This requires a relearning and re-orientation of the workforce towards recovery-oriented competencies. The principles of recovery – freedom of choice, self-determination and empowerment – should be incorporated into areas of routine mental health practice, such as case management, working with homeless people, services for people with dual diagnoses and supported living arrangements. Over the past 12 years, Pat Deegan has worked actively with mental health staff in a variety of US settings in order to convey how the recovery-processes of people with psychiatric conditions can be supported in practice. For her, the most important elements of recovery are preserving hope and sustaining the conviction that people with a psychiatric condition are first of all individuals and should not be reduced to the passive bearers of clinical diagnoses.

Hope

Hope is not just another word for Deegan. She believes that hope is a matter of life and death for herself and for those individuals with a psychiatric diagnosis who have spent much time in psychosocial programmes and services. Hope arises from darkness, much like a water lily whose seed ripens invisibly during the cold and dark winter season. Pat recalls the onset of her illness:

> '... We know this because like the flower, the sea rose, we have known a very cold winter in which all hope seemed to be crushed out of us. It started for most of us in the prime of our youth. At first we could not name it. It came like a thief in the night and robbed us of our youth, our dreams, our

aspirations and our futures. It came upon us like a terrifying nightmare that
we could not awaken from' (Deegan 1996, p 3).

The real 'conspiracy of hope' is tied to the question: what has to change in the environment for a seedling to grow? It isn't about the question what may be wrong with 'the
mentally ill'. What we must begin to ask is: how can we engender a hopeful, humane
environment and relationships that promote growth and development?

In her article, *Recovery as a journey of the heart*, (2005a), Deegan emphasizes that
hope and biological life are inextricably linked to each other, and relates this to a story
that Martin Seligman (1975) mentioned in his well known book about helplessness. It is
a story about a man who was a major and a physician during the war in Vietnam. This
major met a young soldier who was quite resistant to pain and suffering. The soldier had
been interned as a prisoner of war. The reason for his relatively good physical condition
in spite of his extreme weight loss was that he had been told he would be going home
soon. However, as soon as he realized that he had been deceived about this, he stopped
working, developed symptoms of a severe depression and refused all meals. When the
major first met him he was lying in bed in a position like a fetus; he no longer moved.
His comrades were taking care of him and trying to pull him out of his stupor. Eventually
it reached the stage where the soldier was defecating and urinating in his bed. Shortly
before he died, he gave the full address of his parents to the major. What Seligman was
trying to convey through this story was that it had been hope that had kept this young
man alive. As soon as he gave up hope and began to believe that all his endeavours
would fail, he died. What Seligman learned from this was that if animals and human
beings learn that their actions are futile they become more likely to die. And, the opposite
is true: if a person believes they have some control over their environment, then they are
more likely to live.

Deegan sees a connection between this story and the lives of people with psychiatric
histories. She thinks that whenever people feel that all their efforts are in vain; when they
experience that they have no control over their environment and that whatever they do has
no impact whatsoever on their situation; when their treatment team doesn't listen to them;
when all important decisions are made for them; when service providers decide where
and with whom they should be living, how they should spend their money, what time
they should be back at the residence; etc – 'then a deep sense of hopelessness, of despair
begins to settle over the human heart' (Deegan 2005a, p 63). And then they do whatever
anyone else might do to avoid the catastrophic consequences of utter hopelessness. They
develop a tough heart and cease to take care of themselves. Pat thinks it safer to become
helpless than hopeless.

The great danger is that the providers might overlook the intensity of the existential
struggle of a person with a hardened heart. This might mean that the team only notices
negative symptoms and a poor prognosis, without expecting anything further of the
person. Or the team judges the person to be lazy, unmotivated and apathetic, and
consequently lets their own despair take over, dismissing the person as someone with
a low level of functioning. Deegan insists that trainers of the next generation of mental
health professionals make sure not to perpetuate the misunderstandings of today's
students. Students should be helped to understand that states of apathy and lack of
self-care on the part of people with a mental illness are actually highly motivated,

adaptive strategies, which are used by desperate people who are in danger of losing hope altogether (Deegan 2005a).

Pat Deegan says that our task is not simply to pass judgment on whether someone will recover from mental illness, or whether they are likely to overcome the devastating consequences of poverty, stigma, dehumanization, degradation and learned helplessness. 'Our challenge is rather to participate in the "conspiracy of hope". And it is our task to create a "community of hope" for people with psychiatric, to create, in other words, an environment that offers possibilities for further development. It is our task to convey the spirit of hope to mental health teams. We need to ask people with psychiatric problems what they would like and what they need in order to grow, and to provide them with fertile ground where new life can take root. And finally, it is our task to be patient, observe with suspended belief and bear witness with respect, how the life of another human being can unfold' (Deegan 1996, p 8).

Recovery and the necessary shift of attitude among mental health service providers

Pat Deegan maintains a critical attitude towards trendy new labels like 'consumer integration', 'empowerment', 'clubhouse models' and 'partnership' when such positive sounding terms merely denote a superficial change in psychiatric services. She sees the great danger of merely using the newest programme designs and politically correct language. Actually changing the services that truly enable people with mental health problems to grow can be rather difficult and cumbersome. Deegan is convinced that in spite of the changing terminology the basic relationships between those who have been given a diagnosis and those who have not, has not yet really changed significantly.

The way people deal with each other within mental health programmes and in society must be transformed if people are expected to make their way from mere survival to a voyage of recovery. Empathy and supporting the person-hood of a human being are essential, even when it seems that he/she has been lost to him/herself.

In the following, Deegan (1996, p 6f) describes an interesting interaction that happens quite frequently between patients and mental health staff members. Quite often providers attempt, with an eager saviour mentality, to pull patients out of their lethargic and apathetic states. The more the person seems to withdraw, the more service providers encroach on them. The more they seem to be giving up, the more helpers try to motivate them. The more desperate the person appears, the more the service provider succumbs to superficial optimism. The more treatment plans are rejected, the more plans are produced for the person. Finally, service providers find themselves in a state of burnout and become exhausted. Then they start to get angry with the patient. Providers begin to feel used by people who seem to be rejecting their help. They feel as if their identity as providers is being challenged by someone who is lost in pain and indifference. It is not uncommon for the person who is suffering to be blamed and told that he is lazy and hopeless, manipulative rather than sick, and bad rather than mad. It is not that the help itself is considered useless but rather that the patient seems to refuse any help and therefore cannot be helped. He/she should be kicked out of the programme and be left to hit rock bottom, to shake them up so that they will accept the helping hand that is being offered.

Something very interesting takes place during this phase: even the therapeutic team gives up their dedication to helping this person any further. It hurts too much to keep trying to help and failing. The team bows out, some members even quit, others who stay become hard, insensitive and cynical. These are all forms of giving up and of despair, which is what the team is expressing. Just as the person with a mental illness has given up hope, so the mental health service providers are apt to do the same. They spend more time taking people out of the programme than inviting them to join it. Admission criteria become increasingly rigid and inflexible.

If 'power over' people is exerted in this fashion, it produces nothing but unnecessary dependency and learned helplessness. Service providers need to start to share 'power with' the people rather than to keep controlling them. In this way, traditional power-relations that have been historically so oppressive for people with mental health problems would begin to change. In practical terms, this means that service providers should stop making judgments about what is 'in the client's best interest'. Instead, they should ask what the clients want for their own lives, and provide them with the skills and support to achieve it (Deegan 1996, p 10).

According to Deegan (1996) the preconditions for a fundamental transformation of clinical care include service providers making sure that:

- the radical imbalance of power between consumers and providers is given up;
- relationships are based on true mutuality;
- violent practices, such as coercive treatment and isolation, stop;
- basic common humanity is recognized;
- negative consequences of dehumanization in the psychiatry system stop.

Overcoming barriers to recovery

Deegan (1996, p 10f) advocates taking down the barriers that impede the efforts of people who suffer emotionally from getting into recovery. The following abridged critical questions might serve as guidance for studies on this subject:

1. Are the people we work with overmedicated?
2. Are consumers in both community based and hospital programmes involved in evaluating staff work performance?
3. Are programme participants and hospital inpatients receiving peer skills training on how to participate in, and effectively get what they want from, a treatment team?
4. Are there separate toilets or eating space for staff and programme participants?
5. Who can use the phones? Who makes what decisions? Who has the real power in this programme?
6. Do we understand that people with psychiatric disabilities possess valuable knowledge and expertise as a result of their experience?
7. Have we created environments in which it is possible for staff people to be human beings with human hearts?
8. Do we work in a system which rewards passivity, obedience and compliance? Is compliance seen as a desirable outcome?

9. Have we embraced the concept of the 'dignity of risk' and the 'right to failure'?
10. Are there opportunities within the mental health system for people to truly improve their lives?

Recovery versus rehabilitation

Pat Deegan makes an important distinction between recovery and rehabilitation. She states emphatically: 'We are not passive objects which professionals are responsible for 'rehabilitating'. . . . We are not objects to be acted on. Rather we are fully human subjects who can act, and in acting can change our situation' (Deegan 1996, p 11f). In saying this she takes a stand against the oppressive connotation of the term 'rehabilitation'. No one has the power to rehabilitate someone else's life. Even the best and most progressive rehabilitation programmes can fail. Deegan offers an apt quote on this subject: 'You can lead a horse to water but you can't make it drink'. Something more than just good services is needed. This 'something more' she calls recovery.

The recovery-concept distinguishes itself from rehabilitation models by holding that people are responsible for their own lives. Deegan asserts that individuals with psychiatric disabilities are not passive victims, but rather responsible actors in their own recovery-processes. She challenges people to always use person-first language, i.e., 'I am a person labelled with schizophrenia' instead of saying 'I am a schizophrenic'. Mentioning the person first always reminds us 'that first and foremost we are human beings who can take a stand toward what is distressing to us' (Deegan 1996, p 12).

Pat knows from her many years of experience that each journey of recovery is unique to each person. Everyone must discover for themselves what promotes their recovery and what does not. Some find that continuing or interrupting their treatment may be an important aspect of their recovery-process, others realize that it might be better for them to leave psychiatric services behind once and for all, as Ogawa et al. (1987) learned in a Japanese study. Still others, who have experienced drug and alcohol abuse, or grown up in families with drug involvement, or experienced sexual abuse, might find that self-help groups play an important role in their recovery. Developing friendships based on true affection and mutual respect seems very important for most individuals in recovery.

A basic precondition for this process is a permanent, affordable and fully integrated housing situation. Many join a spiritual community of their choice, which provides them with strength and hope. Others find it helpful to become involved in support networks and advocacy groups, led by users. Such networks attempt to transform the mental health system, provide alternatives to traditional services, draw the attention of governments to the needs of people and advocate for full civil rights and collectively for social justice.

Pat Deegan does not see recovery merely as a way of getting well from mental illness, but sees it also as a way to overcome poverty, discrimination, internalized stigma, abuse and traumatization that has been caused by certain 'helping professionals' or by the mental health system as a whole. Social action and self-help cannot be separated from each other. To help ourselves means joining together as a group to fight against an injustice that devalues human beings and keeps them in the position of 'second class citizens'.

Recovery does not refer to an end product or result, neither does it mean that the person is 'cured', nor that he/she is simply 'stabilized' or maintained in the community. Recovery often means a transformation of one's self, whereby a person both accepts their limits and discovers a new world of possibilities. Recovery is also a process, a way of life, an attitude and a way of approaching everyday challenges. It is not a perfectly linear process. Just like the water-lily, recovery has its seasons, its phases of darkness and light. Recovery is certainly a slow, deliberate and sometimes difficult process. But the end result is frequently beautiful and amazing. Why did Pat Deegan choose such a difficult field?

'Because we are part of a conspiracy of hope and we see in the face of each person with a psychiatric disability a life that is just waiting for good soil in which to grow. We are committed to creating that good soil. And so I celebrate you. I celebrate the strong and fiercely tenacious spirit of people with psychiatric disabilities. I celebrate the person within each of us. I celebrate hope. I celebrate our conspiracy. And I think we all deserve a round of applause' (Deegan 1996, p 13).

Further publications by Pat Deegan

Deegan PE (1988). Recovery: the lived experience of rehabilitation. *Psychosocial Rehabilitation Journal* **XI/4**: 11–19.

Deegan PE (1990). Spirit breaking: when the helping professions hurt. *The Humanistic Psychologist* **18/3**: 301–13.

Deegan PE (1997). Recovery and empowerment for people with psychiatric disabilities. *Social Work and Health Care* **25/3**: 11–24.

Deegan PE (2001). Recovery as a self-directed process of healing and transformation. *Occupational Therapy and Mental Health* **17**: 5–21.

Deegan PE, Drake RE (2006). Shared decision-making and medication management in the recovery process. *Psychiatric Services* **57/11**: 1636–9.

Deegan PE (2007). The lived experience of using psychiatric medication in the recovery process and a shared decision-making program to support it. *Psychiatric Rehabilitation Journal* **311**: 62–69.

Deegan PE, Rapp C, Holter M, Riefer M (2008) Best practices: a program to support shared decision making in an outpatient psychiatric medication clinic. *Psychiatric Services* **59**: 603–5.

'HOLDERS OF HOPE' - HELEN GLOVER/AUSTRALIA

Who?

Helen Glover's personal story is extremely impressive. She talks about how, even as a young woman, she already felt frighteningly different and feared that an evil virus controlled by external forces was coursing through her veins. Nevertheless, she managed to have a career as a teacher, to fall in love and get married, and to have a successful social life, before she decided to confide in a psychiatrist. Her initial recommendation of a brief period of hospitalization for diagnostic purposes, was the beginning of a dramatic career as patient, with frequent re-admissions, long-term stays, dire prognostic pronouncements and the recommendation that her husband would be better off getting a divorce and finding himself another partner.

At the other end of this dark chapter in her life, Helen Glover has obtained a social work degree and is now a well known and highly regarded recovery-expert and trainer who has developed and directed peer-run programmes in New Zealand, Australia and the UK.

Helen is a stirring speaker and teacher. She describes a life in recovery that includes psychotic crises, suicidality and vulnerability. However, her identity is mostly shaped by her work and the message of recovery, rather than by chronic illness or disability. One of her main goals is to discourage people from considering her as an exception to the rule. She knows and asserts that recovery is possible for all and not just for the 'happy few' who have reached the pinnacle of international fame like she has.

Basic idea – everyone has the potential to recover

Helen knows from her own experience and from her knowledge about others who were able to find exactly what they needed for their recovery, that everyone is capable of it. It is her desire to make this path accessible to the many millions who have not yet found it.

For over ten years she was confronted with a life as a chronic mental patient and the terror of her psychosis. She still occasionally gets psychotic symptoms, but the resilience she has discovered within herself has helped her to withstand the temptation to succumb to chronicity. The difference between her story and that of others seems to be that in her life there have always been at least one person, and sometimes more, who have 'held hope for her' and – even more important – who have given this hope back to her once again.

> 'I will be your "Holder of Hope" and you will be my "Holder of Hope" . . .
> when difficult times come we will already have planned how we want to
> support each other.' (Glover 2003)

Helen believes that not having hope for people with psychotic experiences has catastrophic implications, only surpassed by the failure to return the hope that has been held for them. The attitude 'I am doing this for you' because 'you can't do it for yourself' is infectious and leads to a state that Glover calls 'mental impotence'. This emotional powerlessness has all the characteristics of a chronic illness.

Psychiatric conditions are mostly episodic and it makes no sense to live every day as if you were mentally ill, even though there are days when you can simply enjoy life. Knowing that you have a tendency towards a chronic condition, you may or may not entertain preventive measures. In either case it does not make sense to doubt that you can nevertheless live, work and love. Glover's dream is to overcome the difference between those 'who have made it' and those who are trapped in a life of chronicity, through a combination of professional efforts and the contribution of peers who have their own experiences in recovery.

'Holders of Hope'

It has been known for some time that hope is an important element in recovery-processes. However, actually transmitting and experiencing hope in life are more complicated matters. When is it actually true to say to someone, you are hopeful for them? How frequently and in spite of assertions to the contrary are we holding onto hope for a particular person because we don't trust them to hold onto it themselves? To find the intuitive balance between holding onto hope for someone and returning hope to them is difficult, and mistakes are unavoidable. Helen Glover considers it to be crucial for mental health service providers to develop a competence she describes as an 'intent of hope'.

She also considers the lack of such competence, malpractice. Mental impotence derives from a failure on the part of mental health professionals in the area of holding and returning hope, and as a result, a human spirit and life can be destroyed. A greater harm to a person is difficult to imagine. But such things do take place. When we encounter people in the midst of a crisis, in dramatic situations that we can barely influence therapeutically, we are frequently convinced that this situation is irremediable, a result of non-compliance, a hopeless scenario, because we cannot imagine how this person, who is at this moment in such great distress, can ever become the holder of their own hope again. In such circumstances the following message is conveyed, and often with good intentions: 'I will do that for you as I don't believe you have the ability to do it yourself'. Examples are provided by situations in which too many things are done for a person who could easily take care of those things by themselves. Glover also identifies several 'privileges' that go along with having an illness or a disability, as equally risky. In her own experience of social work training under 'special consideration' she was shocked at first when these 'special considerations' were rescinded against her will, but she then found she was quite capable of applying her own best efforts. Another way that service providers engender 'mental impotence' instead of hope is through their concern that patients and family members might be driven to disappointment by excessive expectations. Glover dedicates a separate chapter in her book to the risk of creating 'mental impotence' by trying to avoid disappointments.

'Mental impotence'

Glover defines 'mental impotence' as follows: the mental health system and society convey a message to the person with a psychiatric problem that leads them to lose their willpower, their dreams, their desires and their memories of health, all of which are replaced by a conviction of incapacity and forsaken hope, which in turn leads to the inexorable death of the human soul. Glover believes that this can occur in an overt or covert fashion and that the symptoms of 'mental impotence' can arise pretty quickly. The longer a person is confronted with such an environment, the more difficult it becomes to escape the situation.

The treatment for 'mental impotence' consists of rapidly abandoning the 'infectious' environment and an exposure to the virus of 'hope'. For this you need other people who may not have professional training but who believe you have the capacity to recapture your life. Such individuals must act in a way that demonstrates their belief that the person can recover, even if it doesn't seem that way at the time. They have to be persistent and make sure they provide the framework whereby the person can regain control of their life on their own.

Working 'as if' and 'morphism'

Holding on to hope and returning it later requires an ability to believe that the bleakness of despair and suffering is only temporary. To consider it as permanent would lead to hopelessness, a focus on darkness and 'mental impotence'. If we show, on the other hand, that things will be different one day, curiosity and emotional dynamics can develop. Such a view also makes it easier for the therapist to tolerate the current despair and even share its intensity without denying it. Knowing that everything is in flux ('morphing'), and that every condition includes the potential for transformation, makes it possible that darkness can be tolerated and that no one has to be abandoned to it.

Helen also talks about realizing your own role in the 'chronicity journey'. The patient role includes many temptations and the decision to move towards health is not easy. The journey has its downs as well as its ups. Both directions are legitimate. The freedom to fashion your own life can handle both. We should not be taken aback by the fact that life can be a roller-coaster that goes up and down, as many people have survived those ups and downs and many people want to have a share in them. You can take someone along on your roller-coaster ride and keep the fear in check. If you hadn't taken the ride, you would feel rather sorry. Helen does not propose to trade in the roller-coaster for a smooth road. Her recovery involves an ongoing experience of ups and downs without losing control. She has a box full of recovery tools for use in situations that seem to be getting out of hand. This includes hitting the breaks hard with medication, which she obtains from her doctors based on her wishes and precise earlier agreements.

'Journey' and 'vehicle' are key images in Helen's explanations. Ideally, you sit in the driving seat of your own life. Sometimes, however, it is more comfortable and safer to be in the passenger seat, from where you can still determine the direction and speed of your trip. Being locked in the boot has to be avoided at all costs. No effort is too great to stay out of that boot. In addition to your own resilience, which you can discover by going through such a process, you might also find that people who are holding onto hope for you, can help you regain control of the steering wheel, get your driver's licence back and find the right vehicle and the confidence to be able to drive it.

Raising the bar

Helen Glover bemoans the fact that, in spite of the many initiatives to involve people with a lived experience in the planning, implementation and evaluation of psychiatric services, the expectation that each and every service user become actively involved in their own recovery, is often lacking. This is something she missed during her many years of psychiatric treatment. Instead, she was told that if you were leading a quiet and peaceful life, you would somehow automatically become integrated into society. For long periods of time, Helen's life was organized exclusively around her treatment – from one appointment to the next, a day programme in between: the life of a sick person among other sick people. She felt sick, as she acted like a sick person, she was treated as such, and she remained ill. Helen does not believe that recovery can develop in such a vacuum of time and amidst such inertia. Turning over your suffering to the experts does not make anything happen. Recovery is hard work.

You need a reason to become actively involved in such work. If the expectations are too low, and the bar is not set high enough, soon you will find no reason to get up in the morning. Without expectations that challenge you, motivation and interests will be lacking and you will be infected with 'mental impotence'. Helen compares the situation to someone who is going through rehabilitation after an accident, when physiotherapists are challenging the patient to deal with quite a bit of pain and to make an effort in order to achieve something. The physiotherapists would never accept that the prescribed exercises could simply be postponed. The influence of Helen's husband, who refused to accept dire prognosis and the recommendation to separate from her, should not be underestimated. He continued to see her as a whole person.

Concerns about excessive expectations that might be disappointed and could lead to relapses are guiding the actions of many service providers. Yes, Helen says, without expectations there are no failures, but also no achievements. In her experience, professionals often underestimate the resilience of the patients and in doing so prevent them from possible activities and successes.

'Entrapment of chronicity' versus 'Entrapment of recovery'

The fear of over-taxing a person, because this may result in failures, indicates a sceptical attitude towards recovery. Just as it is possible to become trapped in chronicity, you might also get trapped in recovery. Reproaching yourself when things have once again gone wrong, worrying that another episode could throw you back to square one, and fearing the disappointment of those who have supported you in achieving a certain goal should you fail, can all be traps.

To accept that illness and recovery can occur at the same time minimizes this fear. Having a bad day should be just as possible at times when you are feeling healthy. Escaping from a black and white view of chronicity and recovery towards a more complex picture with shades of grey should be the aim. It must be possible to integrate your vulnerability and weaknesses into a self-image that also includes the resilience that comes out of these adversities. You have to recognize that facing your life and yourself every day is essential, and that you can live your dreams and disappointments like everyone else.

Recovery of mental health professionals – the only way out

'So many times we ask our mental health professionals to be our 'Holders of Hope'. Sadly, most of them, however, can't be our 'Holders of Hope' because they come from the mind set that says: 'I do not believe that you can recover, therefore you cannot recover'.' (Glover 2003)

Based on her work with mental health teams that want to change their approach towards a recovery-orientation, Glover concludes that such transformations are quite arduous and require much time. One condition for recovery-oriented work is that providers need to be in a position where they can value their work positively and shape it accordingly. If they themselves doubt the value of their work and their creativity, they are hardly likely to provide motivation for recovery.

She sees a culture of fear as one of the main reasons for the difficult work situation of mental health providers. This fear is projected onto the service users. The desire for protection and safety on the part of professionals blocks their view of the potential of clients. Risks need to be minimized. Below-par conditions are kept going and changes aborted in order to avoid any risk of legal liabilities. There are many reasons for this tradition of risk-aversion at all costs. If a team wants to transform itself, it has to become engaged in a process that puts this culture in question.

One important step would be to replace the dominant history of illness, the revolving door and hopelessness with a different and new history. Any small potential change towards a recovery-orientation should be widely advertised and instituted in such a way that it can sustain itself in spite of the dominant paradigm.

These changes must take place if a great deal of expertise and energy is no longer to be squandered. In the face of the fact that the dominant tradition has taken centuries to develop, much patience and tenacity will be required.

'WELLNESS RECOVERY ACTION PLAN (WRAP)' – MARY ELLEN COPELAND/USA

Who and where?

The Copeland Center for Wellness and Recovery in West Dummerston/Vermont, USA has been in operation since 1995. The Center has a presence on the internet at www.mentalhealthrecovery.com and at www.copelandcenter.com.

Mary Ellen Copeland and her team have been actively and successfully disseminating easy-to-understand and well-structured information about recovery, self-help, relapse prevention and social support in emotional crises for several years. The materials have appeared in the form of books, audio-cassettes, CD-ROMs, newsletters and web-pages. Their quarterly newsletter is available online or by post, free of charge. In addition, Copeland and her team offer well-structured seminars and training programmes for facilitators on recovery and well-being in several US cities. Some thousands of individuals with mental health problems have already been reached through these programmes.

Mary Ellen is an author and trainer for recovery in the mental health field. Her main focus is self-help. The concepts, competencies and strategies that she is promulgating through her publications and seminars come from her personal experiences with extreme mood fluctuations and her dialogues with individuals who have experienced psychiatric symptoms.

Mary Ellen's biography sheds some light on the reasons why she has concentrated on recovery, self-determination and hope in her books and seminars. She tells the story of her mother in an article 'Remembering Kate – A Story of Hope' that is available through her website   (www.healthyplace.com/Communities/Depression/mhrecovery/articles9.htm). Mary Ellen is the middle child of five siblings and grew up in a rural area with a father who worked for the railroad. Her mother was a nutritionist and worked for a few years until she got married and became fully occupied by running a household with five children. She was a great cook, taught her children many practical things in both house and garden and supported their creativity and individuality in their education.

When Mary Ellen was eight, her mother became ill at the age of 36 and spent the next eight years in a state mental institution, diagnosed with a severe manic-depressive condition. The doctors said that she was incurable and would never recover. The children visited their mother every week, even against doctors' advice. During her first major depressive episode, the mother had hardly any support; her closest relatives lived far away, and her husband was often working elsewhere for several weeks at a time. Raising all those children became too much for her. She had no opportunity to meet and converse with other women. Instead of receiving treatment in her familiar environment, she was separated from her family and spent years in an overcrowded, dark and smelly institution of the 1950s – lacking any privacy and sleeping in a dormitory with forty other women who also had serious psychiatric problems. No one expected any of them to get well; patients were simply warehoused until many of them died a lonely death: the total opposite of a recovery-oriented environment.

Against all expectations, her mother did recover and stayed well until her death at the age of 82. Mary Ellen spent many hours with her, trying to find out how she managed to get better. Her mother's recovery became the inspiration for Mary Ellen's research and subsequent publications. She became interested in the ways people diagnosed with depression and bipolar disorder managed their day-to-day life, how they could stabilize after major mood alterations and how they could regain control over their lives.

Mary Ellen assumes that one reason for her mother's improvement might have been the attention she received from a volunteer intern and another hospital worker, who had developed a particular interest in her. They listened to her for many hours and encouraged her to talk. She was not used to opening up with anyone, and always had the feeling that no one was listening to her. One nurse secretly gave her mother high dosages of multivitamins. Before she was discharged from the institution, Mrs Copeland began to look out for some of her fellow patients. Between her episodes of bipolar disorder she participated in a support group that had been instituted as an innovation by a dedicated psychiatrist. It was called the Mental Health Fellowship. She continued to attend these group meetings even after she left the hospital and kept visiting the patients she had befriended over the years. Mary Ellen's mother had a strong need for social exchange and mutual support, along with a great deal of willpower.

By the time she was released back to her home, the children had grown up, were adolescents and largely independent; they did not help her much to come back into the family. She had to struggle to regain her space in the family and when she realized that she couldn't get work after coming out of the hospital, she took educational courses. Quite often, she endured rude comments from people in her environment. Finally, she found a post as a school lunch manager, where she became successful and was much liked. Some of the mothering time she had lost with her own children, she devoted to the very needy kids she met through her work. Systematically, she started to get in touch with people in her community and became an active volunteer in her church. And she helped her son to raise his seven children. Her social net of mutual supports kept expanding, so that by the time she reached her old age she was embedded in loving relationships in her community and had many friends and a large family with 24 grandchildren and 19 great-grandchildren.

Mary Ellen herself suffered for many years from the symptoms of a psychiatric condition. At the age of 37 she was diagnosed as 'manic-depressive' and the psychiatrist told her that she would be 'okay', if only she took her pills regularly. She was told that she had to take medication for the rest of her life. For ten years she was indeed 'okay' until a stomach virus caused her to suffer from serious lithium toxicity. Subsequently, she could no longer take her medication. From this time on she had to learn how to manage the highs and lows by herself. With respect to her mother, she said: 'Because of Kate, I knew that my diagnosis of manic depression was not the end of the road, that I would, like her, get well, and stay well'. And she emphasized: 'Kate's story, and the story of others who have walked in her shoes, needs to be told again and again. Those of us with psychiatric illnesses need to know that there are many, many people who, like Kate, get well, stay well and lead rich, rewarding and valuable lives' (Copeland 2008, p 4).

She criticizes her psychiatrists from that period in her life because they did not give her the option, during ten years of drug treatment, to learn how to cope with her mood swings, and they didn't inform her about certain techniques for relaxation and stress-reduction that would have helped to reduce her symptoms. She could have avoided much personal suffering, if her life had not been as hectic and chaotic as it was, and if she had not stayed as long as she did with an abusive husband. She would have done better had she known that she should have been spending more time with people who cared for and supported her. No one had ever told her that she could learn how to diminish burdensome feelings and perceptions, or even get rid of them altogether. 'Perhaps if I had learned these things and had been exposed to others who were working their way through these kinds of symptoms, I would not have spent weeks, months, and years experiencing extreme psychotic mood swings while doctors searched diligently to find effective medication' (Mead and Copeland 2005, p. 70). Today Mary Ellen writes about the experiences that shaped her life, and it is her desire to inform as many people with psychiatric conditions as possible about the many ways that are available to make these experiences less painful, or even to make them disappear completely.

For whom?

Mary Ellen Copeland addresses herself to people who suffer from psychiatric symptoms and are experiencing emotional crises, as well as their friends and supporters. Beyond this, she also reaches out to open-minded mental health professionals with her training programmes, helping them to introduce the basic ideas of recovery into their services and to foster their implementation. By making use of the centre's facilitator-training programme, a strong and growing network of trainers has been developed in the USA, who pass on their new knowledge as well as their own experiences with mental illness to other service users. By so doing, they convey new methods and instructions for self-help based on hope, empowerment, self-determination, recovery and wellness. Copeland does not offer consulting services, and sees the transmission of her competencies and strategies as a complement to, rather than a replacement of, other mental health treatments.

Basic idea

Because of her own and her mother's life stories, Mary Ellen Copeland has developed the firm conviction that users are not forced by an illness to give up their dreams and aspirations and that they have responsibility for their own lives. She points out that even people who had once suffered from very severe psychiatric symptoms, have become doctors, lawyers, teachers, accountants and social workers. 'We are successfully establishing and maintaining intimate relationships. We are good parents. We have warm relationships with our partners, parents, siblings, friends and colleagues. We are climbing mountains, planting gardens, painting pictures, writing books, making quilts, and creating positive change in the world. And it is only with this vision and belief for all people that we can bring hope for everyone' (Mead and Copeland 2005, p 70).

The key factors of recovery

Below we summarize the most important recovery factors presented by Mead and Copeland (2005, p 71f):

1. *'There is hope.'* Too many people have internalized the message that there is no hope, that they are simply victims of their illness and that the only relationships they can hope for are one-sided and infantilizing. People don't need negative predictions about the course of their symptoms, something that no one else, regardless of their credentials, can ever know. Rather, users of mental health services need assistance, encouragement, and support while they work to relieve their symptoms and get on with their lives. They need a caring environment without feeling the need to be taken care of.
2. *'It's up to each individual to take responsibility for his or her own wellness.'* Nobody else can do this but the person him/herself. It can be rather challenging to take personal responsibility when symptoms are overwhelming and persistent. In such instances it might be most helpful for professionals and other supporters to work with the person, to find a way out of such frightening situations.
3. *'Education is a process that must accompany us on this journey.'* People who suffer from psychiatric symptoms are seeking information that can help them discover what is good for them and which steps they have to take themselves. Many of them would like to have mental health providers at their side along the way, and to collaborate with them in workshops and seminars.
4. *'We must advocate for ourselves.'* Many users have the mistaken belief that they have lost their rights as individuals. As a result, their rights are often violated, and these violations are consistently overlooked. Self-advocacy becomes easier as users' self-esteem, which has been damaged by years of chronic instability, is re-established. It is important that users themselves understand that they are as intelligent, worthwhile and unique as anyone else.
5. *'All people grow through taking positive risks.'* Users should make their own decisions concerning their life and treatment; build their own crisis and treatment plans; have the right to obtain all their records; have access to information around medication side effects; be able to refuse potentially hazardous treatment; choose their own

relationships and spiritual practices; be treated with dignity, respect, and compassion, and create the life of their choice.

6. *'Peer support is a key component of recovery.'* Peer support avoids categories and hierarchical roles (doctor/patient). In a recovery-based environment, support is never a crutch or a situation in which one person defines or dictates the outcome. Peer support is a process in which people strive to use the relationship to become fuller, richer human beings. Support works best when both people are willing to grow and change.

Most commonly, people who suffer from psychiatric symptoms are employing the following recovery-related activities and strategies in order to ameliorate or eliminate certain symptoms. This is according to the findings of Mary Ellen Copeland, for instance in the Vermont Recovery Education Project from 1995–2000 (www.mentalhealthrecovery.com/wrap_research_findings_vermont.php; 21.08.08):

- looking for support consisting of listening, not of receiving advice;
- finding people who are positive and confirming, but also direct and challenging;
- avoiding people who are criticizing, condemning or abusing;
- consulting and exchanging with peers;
- reducing stress and applying relaxation techniques (breathing, visualization);
- taking exercise (walking, bicycling, swimming);
- creative and joyful activities (reading, handicraft, artistic work, music);
- writing a diary;
- changing diet habits (avoiding caffeine, sugar, fat);
- going outdoors;
- transforming negative thoughts into positive ones;
- increasing or decreasing the stimulation in one's environment;
- day structure, particularly in difficult times;
- recognizing and controlling symptoms (maintaining well-being; recognizing triggers and early warning signals; counteracting symptoms which may worsen the situation; establishing a crisis plan to keep control even if the situation is out of control).

Principles of WRAP and training programmes

The Wellness Recovery Action Plan (WRAP) is an individualized system for monitoring and responding to symptoms to achieve the highest possible levels of wellness. The principles of WRAP include a shift of focus in mental health care from symptom control to prevention and recovery. Costly mental health and emergency services should be reduced as people who experience psychiatric symptoms effectively take responsibility for their own wellness and stability, manage and reduce their symptoms using a variety of self-help techniques, and effectively reach out for and use the support of a network of family members, friends and health care professionals. The aims are: increased ability to meet life and vocational goals, significant life enhancement and gains in self-esteem and self-confidence as people become contributing members of the community.

Anyone who participates in the training programme – be they a professional or a lay person – should learn to develop a Wellness Recovery Action Plan (WRAP) for themselves and for others. WRAP is a programme for self-help and a training programme for facilitators on recovery and well-being. Whoever is interested can participate in several modules which build on one another.

1. *Correspondence course:* Everyone who wants to become a facilitator starts with the correspondence course in order to become familiar with the principles of WRAP. It consists of four parts and teaches basic concepts and skills of recovery and the development of a Wellness Recovery Action Plan for oneself or for other people who suffer from psychiatric symptoms. In some regions the participants meet once a week to discuss and work together on the structure. The course includes reading specific literature and articles, projects, activities and discussion with the leader. The leader decides whether, according to his/her evaluation, the participants are able to understand and apply the concepts, strategies and techniques and whether they have completed the course successfully. The goals are the following.
First week: Recovery concepts including hope, personal responsibility, education, advocacy, peer support, family and professional support. Possible physical causes of mental illness, and medication.
Second week: Various simple, safe self-help strategies which people with psychiatric symptoms experience useful in ameliorating symptoms and maintaining well-being. Peer-counselling, exercise, relaxation, stress reduction, diary, leisure activities, regulation of stimulation, diet habits, sleep, day structure.
Third week: Developing a Wellness Recovery Action Plan. Day structuring, recognizing of and reacting to triggers and early warning signs, finding out which symptoms make the situation worse, and effective counteracting. Writing of a crisis plan or an advance directive.
Fourth week: Factors influencing well-being, for example, transforming negative thoughts into positive ones, establishing of self-esteem, suicide prevention, reducing trauma effects, developing a life-style aimed at increased well-being.
2. *Facilitator training:* The facilitator training in mental health recovery consists of five days with Mary Ellen and her team. This programme teaches those on the course how to work directly with people experiencing psychiatric symptoms and how to discover the strengths they have which will support their recovery. Recovery-concepts and self-help strategies are discussed, and a Wellness Recovery Action Plan is developed both with individuals and groups. The participants should be motivated and empowered to find out the way they want to feel, how they would like to create their lives, and what they can do to meet their life-goals. The participants learn methods of interaction and various ways of presentation. At the end each participant has to give an introduction to and a presentation about a recovery topic. Mary Ellen and her team have developed a special manual for this training, entitled the *WRAP and Peer Support Manual: Personal, Group and Programme Development*, which is available on a CD-ROM. Upon successful completion of the training each participant receives a Mental Health Recovery Educator certificate and Continuing Education Credits from the Vermont Secretary of State.
3. *Advanced facilitator training:* The aim of this programme is to teach participants how to conduct groups, to give them the opportunity to do some teaching and also to teach them how to provide support for others. The following people are eligible: a) those who successfully completed the Facilitator Training at least a year earlier;

b) those who have facilitated at least three WRAP groups since the initial facilitator training; c) those who have provided ten evaluation forms from people who have attended groups that the participant has facilitated; and d) those who can provide three references from people who have attended groups that they have facilitated.

Further publications by Mary Ellen Copeland and her team

Copeland ME, Allott PK (Eds.) (2005) *Wellness Recovery Action Plan*. Sefton Recovery Group.

Copans St, Ellen MA, Copeland MS, Copeland ME (2002) *Recovering from Depression. A Workbook for Teens*. Brookers Publishing Company.

Copeland ME, Riddle ML (2002) *The Depression Workbook. A Guide for Living with Depression and Manic Depression*. New Harbinger Publications, Oakland.

Copeland ME (1999) *Winning against Relapse*. New Harbinger Publications, Oakland.

Copeland ME, Harris M (2000) *Healing the Trauma of Abuse. A Woman's Workbook*. New Harbinger Publications, Oakland.

'TWO SIDES OF RECOVERY' – WILMA BOEVINK/THE NETHERLANDS

Where and when?

The involvement and participation of people with psychiatric experiences in the Netherlands is formalized and codified by law. Nevertheless, there is still a great discrepancy between formal regulation and the transfer into practice. Wilma Boevink has worked for several years at the Trimbos-Institute, the Netherlands Institute of Mental Health and Addiction in Utrecht (www.trimbos.nl).

Who?

Wilma Boevink was born in 1963. She is a social scientist in the field of psychiatric care, an active member of the Dutch service user movement and a board member of the European Network of (ex-)Users and Survivors of Psychiatry (ENUSP). As a former long-term user of services, she is currently employed in the research department of the Trimbos-Institute, where she is able to integrate her personal experiences and her research activities. She is the leader of a user-led training and consulting company which works in the area of recovery, empowerment and experiential expertise of people with psychiatric disabilities. Since 2006 she has been the chair of 'Stichting Weerklank', the Dutch organisation for people who hear voices and have psychotic experiences. Wilma is the author of book chapters and journal articles on recovery and related topics in various languages. In 2006, she edited a book with the title, *Stories of Recovery: Working Together towards Experiential Knowledge in Mental Health Care*, in which users of long-term psychiatric care describe how they have worked together towards recovery.

As an active member of the service user movement she lists clearly the limitations affecting the collaboration and participation of users on mental health committees.

Frequently, they are not in a position, or are not enabled, to use the law for their own purpose. There are, for instance, difficulties in recruiting active members, difficulties staying in touch with the general population of users, and difficulties with reviewing the many complicated texts. Users have only limited input into the agenda of meetings, little input on the frequency and the course of consultations and little knowledge of how communication works within the mental health field. Active members of the user movement expend a large portion of their energy on internal affairs and bureaucratic issues. Furthermore, Wilma perceives a lack of people, of financial means and of a 'collective knowledge', all of which are necessary if users are to make a substantive contribution.

Wilma thinks that some input of users exists, i.e., for the development of services or the standard of treatment for schizophrenia, and that users sit at the table in a commission that oversees clinical trials of new rehabilitation methods. However, she does not have much hope of this kind of user involvement, for the following reasons. For the most part, service users are only invited once the key decisions have already been made. Also they are only allowed to work within a framework that steers clear of established power relations, or even affirms them. And users of psychiatric services are frequently isolated people who, while they do have a history and experience as patients, are lacking in knowledge of the political or historical perspectives of the user movement.

Wilma had been hospitalized for the treatment of psychotic episodes. Based on her personal experiences, she knew that the need to regain her strength was an important element in her own recovery-process. She realized that it takes time to once again find strength after a period of psychosis. She was confronted with an overwhelming vulnerability that had to be overcome. The world and everything that pertains to it had to be discovered anew. Her self-confidence was shattered and the journey back to herself and the world came with many dangerous obstacles. She had to find a workable balance between wanting to be alone and to protect herself from the upheavals of life on the one hand and becoming actively involved in the world on the other. She describes some steps in her recovery-process:

> 'You must learn which things can be taken for granted again. You must regain the "normalcy" of everyday life. That is a matter of time, of adding every day without calamities to the previous one. And when things have gone well for a while, you may tentatively relax and think that perhaps the worst is over' (Boevink 2002, p 1).

An important aspect of Wilma's recovery was her attempt to grasp what had actually happened to her. Her recovery began at the moment when she dared to look back on her life and to speak about her psychotic experiences. Until then, there was only one official version of her life-story: she had a mental illness that required hospitalisation. In hospital she received treatment which enabled her to live with the residual effects of the illness, even though she had not been completely 'cured'. Wilma declared vehemently that this was not her story and she does not believe in this version, which is of no use to her. Her own version is very different: 'In my version I am not the carrier of a psychiatric disorder. In my story my admission to hospital was the result of a complex interaction of factors. One of the factors is my vulnerability for psychosis and another is about the physical abuse and violence of which I was a victim' (*ibid* p 1). She states that her psychosis was undoubtedly also a response to these unhealthy circumstances. She wonders why she was never asked about the circumstances of her illness, but she knows that such obvious questions are usually not asked in mental health services. Instead, it is paramount to come up with a diagnosis. And once a diagnosis has been found, the answers to all questions would automatically follow. From that moment on, everything you say and do is seen as the logical manifestation of the diagnosed disorder.

Wilma remembers that she too came to adopt the views and methods of the treating psychiatrists during her illness episodes. She feared that if she departed from the path her doctors advised her to take she would have a relapse. Maybe following this advice was necessary for some of the time, but ultimately it kept her tethered to the role of a mental patient. Consequently, she ascribed many things that were part of life to the illness. To her, recovery means learning to distinguish between the normal irritants of life and events that give a clear cause for concern. It is important to learn not to connect all setbacks with the so-called illness, but rather to see them as part of life in general. A person in recovery has to accept life as it is and take responsibility for it. It does, however, take some time and much patience to once again take charge of your life and trust your own judgment.

For whom?

Through her active involvement in user-run organizations Wilma Boevink aims to strengthen the position of users of psychiatric services. There are many initiatives in the Netherlands that offer a different perspective for dealing with people who have mental health problems: for example, the office for patient affairs in Eindhoven; the 'Wegwijswinkel', a counselling service for users in Utrecht; the patient- or consumer-platform in Amsterdam, and the 'Basisberaad' in Rotterdam. These services develop training programmes for mental health professionals, offer courses by users for users and put in place new self-help groups and discussion circles for psychiatric users. In addition, there are training programmes that support the use of personal experiences with psychiatry in professional mental health settings. At national level there are self-help organizations for example, for voice hearers (Weerklank) and people with borderline disorders, which generate insights that can improve the understanding and treatment of psychiatric conditions.

Basic idea

User-run projects are increasingly gaining popularity. Current and former service users are demonstrating their leadership capabilities in many areas. This wealth of activity is driven by the conviction that their own experiences can open up other perspectives on symptoms and emotional problems, and thereby possibly generate different – or even better – services than those available in traditional psychosocial programmes.

Wilma has a clear perspective for service users: 'Self-help and user-directed initiatives are a response to the fact that our unique nature, our experiences, and our knowledge are hardly represented in mainstream psychosocial services. For service-users, either individually or collectively, the focus is shifting: away from agitating against the powers of others and from reacting to their agenda, towards the recognition of our own increasingly powerful strengths' (Boevink 2003).

Recovery-initiatives

In recent years, Wilma Boevink has participated in a recovery-project for long-term services, in which she collaborated closely with eight of her peers. The results of this project were published in the *Stories of Recovery* (Boevink 2006). They met fortnightly over a number of years to exchange views about their efforts to live with persistent mental health problems. Boevink says that the terminology of mental health professionals, replete as it is with notions of disorders and symptoms, was so familiar to her, that it was rather unusual to participate in discussions about mental distress in a role other than that of a patient. Members of the recovery-project were speaking from the perspective of autonomous initiatives and self-help.

The participants sat at tables arranged in a circle, not unlike what happens at certain management meetings and they held to a previously agreed agenda while minutes were taken at the meetings. The participants reported what they had been thinking about during the preceding weeks. They shared experiences and advice about ways of dealing with the obstacles to their attempts to gain new perspectives on life. Reviewing the notes from the previous meeting created a distance from these personal experiences and facilitated a more systematic understanding. In this fashion, guidelines were developed for subjects such as principles of recovery, supportive resources, dealing with psychotropic medication, relationships with therapists, vacations, caring for pets, etc.

In the course of this project, the participants began to want to disseminate the knowledge they had gained to the public. Several initiatives were developed in this direction, for example presentations and discussion groups for peers; investigations within their own service agencies; seminars for residential support staff, and peer-to-peer training sessions on the subject of 'Making a Start on Recovery'. One participant described her positive experience in this project during a lecture for an audience of caregivers: 'You become aware of your own attempts to grow beyond a crisis, of the techniques that helped you, of the times when you fell down and got back up again. We often recognise similar attempts in each other's stories' (Boevink 2006, p 13).

The project was based on two principles (Boevink 2003, p 38):

1. The participants were provided with tools to enable them to develop a new perspective on their life along with new attributions of meaning.
2. The participants were given the opportunity to relinquish the patient role without blocking discussions about their experiences in mental health services.

This way the participants should become aware of the options they have to help themselves. They learned that the contributions of mental health professionals to their own recovery-process needed to be critically evaluated, and in addition they broadened their knowledge-base. This enabled them to banish the stigmatizing diagnosis and prognosis as well as any related prejudices from their own self-image, thinking and actions. Relinquishing the patient role did not, however, imply a denial of the real mental suffering. On the contrary, the illness-related identity was replaced by an identity they themselves chose to live, a history in their own language which contained their own strategies, and the possibility of living with persistent vulnerabilities.

While not developing 'anything new', the recovery-project brought knowledge and strategies to light that had already been present within the user movement. Boevink recognized many of the things that she had learned herself from incidental, informal or organized contacts with peers, experts-by-experience, and other activists. She recognized subjects such as hope, self-worth, self-determination, and 'the power of the collective' (ibid., p 38), instead of diagnoses and patient characteristics rendered in the language of mental health professionals (i.e. length or severity of illness).

Criticism about the narrow views of mental health professionals

Boevink also has a lot to say about typical defensive and derogatory responses on the part of mental health professionals. They react to her approach with the words: 'It's great what you are doing, but our patients would be overwhelmed'. For most of their patients there was no hope, since they were too ill or too disabled (Boevink 2003, p 38). Wilma has heard this all too often. They say that it is a false conclusion of mental health professionals who frequently say that people who are living in recovery have always belonged to some kind of elite among mental patients. This conclusion, says Wilma, is erroneous, stupid and cowardly. Quite often you see people who have freed themselves from long-standing, catastrophic careers as mental patients, even though they had been given a rather poor prognosis. These people had certainly not belonged to a chosen group that could carry the torch of hope for mental health professionals. Minimizing the suffering of such people and ignoring their paths away from it, is an attempt to deny the value and the courage of these people. In this manner, these professional 'helpers' deprive themselves of their own chances to deliver better work as therapists and supporters.

Boevink argues that the survivor movement should separate itself from the mental health sector and suggests that there are many more things available to members of the movement in society, beyond the psychiatric domain. She does not want to be reduced to a 'disorder with the need for psychiatric care' and claims:

> 'We are whole people with a life that wants to be lived even if there are parts of that life which make it necessary for us to use professional care or services. This necessity transforms us into users of psychiatric services. And it is not important where we get the services we need. Definitely, the continuation of the life that we desire is most important to us, the mental health services play merely a functional role in our lives.' (Boevink 2003, p 39; translation by MS)

She expresses her sceptical view about the role of mental health professionals by saying that while one can declare oneself to be a user of psychiatric services, one would need a qualified partner to be used in the positive sense of the term 'used'. 'We are still light years away from this goal.' (ibid., p 39; translation by MS)

A realistic view of recovery

Boevink highlights the aspects of recovery which come from her own experiences, and also points to certain elements that are not pertinent, for example an unrealistic, exclusively positive attitude. 'Recovery does not mean that everything will get better. It is vital to face and accept this. I must look back on periods in my life when my behaviour was odd – to put it mildly' (Boevink 2002, p 2). Instead, recovery according to the author means:

- looking back on what had happened, rewriting one's history to make it one's own story, and developing a new identity;
- claiming right of ownership over one's subjective experiences;
- the person giving meaning to what has happened, and no one else;
- not only recovering from mental problems but also coping with the fact of having been a patient in a psychiatric hospital, including the negative consequences such as exclusion from society, a difficult financial situation, discrimination in the work-place;
- distancing oneself from the habit of the typical life of an institution to which one becomes accustomed more quickly that one can discard it (ibid., p 2).

Recovery does not mean '. . . that everything will turn out all right. Some things never will and you must learn to live with that. In the literature, these are called handicaps. If you can identify them you can make allowances for yourself. This will save you a lot of misery. And it saves your energy for what you can do' (ibid., p 2). The stigma which goes hand in hand with having a mental disorder makes her angry. If people in recovery compare their life with that of other 'seemingly happy people leading their apparently easy lives' they realize what they have missed and that it is too late to correct many things. But Boevink warns that this view is deceptive, because things are never as they seem. People should not lose themselves in these negative emotions. Instead, it is important to be proud of what you have achieved so far.

Recovery – a political matter

Merely participating in the opportunities provided by mental health professionals does not seem sufficient to Wilma. Talking about and working on recovery with others is a political matter for her. She believes that users of mental health services should be able to support each other to a much greater extent than has been happening so far. Simply learning from the knowledge of others, that they have drawn from so many years of experience, enables users to retell their stories and to recognize themselves in them.

Therefore, Wilma challenges the members of the user movement to keep telling these stories to each other, in order to enable them to recapture their unique identities. Stories that say: this is my life, this is me, and this is the way you can help me. Beyond the value they have for peers in the movement, these stories also offer mental health professionals a chance to learn how to communicate in a language that is understood by service users and providers alike. In the epilogue of her book, the author gives an overview of the growing recovery movement in the Netherlands, which gives rise to an optimistic view of the possibilities for exciting exchange and collaboration between service users and professionals in the mental health field:

'Supporting recovery demands a positive and holistic view of health, which is focused on the possibility of personal growth. Service users, providers and scientists in the Netherlands have united in a national recovery strategy. The aim is the development of a recovery programme with and by people with psychiatric disabilities. New recovery groups have started at several locations around the country. They will all follow the same route, starting with exchanging their own individual stories, then moving on to knowledge transfer to fellow service users and professionals.' (Boevink 2006, p 59)

Further publications by Wilma Boevink

Boevink W (2008) Productivity in terms of recovery from a client's perspective. Paper presented at the 2nd European Psychiatric Symposium, Berlin, March 27, 2008. Internet: www.akp-psychiatrie.de/espb2008.htm (31.08.08).

Boevink W (2007) Survival, the art of living and knowledge to pass on: recovery, empowerment and experiential expertise of people with severe mental health problems. In: Stastny P, Lehmann P (eds.). *Alternatives Beyond Psychiatry* (pp 105–16). Peter Lehmann Publishing, Shrewsbury, UK.

Boevink W (2006) From being a disorder to dealing with life: an experiential exploration of the association between trauma and psychosis. *Schizophrenia Bulletin* **32/1**: 17–19.

Boevink W. Life after psychiatry. On the Website of Alaska Mental Health Consumer Web: Recovery from Mental Illness. Internet: www.akmhcweb.org/recovery/rec.htm (31.08.08).

Boevink W, Kroon H (2005) Living with a psychiatric disability: lessons to learn and to pass on. Internet: www.peter-lehmann-publishing.com/articles/boevink_kroon.pdf (31.08.08).

Boevink W (2004) Monsters from the past. In: Lehmann P (ed.). *Coming off Psychiatric Drugs: Successful Withdrawal from Neuroleptics, Antidepressants, Lithium, Carbamazepine and Tranquilizers*. (pp 79–82) Peter Lehmann Publishing, Shrewsbury, UK.

Boevink W, Beuzekom J van, Gaal E, *et al*. (2002) *Samen werken aan herstel. Van ervaringen delen naar kennis overdragen (Working Together on Recovery: from Sharing Experiences to Implementing Knowledge)*. Trimbos-Institute, Utrecht.

Boevink W, Escher S (2001) *Making Self-harm Understandable*. Stichting Positieve Gezondheidszorg, Bemelen.

'NO EMPOWERMENT WITHOUT RECOVERY' – CHRISTIAN HORVATH/AUSTRIA

Christian Horvath is the leader and project director of the self-help organization 'Crazy Industries' in Vienna and a board member of the Austrian Society for Schizophrenia. Over many years he has advocated against relinquishing the notion of cure as an aim of treatment. Reason enough for the authors to interview him about what he thinks of the recovery-concept:

Mr Horvath, for several years now you have argued, in front of several distinguished conference audiences, that patients can be cured. This view was not always greeted by applause. How come?

Well, that was interesting. Several psychiatrists felt that the notion of a 'cure' was too far-reaching and esoteric. They were concerned about patients who might present them with certain expectations in response to the notion of 'cure', which could not be fulfilled. My primary intent was not to promote cure in a broad sense, but rather to establish a counterweight to the perennial notions of stabilization and relapse-prevention. Dedicating your entire life exclusively to relapse-prevention often leads to a kind of risk-aversion that is not conducive to a person's living his or her life – people tend to go in circles.

If cure is not the ideal term, how would you translate and interpret recovery?
The easiest way might be to contrast recovery with the notion of 'empowerment'. We have had many discussions among our members about this latter term. Recovery means primarily to be concerned with your own convalescence. And empowerment in essence means that your position vis-a-vis psychiatry needs to be destigmatized and improved, even if this requires a great deal of readiness to become engaged in conflict. Empowerment requires recovery. In my opinion, users who live along the lines of recovery, experience greater realization of their intentions. After ten years of empowerment you can see the success it has engendered, but you also need to keep in mind the seemingly unavoidable sacrifices that were made.

When you say empowerment, do you mean self-help and advocacy? How can empowerment be combined with recovery in a way that is advantageous for service users?
The first self-help groups were certainly inspired by the idea of recovery. This meant that people simply wanted to lead a better life (quality of life) – in other words, that they wanted to recover. The notion of peer-to-peer advocacy is more problematic. It is a very challenging task and not always conducive to the health of those involved. Moving overnight from being a little patient who is stigmatized and not sufficiently educated to becoming a counterpart or even a decision-maker in discussions with doctors and politicians, is not like a dive into icy water. It is rather like crashing into a burning Christmas tree.

Are you sensing danger in these new English terms?
Of course! For instance, the term 'compliance'. How this notion was praised and reviled during conferences in the 1990s, only to turn out to be a trailblazer for fostering a dependent and indecisive group of patients! One example: a very compliant woman who was in awe of doctors had not taken the opportunity to provide feedback in her therapy, and was therefore given a cocktail of too many outdated drugs, compared to her fellow self-help group members. A few people thought of empowerment as some sort of battle for a vague notion of autonomy. Recovery sounds better than this, since most people are basically thinking about getting well.

Mr Horvath, your analyses are sounding rather grim. Therefore I am wonderwing what you would say, as a person who has worked quite intensively in the self-help movement over the past 20 years, has changed for the better?
Certainly, the desire for change has been the most important factor. Involving service users and family members; new types of medication; self-help groups for users and relatives; some degree of freeing the communication between psychiatrists and ex-patients from its institutional constraints, and a certain enhancement of mutual respect are things that I consider progress. But to a large extent we are still being stigmatized – the anti-stigma campaigns have not helped that much. Stigmatization and discrimination

are key elements of dealing with people who have a psychiatric diagnosis, and they actually aggravate the illness. Recovery is rather hampered by this.

Throughout the nineties you initiated projects to promote vacation and leisure programmes and artistic activities among users in Austria. These were quite successful in spite of lacking funds. What was your basic idea behind these projects?
Exactly! My friends and I from 'Crazy Industries' have organized 14 vacation trips, one conference, 19 art exhibitions – mostly in galleries – eight concerts and 1200 round-table discussions for service-users. Continuing education for social workers and police officers, and invitations to give talks at 150 seminars and conferences are further areas of activity. These activities have promoted a break-through for self-help in Austria and many important newspapers have written about this in a series of quite in-depth articles. One response to this publicity was that we were attacked by jealous rivals, in particular certain anti-psychiatrically oriented individuals. On the other hand, we had to struggle against hostile takeovers by frustrated doctors and social workers, who wanted to use us for their own benefit. To make up for this, we benefited from the very generous support of psychiatric reformers and other groups, such as journalists. Nevertheless, the statement by Harald Hofer, a founder of the user-movement in Austria, still stands: 'You need to have many characteristics of a rhinoceros in order to survive this'. He believed that it was advantageous to develop a thick skin against discrimination and other forms of maltreatment.

Can you give us a few hints for this book and let us peek into your method of working?
But of course! The most important point was to recognize – even in people who are experiencing very active psychotic symptoms – their creative core and potential, which is of considerable importance to society. I considered it essential to set myself up against the views of traditional doctors, who had predominantly negative things to say about their patients – an orientation towards deficits. We need to create a totally new world for users where they can become organized, pursue artistic interests, conduct research and engage in friendly relations with progressive psychiatrists. They also have to be able to understand their respective past histories and to cope with them. I must admit that I have sometimes been too optimistic. But maybe this was necessary to keep all my activities going.

May I change the subject now? What is helpful in recovery from mental illness, and what is not?
This question sounds simple, but is basically rather difficult to answer. Over the years I have noticed certain rules that seemed to have practical relevance:

- Not to put too much pressure on yourself in the course of your recovery, i.e. by saying 'as of April I am going back to work';
- Not to aim for becoming once again the way you were before you became ill; people don't consider the fact that this period was precisely the time of their life when they became ill;
- It is also wrong to assume that a doctor and medication can solve personal problems;
- Do not blame your family for your illness, especially not in a global fashion;
- It is absolutely unadvisable to retreat into social withdrawal, where you could become your own worst enemy behind your four walls;
- Abandoning old pastimes due to feeling guilty is absurd;

- Stay away from dangerous drugs, which can destroy the emotional immune system;
- It is advantageous to develop the belief that you can get well once again. Choose new tasks that are small and manageable, which have a good chance of success;
- Replace the question 'why am I sick?' with 'what is the point of being sick?';
- Assume a friendly attitude towards your doctor without challenging his/her boundaries, while safeguarding your own;
- Pursue some type of sport, at least once a week, even if only briefly;
- Take vitamins (especially Vitamin B) during periods of excessive emotional stress;
- Never remain awake for more than two days;
- Suicidal thoughts are natural during difficult periods, but suicide never solves these problems;
- Shedding a few tears is often a good sign and should not be suppressed;
- Search for the right type of self-help group on the internet.

There are several explanatory models in psychiatry about the origin and course of psychiatric disorders. What is your opinion about this?
I am not totally familiar with the psychiatric concepts of illness, but they are at least intriguing. Since I rarely read books about mental illnesses, which I consider an advantage, I derive my opinions from the approaches and notions favoured by practitioners and from discussions with experts. The difference is that I don't see people as ill, but rather in search of recovery. I think it is a mistake that psychiatry pays too little attention to anxiety and guilt feelings, and that 'preconsciousness' is basically neglected in Europe. Psychotherapy is rarely offered to people experiencing psychosis and the illness is not seen as a way out, or at least as an attempt to find a way out.

Do you believe that the recovery-orientation will prevail?
I hope that it will not become too difficult, because there is a great deal of entrenched opposition from all sides. It is often said: 'Once crazy – always crazy'. The key will be if both psychiatry and its customers experience recovery as a shared perspective. Harald Hofer, whom I already mentioned once in this interview, said at a conference that he could 'not entirely exclude the possibility that psychiatry might advance from an anaesthetizing organization to an honour student of medicine'. That would be better for us.

I thank you for the interview and wish you good luck!
I wish your book much success!

CHAPTER 5

Recovery – Why Not?

THE SLOW DEMISE OF INCURABILITY

Eugen Bleuler's introduction of the plural term 'Schizophrenias' in 1911 conveyed his realization that these are complex conditions with highly varied trajectories. The appearance of a particular constellation of symptoms that can lead to a diagnosis cannot be used as a guide for the prediction of the further course of a condition and is certainly not tied to assumptions about incurability. At least since the first publication of Eugen Bleuler's book, *Dementia Praecox or the Group of Schizophrenias* (1911), people have been aware of this and have seen the evidence repeatedly: the course of schizophrenia can differ dramatically.

Complete restoration of health is possible, as is an episodic course. Not infrequently, courses are characterized by persistent symptoms and disability over many years. In recognizing this, Bleuler moved on from Emil Kraepelin's pronouncement that the condition he called 'dementia praecox', in contrast to manic-depressive illness, (now known as bipolar disorder), always involved a steadily progressing deterioration. In psychiatry, just as in general medicine, most disorders are not characterized by their course over time, but rather by a particular constellation of symptoms, which are more or less pronounced and have a longer or shorter duration. This applies to anxiety disorders just as much as to depressive reactions, stress-related conditions and obsessive-compulsive disorders. Full recoveries are not rare and a great deal of health is manifest between episodes of dysfunction. A healthy and meaningful life is quite possible in spite of longer lasting difficulties. Psychiatric treatment has developed rapidly in the pharmacological and psychosocial domains, thereby combating dysfunction and promoting well-being.

Incurability

In spite of these facts, the "myth of incurability" (Finzen 2004; Harding and Zahniser 1994) still lives on, especially concerning so called 'severe and disabling mental illnesses', and in particular the group of schizophrenias. The persistence of this myth is hard to understand, given that it has little to do with reality. To this day, individuals who have experienced psychiatric disorders and were given certain diagnoses are still threatened by the Damocletian sword of 'incurability' dangling over them. Unfortunately, the experience of many of them is that the mental health system cannot alleviate the fears

Recovery in Mental Health: Reshaping scientific and clinical responsibilities Michaela Amering and Margit Schmolke
Copyright © 2009 John Wiley & Sons, Ltd

connected to this myth. A looming hopelessness, arising from the erroneous notion of incurability, undermines the forces that could be applied to recovery and subverts the healing process. This situation is misguided and unacceptable. It is high time to effectively challenge the myth of incurability and to curtail its destructive potential. Everyone who is aware of this mischaracterization is called upon to take responsibility for corrective action. Outstanding achievements in the direction of wellness and health must be highlighted and given a chance to develop under favourable circumstances. Recovery-approaches constitute a chance for such a paradigm shift.

Chronicity

'Chronos' is the Greek word for time. Time plays a major role in human lives. When health is being compromised, much thought is given to the course of time. How could this happen so suddenly? How long will it last? When do we need to do something about it? Will it ever end?

The term 'acute' comes from the Latin word 'acutus', meaning sharp or pointed. In a medical context, acute refers to an illness which develops rapidly and lasts only a short time – mostly days or a few weeks. 'Peracute' conditions have an even more rapid onset and shorter duration, often leading to death. 'Chronic' means that a condition develops slowly, followed by a protracted and gradual course. This has both positive and negative consequences. Unlike a peracute onset, gradual developments leave ample time for intervention. There is plenty of time to adjust to the illness and to consider the best course of action. But it also means that everything can become rather drawn out and that there can be a tendency to develop persistent symptoms and disabilities.

However, chronic certainly does not mean incurable. Full recovery is possible even after long lasting illnesses. Over time, the experience gained can help people to manage the symptoms and challenges of protracted illnesses to the point that they have only minimal impact on everyday living. Chronic also means that a risk of recurring acute episodes might persist, as in epilepsy for example. Dealing appropriately with such a known and persistent vulnerability, which may include prophylactic treatment, can limit or even prevent the recurrence of acute episodes. The aim of treatment is a life characterised by health and the absence of further illness episodes. This type of vulnerability-model is frequently applied to psychiatric conditions as well as physical ones.

The chronicity of a disorder or vulnerability in itself does not stand in the way of a healthy life. Quite frequently, however, chronicity does get interpreted as a never ending fateful subjugation to an illness and its inescapable consequences. This is certainly not the case, but rather a misinterpretation with very damaging results. A cycle of hopelessness and inaction sets in and can lead to a drastic weakening of resources, thereby actually becoming a self-fulfilling prophecy of deteriorating health, persisting symptoms and disability.

A 1966 article by the psychiatrists Arnold Ludwig and Frank Farrelly in the *Archives of General Psychiatry* demonstrates rather impressively how a 'code of chronicity' impacts on life in a mental institution and undermines all the usual efforts towards improvement. The authors describe how an entire institution, patients as well as professional helpers, are subject to such a code of conduct. The therapeutic zeal of the staff has fizzled out.

A desire for order and obedience is paramount, as is a reluctance to introduce any type of change. Superficial compliance leads to the vastly reduced life of a model patient in a self-contained setting. Challenges and responsibilities are minimal, as are the risks taken, promoting the balancing act of chronic schizophrenia, which is characterized by a minimum of feelings and thoughts. Patients experience themselves as victims and struggle for the care handed out by others. The few rights they are granted as rewards for well-adjusted behaviour are not tied to duties or responsibilities. The illness becomes a means to an end and any changes in the state of chronicity are threats to calm and predictability for everyone.

Ludwig and Farrelly are describing the dramatic manifestations of institutionalism. Realizing its negative consequences has contributed to the phasing out of old-style mad-houses and asylums (at least in the Western world) which have traditionally promoted such developments. To what extent the phenomena of institutionalism have made their way, during the course of psychiatric reforms, into community mental health settings, remains an important question. There are many indications that extramural services and smaller institutions can be breeding grounds for similar problems. The empowerment movement has taught us much about how people can emerge from actual or perceived situations of powerlessness and, once again, take charge of their lives (www.power2u.org). The danger of promoting a 'code of chronicity', much like the one described above, is great in contexts where change is considered problematic and stability remains the only apparent goal. This can occur in mental health services that do not aim beyond the prevention of relapses and/or rehospitalizations, and in those that are chiefly concerned with the avoidance of risk and any and all sorts of crises.

It is important to recognize that certain terms, concepts and myths can have undesirable consequences whether or not they are scientifically founded. Nils Greve (2007) is quoting Bruno Hildebrand when he says that 'Retrospectively, chronic means long-standing. Prospectively, it means unchangeable'. If we are to successfully implement the concepts of recovery we must be able to face and deal with such phenomena. Successful psychiatric work requires the transformation of wrong and obstructive attitudes and positions. This process starts at the level of each individual person. Integrative and multidimensional concepts of psychiatric treatment must be rooted in positive attitudes and in a reduction of the widespread scepticism about the chances of recovery (Lecic-Tosevski et al. 2003).

The course of almost all mental disorders is variable. Remissions are possible, as are recurrences and long-term disabilities. Research struggles with problems of definitions of types of courses and methodological problems of long-term studies. The clinical use of prognostic indicators and determinants of remission and recurrence and long-term courses for individual patients is limited. Many people hesitate to seek an understanding of their mental health problems within a model of medical care for chronic conditions (Lester and Gask, 2006). As a result a considerable proportion of their efforts towards coping and finding meaning in their struggle for recovery occur outside the patient-clinician relationship. A collaborative model of recovery (Lester and Gask, 2006), allowing for individualized interventions and accommodating hopes, fears and subjective evidence in a personalized context, might be better suited to bundle the resources of patients, their families and friends and professional helpers from different professional backgrounds.

Other misunderstandings

Information about psychiatric disorders for patients and the general public has become much more widely available in recent years. Self-help movements, mental health services, advocacy organizations, individual advocates and the pharmaceutical industry have offered many sources of information, including a panoply of books, pamphlets and web-pages with scientific data on the one hand, and practical information as well as personal accounts and advice, on the other. The information about the possible course of disorders clearly demonstrates that mental illnesses follow a great variety of trajectories and can be favourably influenced.

Nevertheless, the stigma of the incurability of mental disorders lives on, as does the myth that many psychiatric interventions are ineffective. Certain misunderstandings will be hard to combat: the term 'endogenous' illness is often used to suggest that the actual aetiology is unknown. This leads to the conclusion that the causes cannot be treated, which in turn is seen as a deficiency and as evidence of treatment failure. In fact, many illnesses do not have one clear cause whose elimination would lead to a cure. Many factors usually act in concert and result in the appearance of a particular disorder at a particular time affecting a specific person in a unique way.

Clinicians are quite familiar with many of these factors and use this information in both diagnosis and treatment. At times, the weight of individual factors alone is not as significant as the precise interplay among them. In any case, it is certain that not being able to identify one definitive cause of an illness would not stop anyone from solving a problem successfully – for example, by changing the situation in such a way that certain factors can be eliminated or at least curtailed; or by creating situations that promote resilience against pathogenic factors. Experiences both in life and from history demonstrate clearly that it is not only when we can eliminate the causes of situations that we can succeed in mastering such situations. We are often confronted with the notion that as long as the causes are in the psychosocial domain, something can be done about them but if they are biological, nothing can be done. This, again, is not true. It is certainly the case that emotional well-being and distress result from a mixture of biological, social and psychological factors. Therefore, it makes sense not to restrict oneself to interventions from one or the other domain, but rather strive to provide the appropriate mixture for each person.

Another popular belief is the assumption that being well means not receiving treatment, and vice versa, being in treatment means being ill. This erroneous deduction does not make any sense either. Suffering without treatment in order to do justice to this definition of health, benefits no one. Finding the treatment that contributes to the greatest measure of health and resilience is surely the best response and one which helps to keep the illness, or at least its negative consequences, at bay. Everyone knows that genetic factors play a role in many aspects of life. Nevertheless many people tend to believe that when genetic factors play a part in a condition, nothing can be done about it. This also is a fatal misunderstanding. Modern genetics is rather busy and successful today in investigating how genetic predispositions and constellations are being expressed differently, depending on the impact of environmental factors. Research on psychiatric conditions shows that genetic factors certainly do not work in a simple, straightforward way. A great variety of genetic constellations can be associated with similar forms of mental conditions. Individuals with similar patterns of genetic vulnerability can develop rather different conditions, which may, or may not, manifest themselves as stressful or disabling.

This list of misunderstandings that interfere with health and recovery can be extended further. Mostly, it consists of unacceptable simplifications. The latest results in the area of brain research demonstrate the extent of the complexity we are facing. Our brains are rather supple. Life events leave traces that can amount to deficits. Resilience and resistances can develop and contribute to recovery. Cells are replaced, nerve connections are enhanced or wither away, depending on the circumstances. The brain can adapt to all kinds of situations; it is in a constant state of transformation. Recovery-work, measures to repair, secure and reconstruct, occur continually. And we can influence these processes to a certain extent.

It will be a long time before these complex processes can be understood, but one thing is clear already: static models of deficits no longer make any sense.

Is the glass half full or half empty?

There are many times in our lives when we face this question. We dread a misplaced hope. We try to avoid premature resignation. We must stay open-minded and curious and struggle on. Either we repeat mistakes again and again, or find a way to stop once and for all. Our life is full of new errors and surprising experiences. We are optimistic to varying degrees. Sometimes pessimism serves a good purpose, sometimes it saps our energy. Some people take risks, others play it safe. Depending on our view of the situation, our goals and our resources, we see the glass as half full or half empty. Our pessimistic assessments sometimes make sense, either because they conform to reality, or because they give way to pleasant surprises. Our optimism is always being challenged. Would a disappointment turn out to be an important learning experience? A crisis turn into a gain? Generally, we can only know this in hindsight. Which challenges are we up to? Which hurdles make us balk? Everyone must pose these questions for their life, independently of illness or health. And our answers determine how we lead our lives, what we dare to do, what we deny ourselves, what we settle for and what is worth a fight.

A DIAGNOSIS OR A VERDICT – THE EXAMPLE OF SCHIZOPHRENIA

A diagnosis of 'burnout' indicates that someone has become over-extended at work and has pushed too hard for too long, while paying too little attention to themselves. A diagnosis of 'schizophrenia' means something entirely different: 'Capable of anything, but good for nothing', in the formulation of Christian Horvath, user activist, president of the Viennese self-help enterprise 'Crazy Industries' and board member of the Austrian Schizophrenia Association (Amering, Sibitz, Goessler, Katschnig, 2002a; see also the interview with Mr Horvath, page 95)

The term 'schizophrenia' is used to describe a group of psychiatric conditions, the symptoms of which, come closest to the popular concept of 'madness'. Psychoses within the spectrum of schizophrenia are sometimes associated with changes in basic mental functions such as cognition, perception and affect. Schizophrenia can develop along a great variety of trajectories over time. The causes and origins of the condition are unknown. Its reputation is dreadful. Prejudices towards people so diagnosed include the notion of inherent dangerousness, that they are of defective character and intellect, and the judgment that they are incurable. These stubborn and widespread misconceptions about the implications of the schizophrenia diagnosis contribute to the fact that many psychiatrists are not keen to use it and most patients are afraid of being given this diagnosis. A diagnosis of 'schizophrenia' spreads horror and pessimism. Instead of offering orientation, a direction, a treatment plan and recovery, it is often experienced as a verdict. A verdict about character: dangerous and irresponsible; a verdict about social role: fellow citizens are seeking distance; and a verdict about the future: the condition is chronic, disabling, and incurable.

Emil Kraepelin's (1856–1926) description of a group of non-affective psychoses as 'dementia praecox' is now more than a century old. Importantly, it is also nearly a hundred years ago since Eugen Bleuler corrected Kraepelin's concept by insisting that the 'schizophrenias' can follow rather divergent courses over time. In 1911 Bleuler published his seminal paper 'Dementia praecox or the group of Schizophrenias'. The longitudinal studies of Huber, Ciompi, Harrison, Häfner and many others (Warner 2004), as well as the re-analysis of Bleuler's data (Modestin *et al.* 2003) have confirmed Bleuler's assumption repeatedly.

A group of eminent schizophrenia experts in the US formulated remission criteria for schizophrenia in 2005 (Andreasen *et al.* 2005) and there has been an affirmative response from Europe (van Os *et al.* 2006). This represents a formidable challenge to all the statements about schizophrenia as a condition whose symptoms inevitably persist over a lifetime. Such beliefs fly 'in the face of evidence, collected over a century of research, that there is a high level of heterogeneity in the course and outcome of schizophrenia and that symptomatic remission is common' (van Os *et al.* 2006).

Nevertheless, it is still necessary in the 21st century to confront the fact that the myth of incurability is still going strong. And it still appears both novel and revolutionary, in the context of the recovery movement to say that: you can recover in spite of schizophrenia; you can recover from and be healed of schizophrenia; you can regain your health in spite of schizophrenia, and a cure can be found for schizophrenia. The chapter, 'Stigma and discrimination', will focus particularly on opinions and attitudes towards the diagnosis of 'schizophrenia', and will also cover ideas on what can be done about this dismal state of affairs. While we are speaking here about the history of the idea of 'incurability' and the actual scientific evidence about the course of 'schizophrenic' conditions, one essential insight into the way stigma and prejudice work needs to be mentioned. And that is that stereotypical ideas about stigmatized groups tend to assume a great deal of immutability in connection with assumed traits, and thus may well be a crucial element in the prevalent unnecessarily pessimistic attitudes about prognosis and the efficacy of treatment (Corrigan 2007).

Heterogeneity of course over time

People who are given a diagnosis of 'schizophrenia' are mostly young, generally between adolescence and the mid-life years. It is hard to say what such a diagnosis might mean for their future. This insecurity is very distressing for those so labelled, as well as for their service providers. Patients and their relatives obviously want to find out from the treating psychiatrists and the other mental health professionals what they should be expecting. Today, one thing can be said for certain, that those conditions diagnosed as schizophrenia can take rather divergent courses over time: a first episode might be the only one. You might have schizophrenia once, but then never again.

For others, an episodic course might develop, in other words, a person might recover from one episode and experience another one after several months, years, or even decades. Episodes of schizophrenia can occur several times over the course of a life-time. Schizophrenia can also become a chronic condition. An acute episode might be followed by a prolonged period of diminished energy, creativity and emotional life. Perceptual disturbances, such as hallucinations, delusions and certain disabilities can persist for long periods of time, even for a life-time. Research provides evidence about this variability of schizophrenia and scientists engaged in longitudinal studies have distinguished up to ten different types of trajectories (Pull 2002).

Longitudinal studies

Eugen Bleuler's observations in 1911 led to the demise of the diagnosis 'dementia praecox'. He introduced the term 'schizophrenia' to correct Kraepelin's erroneous assumption about the unfavourable course of these conditions. As a result, the notion of 'dementia praecox' as an inherently deteriorating and progressive illness was rather short lived and landed on the rubbish-heap of history more than a century ago. The new term 'schizophrenia' was associated with variations in course and outcome right from the outset.

It is important to realize that longitudinal studies of schizophrenia extended over many years and across periods of time when different forms of treatment were practised. Some of these studies began before the introduction of antipsychotic medication, and most of them preceded the movement of de-institutionalization in the USA and Europe, occurring at a time when people with the diagnosis of schizophrenia were liable to spend years, even decades, in psychiatric institutions far from their communities.

One of Kraepelin's misguided assumptions about the unified concept of a 'dementing' illness with an invariably deteriorating course, was based on the observation of individuals who were part of 'the great majority of asylum inmates; they share the experience of having their unique mental character destroyed and their wholesale exclusion from the spiritual community and their environment' (Kraepelin 1904, in Häfner 2005, p6, translation by the authors). This means that Kraepelin did not observe the natural course or the response of this condition to treatment according to current criteria. Instead, he observed phenomena related to social exclusion and institutionalism.

A possible explanation of why Kraepelin's negative assumptions have persisted this long might be two-fold: namely, that people diagnosed with schizophrenia continued to be institutionalized well beyond his lifetime, and the fact that many outcome studies included mostly subjects with histories of prolonged hospitalization. This opinion is shared by Häfner in his thorough examination of longitudinal studies, regarding their original hypothesis about the unfavourable prognosis of schizophrenia (ibid., p 149, translation by the authors): 'Descriptions pertaining to the medium-term course of this illness already made clear that the wholesale pessimistic prognosis regarding the entirety of the condition and its outcome had lost its significance.' Furthermore, he adds that today's more favourable view of prognosis is also related to changes in treatment and the living circumstances of patients.

Important studies pertaining to the very long-term course of schizophrenia have been carried out by: Manfred Bleuler at the Burghölzli-Hospital in Zürich (1978); Ciompi and Müller in Lausanne (Ciompi 1980); Huber in Bonn (Huber *et al.* 1975); Cortenay Harding and Michael de Sisto in Vermont and by the same authors when they compared the states of Vermont and Maine (1987a, 1987b, 1995), and by Hinterhuber in Austria (1973). The follow-up periods in these studies extend over an average of 20 years and in some cases up to 65 years. Such studies are monumentally difficult undertakings and pose major methodological problems for the researchers themselves as well as for anyone wanting to conduct and interpret a meta-analysis of the findings. Considering the studies and their various contexts it is fair to say that one third of outcomes were clearly positive while one third of the outcomes were unfavourable. The remaining third of the populations studied could not be assigned to either of the other two fairly clear-cut course patterns. If we examine the data to determine the percentage of individuals who after many years no longer have symptoms, nor take psychotropic medication and who are, at the most, limited in one of several functional domains, i.e. working, housing and social life, we find recovery rates between 53 and 68% (Davidson, Harding, Spaniol, 2005). A recent population-based study (Rabinowitz *et al.* 2007) enriches the field in two ways. Not only did the researchers find a course of progressive amelioration for most people who had been diagnosed with schizophrenia at the time of hospitalization – with only a small minority of observations of courses of illness marked by deterioration – they also found support for the hypothesis that a small sub-group of patients with high readmission rates is responsible for research findings and clinical impressions which wrongly assume a deteriorating course of illness.

The large WHO study that followed nearly 1400 patients for up to 25 years in ten countries found significant differences between the participating centres (Hopper, Harrison, Janca, Sartorius 2007). Overall, more than half of the subjects were considered to have improved. Nearly half no longer had any psychotic symptoms. In this study, the most accurate prediction about the outcome of the condition after 25 years was derived from its course during the first two years. This is an important finding because it explains why initial forms of support have such an immense significance.

The interpretation of data about course and outcome is not simple. This is particularly true of any influencing factors. Even the impact of treatment variables is difficult to assess. Today we tend to assume that antipsychotic medication has an important role, but there are data that cast serious doubt on some of the favourable effects that are taken for granted, especially over the long term (Warner 2004). We know that many chronic developments result from social situations, in which people live and receive treatment. It is not clinical variables, but the level of social development at the onset and social life during and along with the condition which have a significant influence on course and outcome. Other factors such as economic conditions are also considered highly relevant (Warner 2004).

All this suggests that it is not symptoms that can inform prognostic considerations, but rather social circumstances that preceded the onset of the condition or resulted from it. These circumstances might be linked to early undetected signs of disturbance, but might also result from factors independent of any illness-related processes. Stigma and discrimination play a central role here. However, these circumstances might also be entirely unrelated to the individual affected, to reactions from the social environment and to the impact of other immediate social factors. The psychiatrist Richard Warner has addressed these issues more thoroughly than anyone else.

Richard Warner, from the University of Colorado at Boulder, was the first we know of to combine the words 'schizophrenia' and 'recovery' in a book title. The first edition of his important book, *Recovery from Schizophrenia. Psychiatry and Political Economy*, appeared in 1985 and it didn't just bring together those two terms, but also referred to the economy in its subtitle. This book is a milestone in the discourse about schizophrenia and is available in its 3rd edition, published in 2004.

Warner's point of departure was his desire to explore the 'natural' course of schizophrenia, i.e. the course prior to the introduction of antipsychotic medication. In dealing with this subject he realized that a number of fundamental and widely accepted assumptions about schizophrenia were simply not correct. Right at the start of his book, in his introduction, Warner points out that we have been too pessimistic concerning the 'natural' course of this condition, and too optimistic about the achievements of our treatment methods. From the very beginning he highlights the misery which characterizes the lives of many patients in the era of community psychiatry and draws our attention to the fact that the course and outcome of this condition in Western industrialized countries, where most money is spent on the treatment of schizophrenia, is no better than in developing countries.

Warner uses the perspectives of anthropologists, historians, economists and political scientists in order to understand how divergent economical and political conditions impact on the number of people diagnosed with 'schizophrenia'; on the way their lives tend to unfold; on what kind of treatments prevail, and on how environmental factors shape the course of the condition. His economic, theoretical approach permits an understanding of the way domestic and political economy impact on the condition of schizophrenia. This includes an evaluation of the kinds of factors that regulate life in communities, for example the labour-market and the distribution of labour; poverty; social class; the relationship between different sections of society, and family structures.

His analysis of over 100 follow-up studies of individuals diagnosed with schizophrenia have shown that the recovery rates for patients who were hospitalized after the introduction of antipsychotics are no better than for those who were admitted around the time of the Second World War or during the first two decades of the 20th century. This suggests that the course and outcome at the end of the 20th century was no better than at its beginning. Antipsychotic drugs have been used widely since 1955, but their introduction has had little effect on the longitudinal course of these conditions, nor on the rates of full recovery (around 20%) or social recovery (35–45%). His data demonstrate that de-institutionalization began before the use of antipsychotics and did contribute to an improvement in recovery-rates, which was not however, enhanced further by the subsequent introduction of neuroleptics. Warner's analyses instead show other relationships, for example between economic downturns and poor outcomes. This pertains especially to the Great Depression of the 1920s and 30s in the USA and the recession of the 1980s. Here too, there are strong correlations with recovery in terms of abatement of symptomatology and social rehabilitation.

The relatively low impact of medication on recovery rates is particularly surprising, since the effects of medication on acute psychosis and on the prevention of relapse are documented in many studies. How Warner arrived at this observation is particularly relevant to our interest in the prognosis of schizophrenia. First of all, Warner reviews studies about the effectiveness of antipsychotics that distinguish between patients with a good prognosis and those whose prognosis is expected to be less favourable. Where there was a good prognosis the social situation prior to being diagnosed was stable and positive, such social situations including individuals who had not had to confront symptoms at a relatively early age, and those who had not (yet) shown signs of chronicity. For individuals with a favourable prognosis (at least 20%), medication seems to have a deleterious rather than a helpful effect, in that it might well interfere with the spontaneous recovery-processes.

Warner considers the lack of awareness and consideration of rebound-phenomena as a further cause for the overly positive assessment of drug effectiveness. He also posits that the overemphasis on medication in the treatment of acute symptoms has led to a neglect of the necessary psychosocial interventions and rehabilitation in community settings. The widespread unavailability of evidence-based psychosocial interventions has led to the proliferation of 'revolving door' patients who keep being returned from the hospital to a completely untenable situation in the community. There, such a person is likely to encounter once again the kind of risk factors that frequently lead to relapse, which in turn prompts another course of medication for acute symptoms, before the person is again placed in the same high-risk environment where supports and rehabilitation are lacking. Warner is especially critical of the glaring absence of vocational integration, notwithstanding the availability of successful interventions in this area. It hardly does justice to Warner's book to say that it is full of highly relevant conceptual considerations, supported by an impressive array of data. This first-class scientific book reads like a detective story and offers reviews and insights that are extremely relevant.

Prognosis – 'from demoralizing pessimism to rational optimism'

Not long ago, I (MA) received a call from a Mrs G, who introduced herself as the grandmother of R. She told me that R had been a patient at the day hospital two years ago. I remembered him as a very young man who had had to interrupt his apprenticeship due to a psychotic episode, but who had recovered quickly and had been able to resume his training. Over the past few weeks, apparently, he had become rather ill once again and had withdrawn from contacts with everyone except his grandparents. His grandparents had not been involved during his first psychosis. Now his grandmother wanted to know how they could be helpful to him. R believed that he had special powers and spoke about experiences when he was able to kill 10,000 people with the snap of a finger and bring them back to life in the same manner. He saw himself at the epicentre of a massive world transformation, no longer went to work, wandered around the city all day long but visited his grandparents twice a day. There he ate, rested, and sometimes talked a bit about his highly responsible and burdensome duties. At other times he took a short nap on the sofa. With his grandparents' agreement, he refused professional help. His grandmother's question was: what can we do for him now?

I emphasized how important it was to insist on professional help for their grandson, and assured her that as grandparents they were already giving him essential support by providing him with predictability, nourishment, rest, positive attention, material back-up, and relaxation. All this meant little to her. Above all she wanted to know: what will happen next? How far will the situation deteriorate? Will there be a plateau at some point? These were the grandparents' most burning questions. Could they hope that the situation would stay as it was now? Or was a deterioration unavoidable, to a point where they could no longer manage? Only slowly did I understand that they had never considered that there was any alternative to the situation remaining as it was or getting worse.

I explained carefully that it was not possible to say anything for sure, but that the paramount goal of treatment would be to bring this phase of the illness to an end, and that we had good means towards helping her grandson to accomplish that. Quite possibly, I continued, this episode might cease on its own, but it would still be very important to support him therapeutically along the way, not least because there were strategies to help prevent further relapses.

Mrs G was surprised and impressed. She repeated the information slowly, making sure that she had understood everything. She said she had never before heard any of this. It was completely new to her that there were more than the two options she had considered: everything stays the way it is, or it gets much worse. It took a while for me to understand that they could not imagine another course of events. Even though I had often had this kind of experience with relatives and have thought much about it, I was once again struck by the way these assumptions play out in real-life situations.

It has always seemed to me that clinicians tend to misjudge the information and opinions prevalent in the general population. Most of the time we try not to sound too pessimistic. Many of us make a great effort to keep hope alive. And we are surprised by all the negative talk. Many of our patients have already learned, in psycho-education (information offered to people who live with a psychological disturbance), that a person can recover from schizophrenia, can live with it, and can learn how to manage the symptoms, and not to be ashamed about the condition. Nevertheless, we are still feared when we make a diagnosis of schizophrenia. Maybe we are afraid of it ourselves? Are patients misunderstanding us most of the time? We often pose these questions to ourselves, while at the same time wondering why it is so hard to convince the public about their misconceptions about our work and the treatments we offer.

The following eye-opening experience still bothers us. It is a story that clearly shows the obstacles we are facing when advocating for the concept of recovery from schizophrenia. In the summer of 2001 a popular TV game show host invited a colleague who had identified herself as a 'community psychiatrist', to say what she meant by that description. She replied that she worked in a community mental health service. To his next question, whether anyone could use the services there, she responded that 'anyone can come, but most don't do it on their own, they are brought in by family or by the police'. A bit put off, the host let the game begin. One of the first quiz questions was about the term for the phase of recovery after an illness (revolution, restitution, reminiscence or convalescence), which prompted the host to comment that this would be much too easy a question for a physician. Our colleague reassured him by asserting that such a thing rarely occurred in her field of psychiatry. It is hard to imagine how much money and planning would have to be invested to reach an audience as large as this one in such an effective manner. Her message was crystal clear: patients in community mental health services have to be forced to show up and there is no such thing as recovery from mental illnesses. Such performances give sad testimony to the fact that psychiatry contributes its share to the stigmatization of and discrimination against people with psychiatric conditions who are seeking help (cf. pp 38). And all this happens in flagrant contradiction of the scientific evidence.

There are hardly any studies considering prognosis and course of illness from the perspective of service users. Those few that do exist deal almost exclusively with individuals who fell ill a long time ago. Nevertheless, users clearly tend to maintain hope and promote positive developments (Holzinger *et al.* 2002). Relatives are more pessimistic and tend towards fatalistic resignation. This might be partly related to their worries about how their relatives might fare once their parents are no longer alive or able to support them. This can go as far as mothers feeling relief when their adult children die before them. Often we hear parents, and especially mothers, who attend support groups reporting that their adult children have threatened to take their life, once the parent(s) have passed on. This tragic situation shows once again, the problems caused by hopelessness and the lack of social support.

In re-asserting that a diagnosis of schizophrenia itself has no significance for its prognosis, we are still left with the question as to what might actually help us to make informed prognostic assessments. Besides common-sense rules of life, such as the fact that conditions which have prevailed for a long time are not likely to disappear over night, some more or less reliable prognostic criteria have emerged from research. The results of the follow-up of the significant ABC (Age, Beginning and Course of Schizophrenia) study sample (Häfner 2005) are quite exciting in this regard. The study followed more than 100 patients over 12 years and interviewed them about their experiences before the onset of illness.

Once again it was clearly demonstrated that schizophrenia is not a gradually progressing condition, but one whose course usually results in the emergence of a relatively stable plateau over the middle- or long-range, even for patients who continue to show symptoms and deficits. However, 44% of the study-subjects had no symptoms or cognitive and social deficits at the final data point. Overall, it became apparent that the most active phase, with the most pronounced social problems, occurred at the onset of mental health problems. Unfortunately, these often appear long before treatment begins. This period of time, the extent of prior social disadvantages, the degree of symptoms and liabilities, and the consequences of these in the social sphere are determining factors for the subsequent course of the condition. As has been said before: 'Bad outcome is not a necessary component of the natural history of schizophrenia; it is a consequence of the interaction between the individual and his or her social and economic world' (Warner 2007). And it is this interaction that needs to be influenced at different levels in order to improve the course of psychotic disorders within the schizophrenia spectrum; there is a lot that can be done. You do not need to know the future in order to influence it.

As 'prognoses are difficult especially when they concern the future' (Nils Bohr) it is wise to understand that 'it is not our job to pass judgment on who will and will not recover from mental illness and the spirit breaking effects of poverty, stigma, dehumanization, degradation and learned helplessness. Rather, our job is to participate in a conspiracy of hope. It is our job to form a community of hope which surrounds people with psychiatric disabilities. It is our job to create rehabilitation environments that are charged with opportunities for self-improvement. It is our job to nurture our staff in their special vocations of hope. It is our job to ask people with psychiatric disabilities what it is they want and need in order to grow and then to provide them with good soil in which a new life can secure its roots and grow. And then, finally, it is our job to wait patiently, to sit with, to watch with wonder, and to witness with reverence the unfolding of another person's life.' (Deegan, 1996)

Diagnosis – 'a century is enough'

'Someone as healthy as you must have been misdiagnosed before.'

This is not a rare comment for user activists to hear. What is being insinuated is that anyone who is capable of working successfully in the user movement and giving brilliant speeches, could not possibly claim to have been diagnosed with schizophrenia. This is an exact replica of Kraepelin's opinion that those who recover could not have been 'schizophrenic' in the first place. 'This person doesn't have schizophrenia at all, he/she is just trying to show off.' Such statements can still be heard today, even from psychiatrists who conduct research on discrimination against individuals diagnosed with schizophrenia. What people making such statements are trying to express, is hard to tell. It is obvious that the old Kraepelinian verdict is easily mobilized whenever a person or a movement is being discredited on the grounds that they justify their engagement with their own record of being diagnosed with schizophrenia and with their experience of psychosis. Those speakers from the user movement who display 'clear signs that they are schizophrenic' are the ones respected by traditional mental health professionals. Not infrequently, we are asked to recommend such individuals, who can then be invited to speak, without any qualms. Should it happen that such a speaker does not display anything that might be considered a symptom of a mental illness on the day of the event, the person who invited them might risk losing face for that very reason. This means that some individuals end up having to fight for their current or former diagnosis. On many occasions we have had to 'defend' friends and acquaintances from the user movement against colleagues, by pointing to the publications which describe their experiences with mental health problems, diagnoses and treatments. Such controversies are not that rare and show quite clearly that in the eyes of many experts intelligence, success and public appearances without obvious symptoms or deficiencies are not compatible with a diagnosis of schizophrenia.

In most parts of the world diagnoses are made according to WHO classifications. The diagnostic criteria are codified in the current edition of the ICD (International Classification of Diseases) – ICD-10. They are regularly brought up to date and adapted to meet the most recent scientific standards. In psychiatry, the DSM (Diagnostic and Statistical Manual) of the American Psychiatric Association, now in its fourth edition (American Psychiatric Association 2000), is internationally highly relevant for research and of course in the USA for clinical and reimbursement purposes.

The diagnosis of schizophrenia is made, like other disorders, on the basis of a combination of symptoms and deficits of a certain intensity that must be present for a certain period of time. Ruling out certain other diagnoses is also fundamentally important. Classic criticism of this approach – 'a convention of unknown validity' (Parnas 2002) – concerns the disregard of aetiological considerations, the lack of biological markers, and accepting the same diagnosis for conditions with widely varying courses and outcomes. For schizophrenia it has been suggested that a variety of conditions might be currently subsumed under the diagnosis of schizophrenia. However, up to now all efforts to resolve this frustrating situation by assigning different diagnoses according to different types of courses, thus taking apart the diagnosis of schizophrenia, have been unsuccessful.

Prognostic issues are rarely addressed in these diagnostic systems. As far as schizophrenia is concerned, we must take note of the differences between the two most prevalent diagnostic systems, the ICD-10 and the DSM-IV, and in particular of the minimum duration required which, according to the DSM-IV is six months, and according to the ICD-10, only one month. In addition to its shorter duration requirement, the ICD states explicitly that the diagnosis has no prognostic significance and that it makes no sense to assume anything about the duration of the illness or its chronicity on the basis of this diagnosis. The DSM-IV, which only permits a diagnosis of schizophrenia for individuals who have been ill already for over six months, has a few things to say about this subject. For example, concerning 'paranoid schizophrenia' it cites evidence suggesting 'that the prognosis for the Paranoid Type may be considerably better than for the other types of Schizophrenia'. Concerning the so-called residual type, DSM-IV suggests that this can either be an ongoing state or 'may be time limited and represent a transition between a full-blown episode and complete remission' (DSM-IV-TR, www.psychiatryonline.org 05.05.08). Reading this, one has to wish that patients as well as everybody working in and acquainted with the mental health field would realize that the residual syndrome, which used to be called a 'defect state' and was treated and experienced as an irreversible deficit, could actually be a transition towards full remission.

Charles Pull's comprehensive review of the diagnosis of schizophrenia, with its fascinating commentaries, in the schizophrenia volume of the WPA's series, *Evidence and Experience in Psychiatry* (Maj and Sartorius 2002) describes a very challenging situation, in which Tim Crow argues for a negative answer to his question: 'Should schizophrenia as a disease entity concept survive into the third millennium?' In the same context Jane Kelly and Robin Murray clearly state that 'A century of schizophrenia is enough'. The term 'schizophrenia' is described as 'misleading' and 'stultifying' for a variety of different reasons by different international experts.

Important discussions about the diagnosis of schizophrenia concern the urgent need to complement the categorical with a dimensional approach (Allardyce J *et al.* 2007). Changing towards a dimensional perspective in order to undermine the stigma of mental illness that is often exacerbated by clinical diagnosis, is also one of the essential remedies suggested by Corrigan (2007). Another essential strategy which Corrigan suggests against the 'structural' stigma of diagnosis in the mental health field, is to provide contact between clinicians and trainees, and people with recovery experiences, and to replace the 'assumptions of poor prognosis with the models of recovery' (Corrigan 2007, p 36). In this regard it is also hoped that users of services and carers would be involved in the processes leading up to the next editions of the diagnostic manuals (Sadler and Fulford 2004).

Scientific and clinical responsibility

One of the first calls to the Birmingham (UK) Home Treatment Team in 2001 that Michaela Amering had joined, came with the following back-story: a general practitioner had visited a family, having been summoned by the mother of an adult son who exhibited signs of a psychotic episode. The young man had been stable and employed for many years, while being monitored by the family doctor. A few weeks earlier, on his 40th birthday, he had decided to stop taking his medication, with the goal of spending the rest of his life without psychiatric drugs. In the following weeks he quit his job, retreated completely, slept little, and sat up in his room day and night writing incessantly. He hardly ate, spoke in a confused manner, and was terrified of being re-admitted to the psychiatric hospital. When we arrived at the house, the mother told us all this; she seemed rather upset and was frightened that an inpatient stay might ensue. There had been a loud dispute between mother and son that day.

She was not afraid of him, since there had never been a physical confrontation, but everything was now just like it had been during his last psychotic episode, many years ago, when he had ended up in hospital. Roger, the team leader, was familiar with the son from that time. First, the two of them exchanged words through the closed door of John's room, but then John emerged. They had told him that the doctor was new, but quite nice. This didn't matter to him. He didn't want to go to the hospital. He was not psychotic, and as long as he kept a meticulous record of everything, it would turn out all right. That was why he could not sleep and had no time to talk to us, or to deal with psychiatry, because he was in a hurry to write everything down.

John was clearly exhausted and could barely keep his thoughts in order but he wanted to make a good impression on me, the new doctor. He would only speak to us when the mother was out of the room. There was no risk to himself nor to others, but even though he desperately needed help, he didn't want it from us. He did not even want something to help him sleep. He conceded that he had to eat, but said that running into his mother at mealtimes stressed him out, and that was why he had not left his room.

We reassured him that hospitalization was not our goal, and that the team was committed to avoiding admissions whenever possible. We agreed on the following plan: over the next few days Roger would call on John and his mother twice a day to see how things were going. The next day, Roger and John would have lunch at a nearby pub. Roger would keep offering John an evening dose of the medication that I recommended, even though John was set against it. It seemed it might be possible for John to take a break from his work for a night. I reiterated my offer of discussing alternatives to a sudden withdrawal from medication, and I expressed the hope that I would have a chance to speak about this to Roger and John in the coming week.

They would let me know, if and when they were ready for such a conversation. John realized that his mother was worrying a lot and needed support herself. We reassured them both that she could call us any time, if she felt that things were not going well.

A crisis team is ideal for such interventions. Over the next few days, John began to trust Roger and slept well for two nights, with the help of medication. In discussion with him we agreed to a switch from his old medication and planned to consider a gradual reduction in the future.

John now understood the risk of sudden discontinuation, after taking medication regularly for such a long time. But we understood something as well: John had remembered that someone told him at the onset of his condition that he would have to take this medication for up to 20 years. Those 20 years had been up on his 40th birthday, and he assumed that this would be the right moment for discontinuing the medication. Could this be possible? Did someone actually give him this information in 1980 when he was first hospitalized for a psychotic episode?

People familiar with psychiatry would have a good idea as to what might have happened. The doctor who saw John initially gave him a diagnosis of schizophrenia. He believed that schizophrenia was a chronic condition. He assumed that as a consequence of this diagnosis, life-long medication would be indicated to protect the patient from relapses. He might even have felt some degree of optimism in saying: if you stick to this regime, to this medication, you might be able to lead a relatively healthy life. But what about those 20 years? It might have been awkward for a psychiatrist to tell a 20-year-old man that he would have to take medication for the rest of his life. Such news might have been too much for the family and the patient to bear. It would have been a rather drastic pronouncement. Even 20 years seemed like a long time for a 20-year old, nearly a life-time. But still, it might have been easier to say, and easier to take.

No one could have predicted that John would proceed calmly and without difficulties to lead an orderly life as a bachelor, living in his parents' flat, to be a reliable worker in his profession, and an amateur athlete, while continuing to take his medication religiously. And certainly no one had thought that John would stop taking the medication suddenly, after 20 years, following his first doctor's recommendation. No one had mentioned discontinuing the medication in the interim. John had realized that psychiatry was not in the business of helping people withdraw, so he took it upon himself to do it, not realizing, or not wanting to realize, that this had made him psychotic.

Roger and I were pleased about the fact that John was back on his medication and that the psychosis was wearing off, enabling him to resume his work and leisure activities. We thought that once everything had settled down for a while, we could again take up the subject of discontinuation. What might be the best advice after 20 years on medication without relapse? What is known about the effects of discontinuation after 20 years? And especially: what do we know about the long-term course of psychotic disorders?

The schizophrenia volume of the WPA Series, *Evidence and Experience in Psychiatry*, concludes its chapter on course and outcome – 'a topic of considerable debate' - with the statement: 'On the whole, follow-up studies of the course of schizophrenia indicate that there may be very different types of courses, ranging from complete cure to severe disabling chronic forms. Some patients experience only one episode of illness, others have several episodes, and still others suffer from chronic symptoms.' (Pull 2002). Furthermore 'we continue to have no answer to the important question of which patients are or are not at risk for relapse' (Fleischhacker 2002) – a fact that must be accepted even if it is hard to bear for scientists as well as clinicians. There are many things that we do not know.

One probable result of this dearth of knowledge is the fact that many people obviously hold onto their assumptions about schizophrenia's unfavourable course, as a kind of 'fall-back position'. There are quite a few theories that try to explain why science has such a hard time dealing with uncertainty and with changes in basic assumptions. The fact is, that the idea that schizophrenia has a progressively deteriorating course, has proved to be rather stubborn and has prevailed for a very long time. Kraepelin still remains the standard against which all follow-up studies are measured, and his misconceptions are reflected in many statements made by schizophrenia-researchers, but those statements are hardly ever in agreement with him. All follow-up studies contradict Kraepelin's assumptions, while still quoting his work reverently.

Luc Ciompi was in the audience a few years ago when we gave a paper about recovery at a conference in Hamburg. Ciompi is the author of the famous Lausanne study (Ciompi 1980) about the course and outcome of schizophrenia. He is the founder of the 'Soteria-House' in Berne, Switzerland (Ciompi and Hoffmann 2004). He congratulated us on our presentation, but it had obviously irritated him quite a bit. It was hard for him to accept that 'recovery' was presented here as a newly emerging concept, while he had been talking and writing about it for over 30 years. Even though he understood the necessity of promoting recovery, it saddened and enraged him that the paradigm-shift with respect to the erroneous assumption of a poor prognosis had still not taken place.

One possible explanation for the halting acceptance of the fact that schizophrenic conditions can also have a favourable course and that long periods of suffering can be turned around, may be found in another story. As part of the First International Conference on Reducing Stigma and Discrimination because of Schizophrenia in Leipzig, Germany, in 2001, a symposium was held that featured some of the most important user activists speaking on behalf of recovery: Ron Coleman, Judi Chamberlin and Christian Horvath. They spoke impressively about their own histories of suffering and recovery, and also mentioned some biographies of others who were known to them from their work in self-help and advocacy services. It was a very moving presentation, capped by a great deal of applause. Heinz Häfner was the first to respond from the floor. He said, in so many words, that he found the presentation very impressive but would like to caution everyone not to underestimate the suffering associated with schizophrenia. He added that this condition can cause severe disabilities and drive people to suicide. I (MA) was struck dumb and found it completely incomprehensible that he would find it necessary to caution about the severity of schizophrenia the very people who had spent many years in hospitals, had survived and witnessed suicide attempts, and were connected to a circle of friends and colleagues who had experienced psychosis, But Häfner was quite serious. He wanted to express his concern that schizophrenia should never be underestimated.

The users and activists were not taken aback by his remark, and they responded patiently and with seriousness that they were most certainly aware about the suffering since they had experienced it themselves, but that it was equally important for them to showcase their successes, their health and their recoveries, since without hope they would never have achieved what they had. I will never forget this. And I believe this to be one of the fundamental questions about our position towards the long-term course of schizophrenia. Is the glass half full or half empty? Which danger is greater? To become overly hopeful and underestimate the severity of the condition, or take the risk involved with promoting hopelessness? Do we believe that hopefulness has a significant impact on the actual course and therefore must never be relinquished, as the recovery-movement demands? Or do we believe that the risk of promoting excessive hope is too great, and that it should therefore not be raised?

These questions must to some extent be decided by each person for themselves. But the task of researchers and physicians is to present the knowledge that does exist in such a manner that people can make autonomous decisions. We should not always 'play it safe' by simply accepting the age-old proposition of an unfavourable course and communicate this to our patients, who would then in turn also stay on the safe side and clear of any unrealistic expectations. Do we really want them to adapt to lifelong disability rather than consider whether they can actually do something to promote their healing or recovery? Once again, we must all be clear about the fact that we have precious little certainty about the long-term prognosis of schizophrenia. But we do know that the course and outcome can vary considerably – from a one-time psychotic episode to a life with varying degrees of disability.

We must be clear about that and acknowledge that our own attitude has an impact on the way we interpret outcome data that do not allow simple conclusions. Probabilities are interpreted differently by different people. For example, there is the opinion that anyone who refrains from playing the lottery has already won, since the chances of actually winning are so slim, one might as well hold onto one's money. However, many people do enjoy this small chance and don't mind paying a small fee for it. How complicated is the decision required of a patient when a doctor says that there is a 20% chance of recovery without medication, but a 20% chance of relapse even with medication? What does it mean to stay on the safe side, given this information? How realistic is it to assume that one would be among the 'fortunate' 20%? These are highly personal decisions which we cannot make for patients. But we are obligated to be familiar with the scientific data and their possible interpretations. Our ability to understand the limits of statistical analyses and their applicability to individual cases is crucial. We must engage in a careful assessment of the data with respect to the evidence, circumstances and causes of recovery. It is our duty to make the existing knowledge and lack thereof, as well as the many different ways of interpreting it, accessible to everyone. We must carefully reflect the fact that hope is crucially important to people who know and speak about recovery. And we must consider what we are doing to promote hope or to shatter it – with intent, but also inadvertently.

In his article '*From demoralizing pessimism to rational optimism*' Knuf (2004) emphasizes the negative impact of viewing patients as 'chronic' and describes how such an opinion can undermine hope and motivation on the part of patients and providers alike. He asserts that we should not leave patients alone in their active attempts to overcome the illness and to develop a sensible outlook. He demands that we should obtain more knowledge about the ways in which recovery-processes occur, and how we might promote these, rather than stand in their way. This means, among other things, that we need to understand the importance of hope and how it can be preserved.

Knuf formulates strong warnings against issuing a negative prognosis for individuals, an occurrence that patients still experience quite frequently, and which can have a traumatizing impact for long periods of time. His reference to people who are given a diagnosis of borderline personality disorder is particularly important, since they are especially affected by therapeutic and prognostic nihilism.

His explanations as to why service providers might be inclined to hold onto pessimistic attitudes are also quite illuminating. Anyone familiar with the psychosocial field knows about the problem of raising false hopes. Most consider this as rather risky, and believe that disappointments should be avoided at all cost. Offering the prospect of health might sometimes encourage patients to discontinue their medication. According to Knuf, this could lead to situations where negative prognostication is used to ensure compliance. Wisely, he points to the dangers of such interventions and warns about the trap of confrontation leading to denial, when a negative prognosis and the associated fears lead straightaway to a denial of illness, resignation and abandonment of compliance. Therefore, Knuf emphasizes those aspects of recovery that demonstrate how even in cases of persistent disorders, their negative effects can be surmounted and a satisfying life of fairly high quality and meaningful perspectives can be attained.

Knuf's description of an acquaintance who was confronted with her premature newborn's fight for survival in a specialty clinic impressed us a great deal. Reports and photographs of successful treatments and healthy children were of great help to her as a source of courage and hope. His question, how such an atmosphere could be promoted in psychiatric facilities, remains, in our opinion, a key issue for the future of psychiatry.

CLASSIC DIMENSIONS OF MADNESS

Insight

Doctors in all medical specialties would wish their patients to accept the models of illness they are offering. The fact that this usually occurs only to a certain extent, is demonstrated by low compliance rates and a huge and growing market for alternatives to modern medicine. Clearly, most people use medicine according to their own cost-benefit analyses. In addition they use complementary interventions, seek spiritual guidance, and 'knock on wood'. Most people have rather subjective views about the causes, meaning and prognoses of their illnesses.

The way someone thinks about certain symptoms can make the difference between life and death – for example whether a 50-year-old woman considers the pain in her left arm and her anxiety as precursors of a heart attack, or believes they should be played down rather than given medical attention. Often it can take a very long time for patients suffering from panic attacks to realize that their problem might be helped by psychiatric treatment. Instead, they pursue inappropriate and even damaging somatic interventions, a behaviour which markedly aggravates the morbidity associated with such problems. Empirical data show that blaming yourself for an illness can have positive effects on coping with paraplegia, whereas this is not the case for people diagnosed with breast cancer (Wüstner 2001).

There is a long tradition of research about the subjective explanatory models that patients have of their illnesses and how these models might impact on the treatment and outcome of various conditions. It deals with theoretical concepts about illnesses that are constructed from ideas or beliefs of individuals based on their experiences and values. Such research also investigates beliefs about causes and their meanings, and about outcomes and the amenability of various conditions to interventions. People develop such beliefs usually before they become involved in treatment and these continue to evolve subsequently. The explanatory and treatment models of mainstream medicine play a variable role in peoples' quest for the optimal intervention. Some people place their full trust in the medical system, while others rely on alternative forms of help, or on their own capacities and treatment ideas. There are many variables that can help us to understand why people favour certain explanations for their illnesses, and whether, for instance, they blame themselves, the environment or fate. Personality and experience play important roles, as does the level of education, the family environment, cultural norms and much else. On the one hand, such theories are themselves a kind of coping mechanism, but they also determine which coping strategies might be favoured over others. Adding further complexity to this field is the fact that subjective theories about illnesses are not stable over time, but adapt and respond to a variety of situations (McCabe and Priebe 2004).

With regard to concepts of illness in psychiatry it is important to remember the multiplicity of concepts that is being offered in integrated services. Ingeborg Schürmann (1997) lays out the following elements of different 'service cultures' that are found in varying degrees and combinations within psychiatric services:

- a culture of caretaking, characterized by well-intentioned help and patronization, along with a curtailment of patients' autonomy;

- a culture of treatment, relying on experts and expecting 'compliance' from patients, wherein psychotherapeutic and bio-medical treatment arise from different, and often mutually contradicting, explanatory models;
- a culture of pedagogy that uses educational methods to achieve normative goals in a friendly and structured manner;
- a culture of empowerment that favours a transfer of power from the experts to the services-users, thereby creating a more level playing-field, and which aims to secure resources and environments that are conducive to the autonomous development of service-users.

Service users are likely to experience a variety of different treatment concepts within these service cultures, in varying degrees of admixture.

Studies of interdisciplinary teams have shown that team members use rather divergent models in order to gain understanding of their clients' situations. Members of different professional disciplines as well as individuals within one of these groups embrace a variety of different models – such as systemic approaches versus bio-medical – to different degrees (Colombo *et al.* 2003). The same holds true for relatives and consumers. Nowadays, helpers and consumers of services are supposed to collaborate within the predominant bio-psycho-social, vulnerability-stress-coping model, and are expected to be capable of regularly arriving at shared interpretations that guide their interventions.

It is also known that patients – and most likely professional helpers as well – may hold quite contradictory opinions, e.g. medical and astrological approaches, concerning the same set of facts. Such opinions can be switched rather quickly, for instance from the conviction that the person bears no responsibility for an illness to the notion that it has been caused by one's own sinful behaviour. Williams and Healy (2001) have proposed, after intensive study of various explanatory models held by depressed patients, that we speak instead about 'exploratory maps'. They believe this would better illustrate the flexibility and multitude of explorations undertaken by patients in order to arrive at an understanding of their problems.

Subjective explanatory models can have an impact on the course of psychiatric disorders and the resulting disabilities. The idea, for instance, that a person can have no control over symptoms whatsoever, does not bode well in terms of future coping. In order to achieve an effective therapeutic alliance it is essential to gain information about the operant explanatory models of clients. Discrepancies between clinicians and patients must be acknowledged and discussed, and, if possible, reconciled.

In summary we can say that psychiatric patients – not unlike the general population – tend to favour psychosocial explanatory models for psychiatric conditions. In Germany, little has changed over recent years with regard to the fact that only few patients assume that biological causes might be responsible for schizophrenia. The same is true for relatives (Holzinger *et al.* 2003). An interesting distinction between the western and eastern parts of Germany appeared in this data set, with the former showing a greater tendency to look for causes within the immediate family, while the latter saw broader societal factors as more relevant. Transcultural differences and similarities of explanatory models in psychiatry are important and have recently been receiving greater attention (Bhui *et al.* 2006).

Most theories about subjective concepts of illness are characterized by the idea that one person behaves in a particular way towards an illness. In psychiatric conditions, where what constitutes the person can appear affected as well in the course of illness, the situation is a bit more complicated. In the case of the panic attacks mentioned earlier, the fact that a certain situation is misinterpreted, is the core of the condition. 'Lack of insight' is often listed as the most common symptom of schizophrenia (www.netdoctor.co.uk/diseases/facts/schizophrenia.htm 05.05.2008), just as 'loss of insight' appears on lists of symptoms of illness (for example, www.mentalhealthcare. org.uk, 05.05.2008). Due to the nature of a condition with frequent distortions of perception, such as hallucinations and delusions, it should not be surprising that some symptoms of psychosis might make it more difficult to gain insight. However, to consider a 'lack of insight' an actual symptom of the disorder, after everything that is known about the complexity of subjective illness concepts, seems to be going too far. The commonality of this ascription might also be due to the notion that anything other than a concept of illness based on a medical model is seen as evidence of lacking insight. Modern research about insight differentiates between a situation when a person fails to realize that there is anything wrong, and the fact that people have their own ideas, including 'incorrect' ones, about the nature and cause of a disorder (Bentall 2003).

Intensive research has been done on the potential consequences of insight in psychosis. Clinical experience and some data support the idea that insight has a positive effect on course of illness and quality of life. However, there are some studies that contradict these findings, suggesting that insight might be associated with depression and a worsening of quality of life and social relationships (Hasson-Ohayon *et al.* 2006). We can only hope that we will soon gain a better understanding of the necessarily complex connections between the cost and benefit of insight concerning diagnoses such as schizophrenia. It is clear that a simple 'denial' of psychiatric problems and illnesses cannot be the key to solving this problem. Developing insight apparently also involves risks, with the timing of insight formation being of particular importance in positive and potentially problematic ways. It is certainly alarming, for example, that a connection has been established between early insight, depression and suicide attempts (Crumlish *et al.* 2005). In a study which tested labelling and psychotherapeutic theories, Warner *et al.* (1989) found that the locus of control could be one clue as to which circumstances can make acceptance of illness an asset in regard to self-esteem and functioning. They suggest that treatment efforts 'should be directed just as stringently towards this goal as they are towards encouraging the patient to accept their diagnosis' (Warner *et al.* 1989, p 407). Pushing for 'insight' or 'acceptance of diagnosis' has the potential to simply and dangerously 'add insight to injury' (McGorry 1992) if the complexities of the individual situation, context and needs are not taken into careful account.

Furthermore, realizing that one might need help is certainly not tied to having 'insight into an illness'. More often, patients turn to mental health services at a time when these services consider them to be lacking insight. One powerful assumption that informs psychiatric practice is that if people had better insight into their conditions, they would stick more faithfully to treatment recommendations. Reality shows that this is not necessarily so. Many people who hang on to their own explanations for an illness might still follow the doctors' instructions. On the other hand, even if people adhere to a medical model of an illness, they might still not comply with doctors' orders and, for example, discontinue their medication repeatedly. Finally, nothing supports the notion that psychiatric patients should be more 'rational', insightful or compliant than individuals dealing with physical health conditions, such as high blood pressure.

Compliance

The term 'compliance' suggests 'faith in treatment' and has been widely used in the international literature. The use of the term in non-medical areas is strongly influenced by its meaning in the sense of being held to an obligation. For this reason, there have been a number of attempts to replace the term compliance with others, in the hope of supporting patients' development towards autonomy to the point where they become 'experts on their own condition'. The term 'treatment adherence' was proposed as one alternative, but seems to evoke similar associations. In 1997 the Royal Pharmaceutical Society of Great Britain decided to replace compliance with the term 'concordance' (Sayce 2000).

In addressing this rather complicated subject we opted for staying with the most commonly used terms – compliance and non-compliance – while acknowledging the controversy that surrounds them. Focusing on compliance with pharmacological therapies, it can be clearly stated that it is rather low. At least one third of all patients can be considered as non-compliant or only partially so. Studies of people diagnosed with schizophrenia show no significant differences from studies of patients with hypertension, asthma or epilepsy: in both sets of studies there is a mean non-compliance rate of 50% and great variation, between 24% and 88% (Puschner *et al.* 2005). Interventions to improve compliance have been around for many years, with psycho-education being the most popular method. However, cognitive-behavioural approaches and Motivational Interviewing are getting increasing attention. Studies looking at interventions have been conducted in the areas of depression, anxiety disorders, addiction, eating disorders, bipolar disorder and schizophrenia. Such studies have also been carried out on traumatic experiences and post-traumatic problems.

There is some evidence as to the effectiveness of psycho-education and other measures of enhancing compliance in individuals diagnosed with bipolar disorders (Vieta 2005). However, most available information is about enhancing compliance among people with a diagnosis of schizophrenia. Generally speaking, these are psycho-educational group-based programmes based on the assumption that obtaining additional information will enhance compliance. It appears that conveying information is indeed the most appreciated element. Also, the need for information is one which patients are entitled to have met. Detailed information about medication is often new to patients and quite well received. Exchanging information with others who have had similar experiences is considered helpful and may lead to important new realizations, manifested by statements such as: 'It's great to meet other young people who are quite normal and who have experienced psychosis'. Common prejudices, such as 'mentally ill people spend all their time in bed' can be eliminated. According to participants, an important factor in explaining the effects of the Viennese programme, 'Knowing-Enjoying-Better Living' (Amering *et al.* 2002b), which offers a curriculum consisting in part of standard psycho-educational topics, was related to the atmosphere in the group, i.e. whether the group members related well to each other. Major cognitive impairments were experienced as rather troubling within a person and in relation to others. It appears that the timing of the intervention was crucial, i.e. participants found it sensible to enroll in such a programme during times of relative stability, in other words not during a crisis or a hospitalization. The fact that the moderators were open and willing to share some of their own personal experiences and opinions was much appreciated. Participants expressed a desire for more information regarding psychosocial interventions and more group activities, such as outings, etc.

Our programme in Vienna aimed to enhance quality of life and knowledge about the illness. This was achieved in many cases. Many participants developed a greater acceptance of medication, an awareness of their specific susceptibilities, as a greater sense of having control over their lives and a reduction of their symptoms. One year later, these changes were still noticeable, independently of any participation in any additional group sessions (Sibitz *et al.* 2006). In general it can be said that psycho-education for individuals with a diagnosis of schizophrenia usually leads to clinical improvement and greater knowledge about the condition, whereas its impact on compliance remains moderate or uncertain. For an intervention to have an impact on compliance it must actually be able to transform attitudes and motivation (Zygmunt *et al.* 2002). Advice and suggestions about how to develop structure and reliably take medication seem effective as well. Obviously, this would only be the case for people who have decided to take their medication regularly, but who are affected by disorganization and forgetfulness.

We know that psychiatrists themselves show little compliance with guidelines in their practice. In recent years, this has improved but is still far from 'good compliance' (Leucht and Heres 2006). This is especially true in the treatment of psychoses, where we also know that psychiatrists and other mental health professionals would not necessarily rely on scientifically proven treatments should they themselves be affected. Only 35% of non-medical staff and 71% of psychiatrists state that they would take a neuroleptic should they be affected by a condition within the schizophrenia group. Twenty-three per cent of mental health professionals stated that they would not recommend antipsychotic medication for a relative (Rettenbacher *et al.* 2004). One third of psychiatric professionals report that they would refuse neuroleptics in an advance directive for the eventuality of an acute psychotic episode (Amering *et al.* 1999).

Compliance defined as unilateral obedience to medical orders remains a rather dubious therapeutic goal. It is about looking for consensus. Consensus can develop within a therapeutic relationship where the decision-making process is shared by patients and clinicians. Factors related to the patient, his/her condition and personality are just as important as the abilities, personality and experience of the doctors. Factors pertaining to the immediate environment, such as time, structure and the reliability of contacts have to be suitable. The whole process of shared decision-making is embedded in a particular culture of expected or actual dealings with each other and with health problems.

The fact that mental health professionals are experienced in maintaining therapeutic relationships in rather challenging situations represents a great opportunity for respecting divergent opinions and arriving at decisions that are acceptable to both parties. The science of shared decision-making, which is devoted to this subject, originated from somatic medicine. Medical sociologists, who have investigated the ways in which therapeutic decisions are made, and what may be required to keep the contact between patients and doctors meaningful, have provided us with a fair amount of data already. In recent years, mental health experts have followed this trend and have begun to publish conceptual papers, which have gradually been followed by scientific studies. Conceptually speaking, it is obvious that psychiatry should lend itself particularly well to shared decision-making. The role of expert in one's own cause, which is being propagated by health planners in several countries, is rather suitable for psychiatric conditions, because frequently they last for some time, and because there is an array of different treatment options (Hamann *et al.* 2003).

Also, the potential value and advantage of non-compliance is being considered and analyzed. Not unlike the discussion about the costs and benefits of 'insight', it is still not clear under which circumstances and for whom compliance or non-compliance might make sense. What matters is understanding and managing situations and therapeutic relationships in such a way that non-compliance can be understood as an expression of setting what may be necessary boundaries or as a manifestation of resilience (Deegan 2007). The psychologist Thomas Bock has addressed this subject extensively for a number of years. The fourth edition of his book (Bock 2006a), *Light-years – Psychoses without Psychiatry – The interpretation of illness and designs for living of individuals with untreated psychoses*, appeared in 2006 as well as *Self-definition and Psychosis. Non-compliance as a Chance* came (Bock 2006b). Unfortunately both books are only available in German.

Capacity

Questions of insight and compliance are especially important and sensitive in psychiatry, since it is charged, under certain circumstances, to intervene against a person's will. The question of capacity to consent to or refuse certain treatments plays a major role. A capacity to exert insight and judgment is required. This involves assessing whether a person is capable of assimilating certain information, evaluating its relevance, considering it judiciously and, based on all this, making a choice or an informed decision. In recent years the scientific basis for such capacity evaluations has become considerably more solid and transparent. Studies have shown that a sizable proportion of non-psychiatric inpatients also frequently lack these capacities. This has recently led to the intriguing possibility that one unified legal code might be capable of regulating all these situations. Currently, most countries have separate legislation that exclusively addresses involuntary treatment and/or admission within the psychiatric realm. Such a separate code would then be superfluous, and an important step towards equal treatment of psychiatric and non-psychiatric patients would have been taken ('Fusion of mental health and incapacity legislation', Dawson and Szmukler 2006).

Coercion

International studies have shown that less than 50% of individuals who are psychiatrically hospitalized for the first time, accept such treatment of their own free will, an experience that is frequently repeated in the course of a patient's career (Pescosolido *et al.* 1998). Openly coercive measures are part of psychiatric treatment worldwide. Most countries have special laws that regulate forced treatment and involuntary hospitalizations, while parallel regulations are established to safeguard patients' rights. There have been frequent concerns regarding the personal and societal impact of forced psychiatric treatment, which have led to the development of alternative interventions. On the one hand, such alternatives can avert or reduce the use of coercion in psychiatry, on the other hand they can limit the negative effects of coercion by employing the greatest possible extent of procedural justice, for example, through advance directives.

The frequency of involuntary hospital admissions ranges internationally from 1% to 50% (Riecher-Rössler, Rössler 1993), and among European countries from 3% to 30% (Dressing and Salize 2004) of all inpatient admissions. On top of the legal requirements, available services and their organization seem also to have an impact on the rate of involuntary admissions, and on the attitudes of the public and of mental health professionals. Most people who are involuntarily admitted fall within the diagnostic group of 'functional psychoses'. Individuals diagnosed with 'schizophrenia' are at greater risk for involuntary commitment. Additional risk factors are the severity of the condition, and being a younger, unemployed man (Riecher et al. 1991).

There are many studies addressing the question of how coercion is perceived and under what circumstances. Several instruments have been developed to help quantify and describe various aspects of coercion and its perception by patients. It is now known that the subjective perception of coercion frequently does not correspond with the formal legal statute that authorizes a coercive measure. In other words, patients are on the books as being treated voluntarily, but experience coercion subjectively, while others who are officially under involuntary procedures, experience little or no coercion. The extent of coercion perceived in a hospital depends not only on perceived threats but also on procedural justice (Monahan et al. 1996).

The so-called 'thank you theory' draws our attention to the fact that many patients who had originally refused to be admitted, and might even have resisted with physical force, change their opinion later to the point of expressing gratitude for the intervention. Several studies show that up to three-quarters of involuntarily admitted patients ultimately accept the treatment and, once discharged, agree that the commitment had been necessary. A large study has shown, similarly, that many patients changed their opinion regarding the necessity of hospitalization in the time period between their admission and four to eight weeks after discharge (Gardner et al. 1999). However, the subjective perception of coercion remained stable over time, and the attitude towards the hospitalization did not change either. Involuntarily admitted patients do not seem to be thankful for the experience in the hospital, even though they might report later that it had been necessary.

Kaltiala-Heino et al. (1997) identified a group of individuals who – irrespective of their legal status or the use of coercive measures – had subjectively felt coerced into the admission to hospital. They referred to them as the 'core group of true involuntary patients'. Compared to those patients who did not report any subjective experiences of coercion, these people felt consistently more negative about their treatment – about the hospitalization as well as their follow-up care – this was independent of their legal status. Interestingly, the authors suggest that for the group of patients who retrospectively accepted the treatment even though it had been forced on them, it should have been possible to convince them in the first place as they seem to have been in agreement with receiving treatment at some level. However, the 'group of true involuntary patients' did not benefit from their treatment, which leads us to ask the question whether it might be possible to find alternative ways of helping these individuals. The suggestions of these authors lead directly to the more complex and methodologically more difficult questions regarding the consequences of coercive measures. These questions don't lend themselves easily to scientific investigation. For example, an experimental design involving randomization, i.e. the random assignment to comparison groups, which is de rigeur in scientific studies, cannot ethically and legally be undertaken to address these type of questions.

The recent laws regulating outpatient commitment in the USA create a particularly interesting situation because due to their newness it is still possible to study random comparison groups in order to assess the effects of this particular coercive measure. Swartz *et al.* (2001) have shown that it is not merely the legal situation that enhances treatment compliance in outpatient settings, but that compliance is enhanced by better and more readily available services and by the administration of long-acting depot medication. This might indicate that it is not actually the legal commitment itself which enables patients to be treated better. Instead, it may well be the case that because of the legal context they are being cared for in a more intensive and consistent manner.

Such findings have led to situations in some states, where outpatient commitment is only permitted in counties that can demonstrate the availability of all treatment options known to be helpful. This enables the system to find out whether patients would refuse to use those treatment options voluntarily. Only if circumstances arise, in spite of all available voluntary options, which make it reasonable to resort to outpatient commitment, does an application for such services become permissible (Appelbaum 2003). This would mean that services had first to be improved, and to broaden what they could offer, before patients could be coerced by law to use them.

Trauma and coercion

It is generally assumed that psychosis in itself (for example, Shaw *et al.* 1997) as well as coercive measures in a psychiatric context, might have traumatic effects (for example, Riecher-Rössler, Rössler 1993). Laura Cohen (1994) describes the traumatic aftereffects of an involuntary commitment based on Judith Lewis Herman's (1997) work about the conceptualization of psychological trauma. Cohen also emphasized the traumatic effects of psychotic experiences themselves and considered the possible sequelae of retraumatization for individuals who not infrequently have been traumatized by physical and sexual abuse in their earlier years. Several more recent studies (for example, Read *et al.* 2001) have made it necessary to face the fact that a considerable proportion of patients with a diagnosis of 'psychosis' have experienced trauma in their lives – this is particularly pronounced in women (50%) – and that a far from negligible proportion of them also suffer from post-traumatic disturbances. In a study of involuntary commitment and post-traumatic disturbances of patients diagnosed with schizophrenia Priebe *at al*. (1998) found that patients who had experienced involuntary commitment in the past, report significantly more often about negative aspects of treatment, such as coercion; excessive noise; overcrowding and monotony within the institution; unfriendly, rigid and impersonal treatment, and a lack of empathy and support from professional helpers, than those who were never forcibly hospitalized. The two were not, however, different in terms of sociodemographic and clinical variables, in the degree of psychopathology and in their diagnosis of post-traumatic disturbances.

The review of Frueh *et al.* (2000) provides pointers that help distinguish between 'traumatic' and 'harmful' events. Events that occur within a psychiatric setting and lead to the typical symptoms of post-traumatic stress disorder (PTSD) should be considered as 'sanctuary trauma'. Other events that are stressful, anxiety-inducing, and humiliating, such as restraint, seclusion and encountering violent behaviour, should be considered 'sanctuary harm'. The authors of this study advocate a systematic investigation into the occurrence of such events. Such an investigation should include the prevalence, perception and consequences and prevention of coercive measures.

Open questions

Whether involuntary and voluntary treatment are equally effective, remains a burning question. So far, research has shown that far from all patients (33-81%) report after the fact, that legally enforced treatment had been helpful or necessary, compared to a substantial group that experienced it as harmful (Katsakou and Priebe 2006), despite evidence of clinical improvement.

Further urgent questions relate to the individuals who have been exposed to coercive measures: How do such measures influence the way they think about themselves, their self-assessment and self-esteem? How do they impact their attitudes towards the illness, and their explanatory models? What is the impact on their view of the available mental health services, and consequently, how do coercive measures influence treatment compliance. Are coercive measures affecting interpersonal relations, in particular with family members? How long are such influences likely to last? Are they relevant for perceived and actual stigma and discrimination?

Understanding the way involuntary treatment impacts on individual patients is an essential step towards conceptualizing and planning of further studies on the short- and long-term effects of coercive measures. Clinical experience and research findings have shown that short-term responses of patients range from relief to anxiety, defeat and humiliation. Attempts at capturing the ethical benefits and costs of coercive measures during short-term inpatient stays have shown that the subjective cost-benefit ratio impacts on the effectiveness of treatment (Kjellin *et al.* 1997). The association between perceived respect for autonomy and self-reported improvement in mental health was found for committed as well as for voluntary patients.

Reducing coercion

In recent years, situations involving physical restraint and seclusion in the context of psychiatric treatment have attracted considerable interest among researchers. The opinion has taken hold that efforts towards limiting such interventions are desirable and that considerable curtailment is possible. It was important to clarify that a reduction of physically coercive measures would not incur additional costs, as had been widely assumed (Lebel and Goldstein 2005). Also, the hypothesis that a reduction in physical coercion would lead to an increase in violent acts on psychiatric units has not held true. The essential ingredients of successful programmes to reduce physical coercion are improved documentation and enhanced transparency, collaboration with patient advocates and training curricula for staff focusing on de-escalation strategies (for example, Smith *et al.* 2005).

There are qualitative studies of the potential contribution of users of services towards the reduction of coercive measures by using alternatives such as advance directives (Amering *et al.* 2005) and towards curtailing physical coercion and its negative consequences (Robins *et al.* 2005). These studies point out that next to system-variables such as continuity of care and the quality of record-keeping, the actual way in which mental health staff communicate plays an important role.

Violence and mental illness

The greatest and most regrettable discrepancy remains between the popular assessments of how dangerous individuals with mental illness might be, and the factual reality of this situation (Angermeyer *et al*. 1998). The existing stereotype of dangerousness associated with mental illness in the general public (Phelan and Link 1998) in no way corresponds to the risk to which the public is exposed. Even those links that can be found between some forms of psychiatric disorders and violent acts are not usually of direct causal relevance. Factors other than the diagnosis show the greatest correlation with proneness towards violence and need to be understood in the context of a complex multidimensional system. Just as in the general population, personality factors are much more likely than illness-related variables to be associated with greater risk. Social neglect and dangerous behaviour in the past are as important as alcohol and substance abuse, which are in general the most important risk factors for delinquency.

Finally, the fact that individuals diagnosed as mentally ill are frequently victims of violent crimes, is also related to many factors that have little to do with the illness itself. Poverty, isolation, homelessness and substance use are again important risk-factors, which are only somewhat reduced by psychiatric treatment (Lovell *et al*. 2008). The common occurrence of violent trauma in the biography of psychiatric patients (Hanson *et al*. 2006) and their relevance for illness, treatment, and outcome, is far from sufficiently investigated and understood. There is still much to do before we can do justice to the role of violence in the lives of individuals who are receiving psychiatric treatment.

PSYCHIATRIC TREATMENT AND SERVICES

State of the art

While the great reforms in psychiatric services and treatment of the past decades are far from completed, community-based, integrated service models have by and large replaced the institutional psychiatry that had been dominant in earlier years, at least in the Western industrial nations. Psychiatric inpatient treatment increasingly takes place in general hospital units and is essentially restricted to the provision of crisis intervention over a few days or weeks. While the 1960s where still dominated by the aim of avoiding 'institutionalism', i.e. the negative consequences of long institutional stays, nowadays these concerns are confounded by economic considerations calling for ever shorter inpatient stays.

What form acute services should ideally take and what role hospital beds and their location might play, are questions that remain at the forefront of service planners' concerns. The day-hospital as a support service in acute situations is being looked at as a significant alternative to inpatient treatment, as are models of acute home treatment. Many areas in medicine are currently promoting the expansion of day-treatment services. The possibility of providing diagnostic and treatment services in collaboration with large medical centres underscores the expectation that day-treatment slots could be used for acute interventions and, depending on local situations, may actually replace inpatient beds. From a scientific perspective, the minimal number of hospital beds needed remains undetermined, as do questions about effectiveness, suitability and possible adverse effects of community-integrated acute interventions, and the 'dosage', i.e. the intensity of the required community-integrated services that are capable of preventing hospitalization.

The fact is, hospital stays take up only a tiny fraction of time in few patients' lives. Psychiatric treatment occurs essentially in the community. The type, mix, funding, organization and use of psychiatric services is rather variable from one area to another. Even within Europe, Australia and the USA – countries with comparatively well developed and equipped health care systems – there are marked regional differences.

Integrative treatment

It has become clear that state-of-the-art treatment must be integrative, working towards a concept of disorder using a combination of person-centred, phase-specific supports from the following domains:

- pharmacotherapy
- problem-specific psychotherapies
- rehabilitative services
- psycho-education
- social supports
- self-help
- working with significant others

Remarkable progress has been made in each of these areas over recent years. Treatment options have increased and improved, as have policies and operational and organizational structures. Many psychiatric problems call for complex interventions. This means that diverse methods and practitioners have to provide their input in a co-ordinated fashion. Psychiatrists, psychologists, nurses, social workers, occupational therapists, physiotherapists, lay helpers, and peer specialists need to work collaboratively in multidisciplinary teams. Multidisciplinary team-work poses new challenges to all professional disciplines. The task of developing the team and the larger service organization require adequate expertise. Division of labour and any specialization within teams need to be adapted to the requirements and contexts of local situations, thereby enabling the optimal application of different skills among team-members and, if necessary, adding new sources of expertise. Most community mental health teams are continually trying to determine the optimal relationship between 'generalists' and 'specialists', as well as the optimal delineation of boundaries within the team. Needless to say, there are differences between various countries and various local traditions, concerning professional formation and identities.

A person-centred approach in real life

Clearly there is a development away from an institutional basis of service delivery. Person-centred services are being widely propagated. In psychiatry, such services must be adapted to the needs of individual patients – and not the other way round. Frequently, the needs of relatives and other members of the immediate network also require consideration. Family and friends have needs of their own. Community mental health professionals work *in vivo*, for example by visiting a home, and meeting family members, friends, and neighbors, in order to use their resources and to meet their needs regarding information and contact with self-help and advocacy organizations.

Doing justice to the requirements of community-integrated services also means providing training at locations where the treatment primarily takes place – in the community. Community mental health workers must have the capacity to act in a mobile and flexible fashion and to become familiar with a variety of settings, such as outpatient clinics, emergency services, rehabilitation facilities and hospitals. They need to understand the legal basis of their activities as well as those of other professional groups within the multidisciplinary team in a variety of settings.

New demands are placed on the capacity of community mental health workers to assess risks, for instance, in connection with whether a person can still be treated in the community, whether they might benefit from a hospital or crisis centre stay, or when and under what circumstances a home visit might be appropriate. The new role of being a 'guest' in the home of the person receiving services must be practised in order to achieve an accommodation to the environment that fits best with diverse treatment needs. It is certainly clear that we are not always dealing with the patient alone, but often also we are dealing with other people who are present at the place where services are rendered, such as family members, friends, neighbours and volunteer helpers. In many locations, the responsibilities, competencies and legal underpinnings of services and individual providers are still rather poorly defined. Also, the correct balance between support, control and neglect of people receiving services remains an ongoing dilemma when operating in the community.

Participating in the world of employment continues to be an essential element in coping with everyday life and the risk of mental health crises. Services that support a person who wishes to enter or re-enter training or employment constitute an important step towards improving quality of life and preventing relapses, both from the perspective of service providers and patients themselves. Even healthy individuals experience the loss of a job or a training opportunity as a serious emotional set-back. Aside from constituting a direct threat to their livelihood, self-worth and confidence in their capacities are often compromised. Social networks and social integration – variables that are known to contribute substantially to a reduction of pathology and an enhancement of quality of life – are directly linked to the ability to maintain employment.

The exceedingly important role that work opportunities play in ensuring successful treatment, is contrasted by a sad reality. Frequent disruptions of education and high unemployment rates are aggravated by the fact that many young people are receiving disability pensions, which creates a rather disadvantageous social situation, even though such support is often the only possible way to ensure self-sufficiency in a case of a reduced work capacity. Several rehabilitation models have been sufficiently developed over recent years to the point where their influence on this unfortunate situation can now be the subject of research studies.

Regarding the question of 'train and place' versus 'place and train' (Burns *et al.* 2008), most recent data show that it might be more advantageous to identify and sustain employment and apprenticeship opportunities, and support individuals with particular disabilities in those positions, rather than them going through separate training programmes before they are placed in jobs. Of course this makes sense with respect to a reality-orientation within actual life contexts, but only works well when close co-operation exists between the clinical and the rehabilitative domains. Multidisciplinary teams can include specially trained vocational and educational counsellors. Their interventions are not just centred on the clients, but encompass the employment situation as a whole. Employers must be motivated to safeguard the job of a worker who may have fallen ill and, in general, to participate in vocational integration projects; fellow workers also need support in these kinds of situations. The success of social firms and affirmative businesses most likely relies, to a significant degree, on the development of a feeling of community (Warner 2004).

It is not at all surprising that person-centred approaches in life in general and work environments in particular, appear most promising for the vocational rehabilitation of people with severe mental disorders. However, the various options for vocational integration, for instance considering whether someone should aim for a job in the private sector, in the public sector or in a special needs setting, are rather dependent on the general status of local and national employment opportunities. Regulations concerning worker's rights (i.e. disability-related protections) and anti-discrimination laws are also important factors. The type of regulations that seem to emphasize the risk to one's livelihood presented by a trial period of work (i.e. that a person might be cut off from a disability pension without having secured permanent employment with adequate health benefits), or that lack flexibility when it comes to supporting part-time work and additional earnings, are experienced as rather unfavourable when it comes to considering employment. Not only do these unfortunate regulations reduce motivation, they might actually induce additional stress and fear for all concerned.

The collaboration between clinical disciplines and those working in the social sphere is of essential importance when it comes to finding out what kind of help is needed and how to best provide it. Ideally, here too, all participants should be part of a multidisciplinary team, which works in a flexible and easily responsive way across the boundaries between inpatient and community-based services.

Shortcomings

The primary aims of psychiatric reforms – closure of institutions, development of community-based services, integration of psychiatric services within the provision of general health care, and integration of social and medical services – have been accomplished to different degrees in Western European countries. Countries have achieved 30%-70% of the reform goals (Becker and Kilian 2006). Reform is not only about services. Becker and Vazquez-Barquero (2001) noted that most unmet needs were in the areas of access to employment opportunities, the integration of psychiatric and general medical services, and the support of relatives and friends.

For the USA, data show that fewer than 25% of all patients with severe mental illness receive the kind of treatments which correspond to evidence-based recommendations (Anthony *et al.* 2003). The causes of this state of affairs are varied. Many interventions whose benefits are already scientifically proven are barely available. Examples include psycho-educational groups and diagnosis-specific cognitive therapies that may be useful for the treatment of persistent psychotic symptoms such as delusions, voice-hearing, and cognitive dysfunctions. Many treatments are not widely known among practitioners, and few referrals are being made, for example, to self-help and advocacy groups for families and friends or to employment programmes for mental health service users. Frequently, an accurate assessment that is required as the basis of a person-centred integrative treatment plan cannot be completed because of time constraints. In many instances, there is simply a lack of the resources that are required to provide a complex set of supports and services. And in many parts of the world there is not only a lack of acknowledgement of both human rights and patients' rights but a lack of resources for mental health services, which are scarce, inequitable and inefficient (Saxena *et al.* 2007).

Even in rather well resourced areas, interventions based on the old established types of services are still predominant. We are still thinking in categories such as hospital, day treatment, residential facility, sheltered workshop, and expecting the patients to adapt to the available institutions, frequently one after the other. However, significant disadvantages become apparent when patients are asked to adapt to every change of service-needs. The required changes from one homogeneous 'intervention cubby-hole' to another should not be expected of individuals with a mental illness at every juncture of improvement or deterioration, without considering the risks. Besides, the working of many services is hampered by the fact that they are situated outside the person's living environment and therefore can have little direct impact on their social network.

If services are to be provided which are tailor-made for the individual and can be delivered over a longer period of time within the social environment, both the problem of the fragmentation of services, and that of funding, will have to be remedied. Ideally, models that offer an integrated approach, are financed by a composite budget which includes both social and health-related services, and which can be allocated flexibly according to the various needs. For example, investments in community-based services can offset the need for hospital beds, which in turn would make more funds available for non-hospital support. Also, such a funding strategy can ensure that sufficient beds remain available in each region, without compromising the resources in the community.

An orientation based on the actual and fluctuating needs of service users not only leads to a more encompassing planning effort with respect to services and funding sources, but also to an optimally efficient use of the resources provided by the various professional disciplines. One important consequence of engaging service users within their primary environment is the greater use and application of their own resources, and of the supports offered by their personal and work associates.

This is especially important because we have learned that any improvement in the quality of life of service users depends heavily on the way their social life develops. Only certain symptoms, such as depression and anxiety – independent from the diagnosis – have a tendency to diminish the quality of life. The number and quality of social contacts, however, have a much greater bearing on quality of life. Social interactions that stigmatize tend to have adverse effects. Self-esteem and trust in one's own capacities enhance quality of life. Thus it is not surprising that service programmes which provide little support in the areas of occupation and social connection have a rather unfavourable impact on quality of life (Hansson 2006).

Studies that look at whether certain areas of need are met or not show that unmet needs have the greatest adverse effect on quality of life (Wiersma 2006). In these situations, met needs in other areas do not seem to compensate for a specific unmet need as much as one would like. Therefore, it is crucial to continually assess what kinds of services are lacking in a particular region, but even more importantly, during a specific episode of treatment. It seems to us that a global estimate would probably reach the conclusion that a minimum of 25–50% of service users are being negatively affected by a lack of support in various essential domains.

It is not possible here to adequately address the widespread lack of financial resources that individuals with psychiatric disabilities frequently endure. Certainly, such deprivations should not be underestimated. Poverty is an additional burden for many people with mental health problems and must be one of the more cruel hindrances on the path towards recovery.

The neglect of physical health issues among individuals with psychiatric disabilities is another area of great concern. Its causes are manifold and include personal neglect, avoidance of help, and minimization of the expressed complaints by mental health professionals who are treating the person for depression or schizophrenia. The consequences are dramatic and are demonstrated by a significant reduction in life expectancy. It looks as if it would be more beneficial to integrate psychosocial and general medical services, (including, for example, routine monitoring via certain blood tests and other diagnostic examinations) and to promote greater collaboration with other medical specialists.

Support for individuals with mental health problems who have or desire to have children, is another area that is significantly underserved. Specialized services dealing with family planning, support throughout pregnancy and birth, and specific support for parents with psychiatric conditions have shown promising results, but are hardly ever available. The same applies to the needs of children of parents with mental health problems.

Even though the list of underserved areas could be extended considerably, it is important to say that overly extensive care could also be a problem. Excessive services can clearly have negative consequences beyond the squandering of valuable resources. The most common areas where there is a surfeit of resources that are no longer needed – or only needed to a lesser extent – are pharmacotherapy and supported living (Wiersma 2006).

It is unfortunate that psychiatric help is often sought rather late in the game, mainly because of perceptions of the stigma associated with psychiatric illness and treatment. There have been recent developments in this area, such as specialized early detection and intervention services.

Recent developments

Early detection and intervention

In spite of the rather unclear research base, attempts at the early detection and treatment of individuals with psychotic symptoms and of those who may be at greater risk for developing psychosis, have led to the development of specialized services. Even though it seems quite clear that the course of psychotic conditions is adversely affected by a prolonged lack of information and help when suffering such experiences, the indication, type, extent and timing of early interventions remains a controversial topic (Riecher-Rössler *et al.* 2006).

The kind of interventions that have shown positive results in scientific studies consist of step-wise and integrated service-offers. The international consensus regarding early treatment of psychotic conditions (International Early Psychosis Association Writing Group 2005) demands that interventions should be:

- person-centred;
- recovery-oriented;
- phase-specific;
- integrative;
- integrated.

Treatment should take place in an atmosphere of

- precaution and circumspection;
- accompanied by evaluation and research of new concepts and ideas;
- without stigmatization or discrimination.

This prudent consensus reflects the fact that we are dealing here with rather young individuals. It is also influenced by the controversy about possible adverse effects of early or premature treatment. This includes the possibility of stigmatization, excessive treatment, 'unnecessary patient-careers', but especially the risk of specific harm caused by medication and by psycho-educational, psychological and psychosocial interventions. Our proposal in this context is to extend the creativity and strong motivation of people working in, and concerned with, this crucial area as a model in order to maintain and encourage caution, prudence and respect for complexity with all age-groups and in all treatment situations.

Other specializations

Other specializations are concerned with services for individuals with 'dual diagnoses'. The people most active in this area are mostly those who deal with serious psychiatric conditions as well as the abuse of and/or dependency on substances or alcohol. Most general psychiatry services and specialized addiction programmes are overly taxed by the frequently unfavourable collision of these type of problems. Consequently, an increasing number of specialized teams for the treatment of these challenging dual problems are being formed. Patients who are particularly deserving of treatment, but who have a history of forced interventions and disrupted treatment, are being served by specialized Assertive Outreach Teams (Burns and Firn 2002). The therapeutic challenge posed by patients diagnosed with borderline personality disorder provides yet another example of a need for new and specialized interventions. Specialized services for women and men, as well as culturally relevant and age-appropriate interventions are being evaluated, as they are expanding. It remains to be seen to what extent and in what circumstances such specialized services might be superior to general treatment programmes. Another area of specialization manifested by the expansion of forensic beds, needs to be followed with concern. The same goes for other areas of potential re-institutionalization, such as residential facilities.

The need-adapted treatment model

The spectacular successes of the Scandinavian teams with their need-adapted model (Alanen 1997; Lehtinen 2002) has prompted a fair amount of interest internationally. This model is characterized by prompt intervention in the setting of the people's own lives, which involves the social network from the very beginning. Teams which work with individuals experiencing psychosis are clearly committed to those individuals and remain involved over the long term and offer ongoing individual treatment and systemically oriented psychotherapy, while at the same time practising great restraint in the prescribing and dosage levels of psychotropic medication. These conditions are likely to be the ones that contribute to the exceptionally positive outcomes. In a considerable proportion of interventions, antipsychotic medication is not used at all, and in many other instances only in low dosages. Long-term relapse rates and functional outcomes of the experimental groups enrolled in this approach appear superior to those of traditional treatment models (Seikkula *et al.* 2006).

New roles

The concepts of patients as experts (Tyreman 2005), illness self-management (Drake *et al.* 2000), shared decision-making (Deegan and Drake 2006), participatory psychopharmacotherapy (Aderhold and Stastny 2007), advance agreements (Henderson *et al.* 2008), psychiatric advance directives (Amering *et al.* 2005), trialogue (Amering *et al.* 2002) and psychosis seminars (Bock and Priebe 2005) all represent relatively recent developments that have changed the traditional roles of clinicians and patients.

Patients are assuming a more active consumer-role in a service relationship (Priebe 2003). At the level of therapeutic relationships, participatory models strive for 'shared decision-making' rather than paternalistically tainted compliance-models. Needless to say, this demands new skills of both clinicians and service users. In situations that call for ongoing support over long periods, joint planning and decision-making is absolutely essential. Ongoing medication also calls for much co-operation and exchange of views. To find the most suitable medication regimen for a particular individual, it is not sufficient for the doctor to be familiar with the intended and the untoward effects. A close collaboration is required. Patients must bring their knowledge and experience to the table. The scientific basis of the professionals' knowledge and their experience with large numbers of diverse patients must be combined with the subjective and frequently quite individualistic experiences of service users. This not only requires considerable respect for each other, but also a fair amount of time and effort on both sides.

We can assume that approximately 50% of today's mental health service users are using the internet, and we know that about half of all internet-users are seeking and finding health-related information there. Approximately one third of internet-users are pursuing questions about psychiatry. The information they obtain is rarely satisfying, and many service users discuss what they have found with their doctors (Schrank *et al.* 2006). We need to take time for these discussions. Simultaneously, there is also a development towards quality control regarding health-related information on the internet. Other publications, such as guidebooks that provide information and assist in making decisions are also increasingly available. Such materials enable service users and professional helpers alike to deal with the users' conditions and treatments in a self-determined and assertive fashion. We need to take the time to become familiar with these types of materials, so we can keep up with clients and make sensible recommendations.

The scientific findings about treatment contracts and crisis plans (Henderson *et al.* 2004) are impressive. Such pre-arrangements must be well thought out if they are to be useful in a future crisis and helpful to service users in communicating their informed decisions to the professionals. It appears evident that neutral people such as mediators can play an important role in helping negotiate such agreements.

My own research on the subject of psychiatric advance directives in New York (Amering *et al.* 2005) has shown that even users with a long history of forced treatment and disappointments are willing to enter into a process that challenges them by demanding they take a great deal of personal responsibility. Those who are engaged in this process are doing so with much respect for the process and are committed and ready to make considerable efforts. It was most impressive to find that people who were drafting an advance directive clearly took into account the scope of professional helpers and institutions and aimed to achieve a balance between their scientific, legal, and professional standards and regulations on the one hand, and their own experience on the other, with the aim of avoiding mistakes and optimizing their treatments. These are exciting prerequisites for new forms of collaboration. However, currently we continue to share the concern of many consumers as to whether the mental health system can actually meet these new expectations.

STIGMA AND DISCRIMINATION

Today stigmatization and discrimination are clearly seen as major problems in treatment, coping and living with mental health problems. Stigmatization makes people suffer from a 'second illness' (Finzen 2001). It keeps people away from help and services. Stigma and discrimination interfere with and hinder interventions that might be curative, minimize suffering and promote social integration. Those who are suffering and their families are brought to despair by stigmatization, which also causes resignation among service providers. Stigmatization is one of the major obstacles to recovery.

Stigmatization can be a result of symptoms. For example, when someone talks about hearing voices, this might be taken as a sign of a serious mental illness. In such situations, people might actually believe that the voices are uttering threats towards them and that hearing voices might be a sign of danger. Depression and negative symptoms might lead people to assume that there is a character deficit. Even within families it is hard to accept that a relative might sometimes lack the energy to complete his/her tasks. These faulty assumptions can have rather unpleasant consequences, for example suggestions such as 'pull yourself together' or 'just keep things going as usual'. Such suggestions show how certain observable behaviours can lead to stigmatization. Fortunately, the newer forms of medication have had some positive impact in this area. Many earlier psychiatric drugs caused visible side effects which then became associated with the illness and contributed to labelling and exclusion. Even the diagnosis alone is frequently a source of stigmatization. A diagnosis of schizophrenia has particularly nasty effects in this regard, a fact that will be addressed further in comparison with depression.

As a medical specialty, psychiatry is also subject to some stigmatization. An obvious example of this is shown in the representation of psychiatry in feature films, where psychiatrists generally are either shown as criminal masterminds, friendly losers, or sex fiends who have sexual relationships with their patients. Psychiatrists' explanation for the widespread prejudice towards their work is often that the stigma of the patients rubs off on the doctors. On the other hand, looking at the data on popular opinion about psychiatric treatment might explain why users of services often feel that the negative reputation of psychiatry rubs off on them, whenever they admit to receiving such treatment. This is especially true about psychopharmacological treatment, which is essentially seen as unhelpful, causing dependency and making the person see the world through rose-tinted spectacles. Popular opinion about psychiatric treatment also includes bizarre visions of what happens in psychotherapy sessions. To achieve any kind of change in this area it is advisable to abstain from mutual accusations and instead to join forces to fight stigma and discrimination.

Stigma research characteristically has an essential focus on the attitudes of various populations towards psychiatric conditions such as dementia, depression and schizophrenia. The processes leading to stigma as well as the possibility of ameliorating this situation are also the subjects of research – at the individual level with respect to personal anti-stigma convictions and activities, and at the policy and societal level in general.

Individual stigmatization and discrimination are often measured by determining the degree of 'social distance', that people claim to seek. Structural discrimination can be assessed by examining whether certain social structures, legal regulations and political decisions are more likely to increase or decrease discrimination. Finally, the concept of self-stigmatization merits our attention. Service users are part of the general population and often share these opinions. It is not easy for them to distance themselves from those opinions, and is extremely difficult for them to develop counteracting positions. The following are some typical stigmatizing assumptions about mental illnesses:

- guilt – mentally ill individuals are themselves responsible for their conditions, or their families are to blame;
- incurability – a chronic course, unfavourable prognosis, ineffective treatments (stigmatization also of the specialty of psychiatry);
- unpredictability and dangerousness of mentally ill individuals, breaking of social conventions.

There are many sources of incorrect and negative ideas about mental illness:

- lack of information – 'I don't know anyone who has a mental illness'; 'Mental illnesses do not respond to treatment';

- misinformation from the press, movies, TV – 'psychopathic murderer', 'split personality';
- defensive positions – 'I can't imagine ever becoming mentally ill'; 'things like this don't happen in our family'.

Ignorance and the formation of myths do not merely influence the general population with respect to mental illness, but also shape the attitudes of medical practitioners, insurance companies, teachers, and many key opinion-makers in society.

Link and Phelan (2001) conceptualized the stigma-process as follows:

1. A difference is noted (for example, a symptom);
2. A label is applied ('mentally ill');
3. A connection with negative stereotypes in society is established (for example, unpredictable, incurable);
4. Social distance is sought;
5. Discrimination follows.

The group of researchers around Pat Corrigan (Rüsch *et al*. 2005a and b) are focusing on the identification of, and the connections among, the following stigma-components: People who hold prejudices feel reinforced by stereotypical images in society and respond with discrimination.

It is not at all easy to understand these types of processes, but to try to counter them – or even to attempt to end them altogether, is even more challenging. Albert Einstein offers his own sad conclusion: 'It is harder to crack a prejudice than an atom'. However, both goals must be considered feasible. But before we report about the possibilities and successes of the empowerment and recovery movement against stigma and discrimination, we will take a brief excursion into the research on stigma and discrimination in mental health.

Attitude research

One of the most popular methods in attitude research is based on the use of case-vignettes. Subjects are shown a written short story that recounts a typical psychotic episode from the schizophrenia spectrum or a depressive condition in an animated and naturalistic fashion. They are then questioned with respect to their opinions about: the nature of the described difficulties (for example, whether it should be considered an illness); its causes and prognosis (with and without treatment); the qualities that are ascribed to the portrayed person, and about any emotional responses that may have been elicited by the person and their story. Finally, they are asked about the extent of social distance they would like to have between themselves and the person in the story.

A representative survey of the population in unified Germany from the year 2001 that uses such a methodology (Angermeyer and Matschinger 2003) gives us a good idea about the situation. Five thousand and twenty-five subjects were confronted with two vignettes of the kind just mentioned. Seventy-one per cent recognized one of them as an episode of a schizophrenic psychosis. Sixty-two per cent identified a depressive episode as an illness.

When looking at the stated causes, it is possible to infer what the remaining subjects had considered. Nearly one fifth of the subjects were thinking about an 'immoral lifestyle' as a cause for such situations; about half considered alcohol use (which is not mentioned in the vignettes) and 40% a 'lack of willpower' as being related to the causes of the depicted situations. We have to acknowledge this as a rather sad state of affairs before we can consider other interesting results that might well have influenced the treatment recommendations later elicited. Between 30-40% of the subjects considered a lack of parental affection and a broken home as possible causes. There was a high correlation with stress at work, revealing rather substantial differences between the 'schizophrenia situation' and the depressive episode. Fifty-nine per cent assumed that work-related stress might play a role in causing schizophrenia, an opinion that was found among 78% of subjects with respect to depression. Comparably similar results for stressful life-events are reported for schizophrenia (73%) and depression (81%). On the other hand, genetic causes (59% for schizophrenia and 44% for depression) and defining it as a brain disease (69% vs. 44%), reveal greater differences. We will deal below, in more detail, with the description of psychiatric conditions as 'brain diseases' and its relevance for stigma and discrimination.

The attributes ascribed to the individuals in the vignettes can be divided into two groups. The first concerns being seen as needy, dependent on others and helpless, and were reported most frequently (60-90%), without any differences between the two diagnoses. In contrast, representing a threat, danger or lack of self-control was mentioned nearly twice as often for schizophrenia (about 40%) than for depression (about 20%).

The assumptions about course and outcome of these conditions are particularly relevant for our subject of 'recovery'. Only a minuscule proportion of subjects believes in a cure without treatment for schizophrenia (1%) and depression (2%); full recovery with a risk of relapse (3% vs. 4%), and partial recovery (6% and 7%). Fifty-nine per cent (or 50% for depression) believe that the natural course of these conditions consists of deterioration. Remarkably, only 10% (and 11% for depression) came to the sensible conclusion that they actually knew nothing about the natural course of these conditions. Opinions about the course of these conditions with treatment were certainly more optimistic: the largest proportion of subjects (40%) opted for full recovery with a risk of relapse; 25% (19% for depression) believed in the possibility of a partial recovery, and 16% and 22% in full recovery.

We do find significant differences in the emotional responses towards individuals diagnosed with schizophrenia and depression. Sixty per cent of those questioned reported feeling pity and a desire to help in response to both conditions. Several emotional reactions such as uneasiness (48% vs. 32%), insecurity (34% vs. 24%) and fear (34% vs. 21%) were clearly more frequent with regard to schizophrenia than depression, while empathy, i.e. the sense of relating emotionally to the experience of the individual with the diagnosis, was considerably lower for schizophrenia (25%) than for depression (34%). A lack of understanding, anger, and irritation were reported by fewer than one fifth of the subjects. Thirty per cent wanted to keep their distance from individuals with schizophrenia; fewer, (23%), wanted a distance from people with depression.

When we analyze this complex data set, additional enlightening information is revealed (Angermeyer and Matschinger 2003). Women report somewhat more fear and pity, and somewhat less anger. Higher education correlates with less fear. Familiarity with individuals who have or had had a mental illness lowers the desire for social distance. When a subject identifies a 'schizophrenia-vignette' as reflecting a mental illness, their attitude towards the person becomes less favourable. The idea that a diagnosis might suggest a brain disease leads to an association with dangerousness. This, in turn, creates fear, which leads to a more pronounced reduction of pity. On the other hand, identifying the vignette 'depression' as reflecting a mental illness has rather favourable consequences. In this case, a psychosocial model is preferred over a biological one and leads to pity and less anger with no further adverse implications.

Across both diagnoses it seems that a psychosocial model limits anger and promotes pity. On the other hand, a biological understanding – especially for schizophrenia – promotes an association with danger and unpredictability, fanning anger and fear, while reducing pity. These results are important to keep in mind when considering more or less suitable methods of combating stigmatization and discrimination. Assumptions about poor prognosis and an unfavourable course promote anger, which is especially relevant to the notion of recovery. Apparently, the idea which we have come to know as Kraepelinian – 100 years old, outdated for almost as long, but still quite potent – evokes anger among the general population. A model that is predetermined and implies that nothing can be changed seems to make people angry.

The large international anti-stigmatization campaign that has been carried out for a number of years by the World Psychiatric Association (WPA) and the pharmaceutical company Eli Lilly, with the goal of combating the stigma of schizophrenia had as its primary slogan the statement: 'Schizophrenia is a brain disease!', while also offering a number of rewarding small local projects which included service users and relatives. As described above, such a biological model has quite a few unfavourable effects, which we will be describing in more detail below. Apparently, not much has changed in Germany between the major studies of 1990 and 2001: the assumption that schizophrenia has biological causes has tended to become more widespread, along with the wish for social distance (Angermeyer and Matschinger 2005). As for depression, there seems to be a bit more pity in addition to anger (Angermeyer and Matschinger 2004). That is all that has changed.

An elegant study by colleagues from Leipzig, Germany, in collaboration with researchers in Russia and Mongolia, has shown, not surprisingly, that identifying someone as mentally ill in Novosibirsk and Ulan Baator leads to associations with a need for help, dependency and the desire for social distance. But in those locations these opinions were not associated with dangerousness. The authors, Angermeyer, Buyantugs, Kenzine and Matschinger (2004) speculate that this might be connected with the representation of people with a mental illness in the media, and with the role of the media in general. Whatever the cause, clearly the situation differs from place to place.

Iatrogenic stigma

Returning to the measurement of the desire for social distance in general, the researchers inquired of their subjects whether they would, for example, accept a person with schizophrenia as a tenant, co-worker, neighbour or babysitter. Further questions address whether the subject would marry into a family in which a member had schizophrenia, accept such a person into the social circle, or recommend them for a job as a co-worker. Here are some of the results. Researchers in Nigeria used the same questionnaire to measure social distance in their country as the one used in Germany (Gaebel *et al.* 2002). They discovered that the desire for social distance and the feeling of being ashamed of a person with a mental illness was much greater in Nigeria than in Germany (Adewuya and Makanjuola 2004).

It might be tempting to assume that this result can be attributed to greater education and awareness in Germany. Many people are of the opinion that the more is known among the general population about mental illness, the less stigma and social distance there should be. However, a research team in Zurich, Switzerland, has published data in this regard that are rather thought-provoking (Lauber *et al.* 2006). They have shown that psychiatrists are more favourably inclined than the general population towards establishing mental health services in the community, but they, that is to say, the psychiatrists, are equally concerned that such services might lower the real estate values in their vicinity. This attitude has been described as 'nimby' – 'not in my backyard'. In this case, people were saying that they were in favour of supported living in the community for those with mental illness, but preferably not in the property next door to them. But their main finding was that psychiatrists are no different from the general population when it comes to social distance. The implication should be obvious: the role of psychiatrists as inspiring examples in anti-stigma campaigns needs rethinking (Lauber *et al.* 2006). Norman Sartorius (2002, p 1470) picked up on the issue of iatrogenic stigma, i.e. stigma caused by the actions and attitudes of physicians. He expressed it rather clearly: 'Iatrogenic stigma of mental illness begins with the behaviour and attitudes of medical professionals, especially psychiatrists'.

One source of iatrogenic stigma might be the fact that psychiatrists themselves experience stigmatization and discrimination. Beyond the rather offensive public image and myths circulating about the psychiatric profession, there is certainly ample information which demonstrates that the investments in mental health services that psychiatrists are recommending, are hardly seen as priorities. Beck *et al.* (2003) questioned community members about the areas of health care they would like to see funded. A majority of 80% insisted that there should be no reduction in funding for cancer treatment. Forty per cent were of the opinion that AIDS and cardiovascular disorders should suffer no budget cuts. According to this survey, funding for diabetes, Alzheimer's disease and rheumatoid arthritis is already quite compromised. Only a quarter of the subjects expressed the opinion that there should be no savings in these areas. Only a small proportion of respondents (less than 10%) expressed support for funding in the areas of schizophrenia, depression and alcohol-related conditions. The same view applies to funding for research in these areas. For mental health professionals these opinions are rather hurtful and show that our work is far less valued among the general population than we would like.

When we consider the data that reveal how the public thinks about the actual services we offer, we can hardly feel comforted either. Even though approximately three-quarters of the respondents recommend professional help for depression and schizophrenia, they are primarily thinking about psychotherapy, and would favour medication only when this fails. Only 10% recommend medication as the first choice – the same number as those who favour natural healing methods. When looking more closely at the data, it turns out that psychotherapy is seen as a treatment which deals with the causes of an illness because of its assumed psychoanalytic foundations. Medication is seen as a purely symptomatic intervention which carries a high risk of dependency and drug-induced personality changes (Riedel-Heller 2005). Many anti-stigma campaigns have addressed ways to change this situation and to rehabilitate psychiatric treatment, without too much success.

One strategy that psychiatrists use in an attempt to change this situation is to seek to persuade both patients and public to endorse the medical model. However, we have already seen that large proportions of the population continue to 'lack insight' on this subject. What do the people who seek help for mental health problems think?

Roessler et al. (1999) investigated whether quality of life is better outside or inside the hospital, and found out that it is not the location as such which accounts for the difference, but rather the extent of social support that is available to the person. A high educational level decreases quality of life, as does a very severe illness and high subjective susceptibility. Interestingly, they also found that negative assumptions about prescribed medication correlate with a higher quality of life. This is not merely surprising, but also irritating, considering that therapeutic and psycho-educational efforts aim to promote more positive attitudes towards medication, and are judged accordingly. The next surprising result of this study follows the same line: idiosyncratic – individual, rather than conforming to the medical model – assumptions about one's own condition are associated with a better quality of life. It would not be far off the mark to assume that this is due to the fact that in our culture, people who have their own opinions feel better about their lives. At the same time it should be good for how you feel about yourself if your opinions are not too different from the general public's. Psychiatric patients are part of the general population. It might be that sharing the critical opinions of the general population towards psychotropic drugs and the medical illness model, in other words being part of the general public, results in a better quality of life, than toeing the line of mental health professionals and thereby being set apart from one's social environment.

Sibitz et al. (2005) found that those patients who had experienced between two and five hospitalizations expressed favourable attitudes towards medication, while those with none, one, or more than five hospitalizations were rather critical. It appears that at first, patients share the opinions of the general population of which they are part, and therefore have a negative opinion of psychotropics. If they experience benefits from the medication and are not hampered by them in everyday life, they move towards a more favourable assessment. When things do not seem to improve after some time and several further hospitalizations, they return to their critical opinions. The optimal position might be to use medication, but remain critical towards it. Even if taking medication, a person might feel better sharing the public opinion about it, rather than positioning him/herself beside the mental health professionals and against the general public. After all, life means living in society, not in the mental health system.

Stigma – experiences and expectations

Individuals diagnosed with mental illness have frequent and painful experiences of stigmatization. The experience of devaluation occurs most often in direct contacts with others. Such experiences of devaluation can be anything from avoidance or retreat by others, to outright insults and disparaging remarks about mental illnesses and their treatment. Individuals who are known to have a diagnosis or to receive treatment are treated as being less competent than they actually are. Stigmatizing representations in the media are also often experienced as irritating. One third of all service users report that they have been rejected as job applicants or potential tenants (Wahl 1999).

While rejection as job applicants or potential tenants occur far more often than they should, they are reported much less than the experience of being stigmatized when in direct personal contact with someone. One reason for this could be that individuals with psychiatric disabilities might have given up on achieving certain roles in the work-world since they expect to be treated in a stigmatizing and discriminatory fashion, and therefore have little chance of succeeding. Most patients with a diagnosis of 'schizophrenia' or 'depression' apparently expect negative reactions from their environment (Angermeyer *et al.* 2004). This applies to around 75% of all respondents with regard to applying for a job. Nearly two-thirds of all patients assume that others would avoid contact with them because of their psychiatric diagnosis. Again, no difference was found between persons diagnosed with schizophrenia and depression, even though in actuality those with schizophrenia experience such slights more frequently. Unfortunately, an even higher proportion of the general population expects stigmatization of patients (Freidl *et al.* 2003). Alas, it is also known that a majority of stigmatizing interactions occur in contacts with mental health service providers. This is of particular concern, and quite possibly can explain why stigma is often an obstacle for those seeking professional help. In a study of students with pronounced clinical symptomatology, the medical students in the group were least likely to seek help. The main reason for this surprising result was fear of stigmatization and discrimination (Rüsch *et al.* 2005b).

Basically, three main strategies predominate among the methods of personal coping with stigmatizing experiences in the social domain: an active one – educating others – and two defensive ones – avoiding contact and secrecy. Most patients, both current and former, use all three. They each have considerable disadvantages beyond any immediate results. Avoidance and retreat interfere with social integration and limit social support. Disclosure and education must be used carefully, since they might actually lead to an increased experience of rejection (Rüsch *et al.* 2005b). Everything suggested by these data makes it clear how much of an obstacle stigma can be for recovery.

Internalized stigma and stigma resistance

At times stigma leads to especially dire consequences, when persons with a mental illness get the sense that they are not fully fledged members of society. Aside from the objective discrimination that individuals so diagnosed are exposed to, low self-esteem and other burdens result from the subjective experience of devaluation and marginalization. These subjective aspects of stigmatization and their psychological consequences make it even more difficult to deal with the already existing obstacles relating to employment, housing and relationships. These psychological phenomena are contained in the construct of 'internalized stigma' (Ritsher *et al.* 2003). Internalizing stigma ('self-stigmatization') leads to self-deprecation, shame, concealment and social withdrawal, thereby seriously hindering the recovery process.

Link and Phelan (2001) have described how the internalization of stigmatizing events in society turns into damage to a person's sense of identity. As members of society, people with psychiatric disabilities are likely to encounter the prevalent prejudices. As soon as a person has identified him/herself as being mentally ill, or has been considered mentally ill, they are bound to become part of a group which is subjected to prejudice. Individuals who are dealing with stigmatization in psychological ways, have a greater tendency to become wrapped up in these stereotypes, assuming that they are indeed appropriate for themselves, and will suffer from feelings of shame. Feelings of shame play a major role in situations when, following an acute psychotic episode, a person fails to recover fully, and continues to suffer from persistent problems.

Internalized stigma thus constitutes an important aspect of stigma, which should be taken into consideration in all psychiatric and psychotherapeutic clinical work. Interventions that go beyond reducing the symptoms of an illness by alleviating internalized stigma, are likely to be more effective and enduring. Clinicians might be encouraged by a valid assessment of internalized stigma to include the reduction of stigmatization as a verifiable treatment goal, after symptom-reduction. Shin and Lukens (2002) were able to show that patients with a diagnosis of schizophrenia benefited from psycho-education by experiencing a reduction of symptoms and perceived stigma, as well as by an increase in their coping mechanisms. This study employed the Devaluation-Discrimination Scale developed by Link (Matschinger *et al.* 1991, Link *et al.* 1989), which measures the perception of general attitudes towards people with a mental illness 'What would most people say?' Ritsher *et al.* (2003) developed the Internal Stigma Mental Illness Inventory (ISMI) for the purpose of measuring individual internalized stigma.

It includes statements such as the following:

- I feel out of place in the world because I have a mental illness;
- Mentally ill people tend to be violent;
- People discriminate against me because I have a mental illness;
- I avoid getting close to people who don't have a mental illness to avoid rejection;
- People often patronize me, or treat me like a child, just because I have a mental illness;
- I am disappointed in myself for having a mental illness;
- Having a mental illness has spoiled my life;
- People can tell that I have a mental illness by the way I look;
- I stay away from social situations in order to protect my family or friends from embarrassment;
- I can't contribute anything to society because I have a mental illness;
- Because I have a mental illness, I need others to make most decisions for me.

Nearly half the patients diagnosed with schizophrenia score high on discrimination experience and social withdrawal. Alienation and stereotype endorsement occurred in one third of respondents. The self-stigmatizing attitudes that are included in the cluster 'alienation' are particularly undermining of emotional and psychological well-being and of morale, in the struggle for recovery and against the negative fall-out of the illness (Ritsher and Phelan 2004). Anti-stigma convictions that indicate an active struggle with statements like 'People with a mental illness are making important contributions to society' or 'Living with mental illness has made me a tough survivor' could only be found among 24% of the respondents. Stigma convictions were positively correlated with depressive symptoms, and negatively correlated with high self-esteem, empowerment and a focus on the recovery process. In their follow-up study, Ritsher and Phelan (2004) found that high values on ISMI at baseline predicted a worsening of depressive symptoms and a decrease in self-esteem at the point of re-examination. ISMI showed a greater capacity to predict changes in depressive symptoms and self-esteem than the Devaluation Discrimination Scale. Thus, clinicians can now use the ISMI as a valid instrument to measure internalized stigma. This makes it possible to define a reduction of stigma along with symptoms as a verifiable treatment goal.

This is important, since it might help people escape from the trap of self-stigma. Not everyone who is subjected to public stigmatization responds with self-stigmatization and loss of self-esteem. Indifference or an active struggle are also possible responses. Patrick Corrigan addresses these issues in his model of personal responses to the stigma of mental illness (Rüsch *et al.* 2005a and b). First of all, it is important whether and to what extent a person is identified with the stigmatized group of 'the mentally ill'. When the degree of identification is low, it is easier to stay nonchalant about the negative responses of others.

Whenever a person clearly feels associated with the stigmatized group of 'the mentally ill', he or she is much more likely to feel hurt. But here too, there are at least two ways of responding: If the stigmatization by others is considered to be justified, self-esteem might plummet. The response would be quite different, however, if the person clearly felt that these stigmatizing attitudes and negative responses didn't have a legitimate leg to stand on. The energy associated with righteous anger can be quite useful – both for the individual and at the larger social and political levels – as they mobilize against stigma and discrimination, aiming for change in the status quo.

Positive stigma and stigma-resilience

Individuals and groups with the capacity to counteract the stigma of mental health can play a crucial role in the fight against stigma and discrimination. Clearly, people from all spheres of life have shown that they can be unaffected by stigmatizing and discriminating environments and can generate strength through surviving in the face of such adversities. Stigma resistance can be conceptualized as a form of resilience and possible determinants can be explored. Among them are the concept of exposure versus avoidance and the role of turning-point experiences. Finding out more about stigma resistance could be a crucial step in improving both the situation of people and the effectiveness of interventions targeting stigma and social exclusion. Data on stigma resistance in patients with severe mental illness point to the special relevance of the concept of stigma resistance in the context of other perspectives on stigma and discrimination. Research should focus on stigma resistance and its possible value as an independent variable, as well as an outcome variable of specific and non-specific interventions in mental health care.

Margret Shih (2004) at the University of Michigan investigates successful coping with stigma. Her goal is to explain how certain people who are being stigmatized still manage to fare well in our society. This is not rare at all. Fortunately, there are an increasing number of people who are not merely discussing their diagnosis and suffering in public, but who are also reporting how they have managed to thrive while coping with their difficulties, and how they are leading a good life afterwards, in spite of, or in between, disabling experiences. Some of the many examples are books by: Rolf Lyssy, *Swiss*

Paradise; Kay Redfield Jamison, *An Unquiet Mind*, and Daniel Tammet, *Born on a Blue Day*. The pop star Paula Abdul has revealed her bulimic eating disorder and has said she is stronger and happier today as a result of her active struggle against her illness. And of course there is John Nash, the Nobel laureate diagnosed with schizophrenia, who is known to us from the film, *A Beautiful Mind*, and the documentary, *A Brilliant Madness*, who tells us that he took his delusional ideas seriously for so long because he believed they came from the same source as his stupendous mathematical discoveries.

Even though stigma leads to many difficulties and much stress in the lives of those on the receiving end of it, these additional problems don't always have negative consequences. 'People who experience stigma frequently function as well as those who are not stigmatized'- Margaret Shih (2004) examines the processes that help overcome the negative consequences of stigma. She discusses the processes she has found in the literature which contribute to the fact that certain stigmatized individuals can successfully manage the results of prejudice and discrimination.

Resilience: auto-protective strategies for overcoming stigma

Stigmatization can be influenced by several different means (Shih 2004):

Compensation: One strategy might be that people develop capacities to compensate for the stigma by trying extra hard or by developing extra interpersonal skills and/or by specifically disconfirming stereotypes.

Strategic interpretation of the social environment: In order to protect their self-worth, stigmatized individuals might opt for selective social comparisons, for example, measuring up against people in equally bad or worse situations rather than against people in more favoured groups. Stigmatized subjects can also attribute mistakes to being discriminated against, which might help protect self-worth, or deny or minimize prejudice and discrimination.

Multiple identities: People do have multiple identities, for example, a female, older, Christian book-keeper (gender, age, religion, profession) and can switch identities to safeguard psychological well-being as certain identities can be subjected to stigma in certain social domains, but not in others.

Shih distinguishes between *coping model* strategies used by stigmatized individuals to help avert the negative consequences of stigma, which can become rather exhausting over time, and an *empowerment model* whereby active members of society overcome the adversities of stigma and feel energized and experience self-efficacy based on their deeds. She hypothesizes that individuals who are leading a successful life in spite of their stigmatized status are more likely to rely on the empowerment rather than on the coping model. She suggests perceived justification of stigma and degree of identification with peer group as factors that predict whether someone is likely to use the empowerment or the coping model. Individuals who identify with and are frequently in touch with their peer group are more cognizant of the positive aspects associated with belonging to, being part of, their peer group and also more active on the collective level of action, for example they undertake activities that might reduce the impact of social stigma as well as structural discrimination.

Social inclusion

The most impressive compendium of all strategies in the struggle for full social acceptance and participation of individuals with a psychiatric diagnosis is Liz Sayce's amazing book *From Psychiatric Patient to Citizen. Overcoming Discrimination and Social Exclusion* (2000). The author impresses the reader with her immense attention to detail and she does not shirk from any complex or paradoxical situation. We highly recommend this book. Sayce's major strength is the way she fits a vast amount of data and many stories into a clear-cut framework, which we would like to present briefly. She distinguishes and describes four conceptual models, which are used to overcome stigmatization and discrimination.

The brain disease model

The brain disease model is characterized by the medicalization of mental conditions ('illnesses'). This implies parity between people with psychiatric illnesses and those who suffer from physical illnesses, which means, above all, an equal footing with respect to accessing therapies and third party payments. Furthermore, this model promotes ceasing to attribute guilt to the person with the illness and to their families. Critics of the brain disease model fear that this approach abrogates all responsibility under the guise of guilt, while also weakening the efforts to increase acknowledgement of the rights and social responsibilities of people with psychiatric diagnoses. Finally, it remains to be seen whether this model is acceptable to large portions of society and policy-makers.

The individual growth model

The individual growth model conceptualizes mental illness and health as being on a continuum along which all people move up or down throughout their lives. This would suggest that a great number of people are affected by compromised mental health at one point or another. Such a view makes the distinction between 'us' (the healthy) and 'them' (the sick) irrelevant and thereby does away with a substantial source of stigmatization. Not unlike the 'brain disease' model, this perspective also encourages people to seek help. Whether those individualized alternative forms of treatment that are being considered within this framework actually address everyone's needs, remains to be seen. Furthermore, this model harbours the risk of an excessive focus on individual responsibility for the chosen life-path and for the methods of overcoming crises and handicaps, which in turn promotes the marginalization and isolation of those, who cannot be helped with the methods suggested in this framework.

The libertarian model

A large proportion of the classic anti-psychiatry movement follows this model, which questions the justification for psychiatric diagnoses and the medicalization of altered emotional and mental states. The model calls for full responsibility and rights for people who have been labelled with psychiatric diagnoses. In practical terms, this means that any special laws about psychiatric treatment that are on the books practically everywhere must be rejected, especially those concerning involuntary treatment under circumstances that may pose a risk of harm to a person or to others. It also means that a mental illness can never be invoked as an excuse for disturbing behaviour and that there should be no special legal provisions for so-called mentally ill offenders. The downside of this model is the resulting lack of special support on the part of society and its health and social service systems for people who exhibit mental problems, peculiarities or disorders.

The disability inclusion model

The disability inclusion model clearly aims for full participation in all spheres of society. The greatest advantage of this model is that all people who are motivated to do so, regardless of which of the aforementioned models they may be favouring, can join forces under this banner and fight together against discrimination and stigma. A medical model of mental illness is just as compatible with the goal of social inclusion as the idea of a life 'in recovery' without psychiatric treatment. Accepting a label of disability can be a helpful strategy in the struggle against discrimination and stigma. Even a position that defines mental peculiarities as attributes of a cultural minority would endorse the struggle for social inclusion. Initiatives with clearly stated and delineated goals can be undertaken without dissipating the ability to engage in other (broader or differently focused) efforts. Discrimination can be described and attacked on all levels of society. Furthermore, this model facilitates the collaboration among various groups who may be affected by discrimination for different reasons. It takes into consideration the demands of people, who are simultaneously being discriminated against for a number of reasons, for example individuals with sensory disabilities and mental health problems, or people who are also facing ethnic or religious prejudices. For these reasons, the movement increases in strength and appeals to a much greater number of people than other models. Such openness, along with the ability to master the complex field of mental illness and health, offers considerable chances of success for the efforts guided by this model, especially in Western societies, where the political climate is currently not averse to anti-discrimination measures and laws.

Above all, it is important to promote measures against structural discrimination – actually, for 'demolishing structural discrimination' (Thornicroft 2006). These essentially include anti-discrimination laws which protect human rights in general and patient rights in particular. On the one hand, this involves access to optimal care and services for everyone. On the other hand, the circumstances under which someone might be treated against their will must be rigorously regulated, overseen, and curtailed whenever possible. The demands address the right to optimal treatment as well as to being protected from any undesired intervention. From a recovery-perspective this implies the right to determine the timing, extent and type of intervention to the greatest extent possible.

From everything that has been said so far, the importance of active user-involvement in the fight against stigma and discrimination should be obvious, but it cannot be emphasized enough. One impressive example are data from projects in schools that aim to reach young people. When professionals give lectures and facilitate discussion groups with high school students in order to raise the awareness of psychiatric crisis situations and illnesses, they do manage to enhance the knowledge-base of the students, but they cannot diminish the social distance that the students may wish to have between themselves and those with mental health problems. However, if such training is provided by service users in collaboration with professionals, it increases the knowledge-base while also reducing social distance (Meise *et al.* 2000). From this and other studies (Spagnolo *et al.* 2008) it becomes clear that service users have to become visible, and show themselves to others, in order to help to reduce fears and social distance. Many international projects organize such collaborations. Unfortunately, the success of anti-stigma campaigns cannot be measured easily and the risk of messages being misunderstood or timed poorly is considerable. The message that 'schizophrenia is a brain disease', was, to some extent, intended to reduce the prejudice that the person him/herself bears responsibility for the illness, either by virtue of their own character or through the influence of their families. This was meant to banish feelings of guilt and shame. But the idea of a biological aetiology which is implied by this message also had other less favourable consequences, such as increasing the desire for social distance between 'us' and 'them' (Rüsch *et al.* 2005a).

In general it appears that stigmatizing attitudes – at least among the public in the USA (Phelan 2002) and in Germany – have actually increased over the recent past. Nor does it seem that depictions in the media have changed for the better. All of which makes it even more important to press on with positive advocacy and the kind of studies that might demonstrate which strategies are effective, and which it might be better to leave by the wayside.

Rüsch *et al.* (2005a) along with Corrigan and Penn (1999) describe three primary strategies for combating stigma: protest, education and contact. Protest can be a successful way of working against stigmatizing representations that appear both among the public and in the media. The German initiative, BASTA, (www.openthedoors.de 20.08.08) facilitates joining forces with others for an on-the-spot protest action whenever necessary, in a similar way to NAMI's (National Alliance on Mental Illness) stigma-busting operations. Any public education campaign naturally depends on its content. As already stated, the current strategy of using a biological model of mental illness has not succeeded in reducing fear and the need for distance from those with mental health problems, among the general population (Dietrich *et al.* 2006).

An example of successful educational interventions against stigma are school-based projects, for example, 'Madly Human' (www.irrsinnig-menschlich.de 20.08.08; Bock and Naber 2003) in Germany, which use a trialogic format and facilitate contacts between service users, family members and students. Such contacts are precisely the type of strategy that has been shown to change perceptions and attitudes. Knowing a member of a stigmatized group personally is likely to reduce the tendency of stigmatizing the entire group. In projects that combine education with direct contact, the latter seems to make the greater contribution. The entertainment media, and especially soap operas, can also enable many people to get to know about people with mental health disorders, and help them to share their fears and problems as well as their recovery experiences. In this way myths can be dispelled and interest and appreciation can be fostered (Warner 2002).

Protest, education and new forms of direct contact are also the primary strategies of the international hearing voices movement, which we want to introduce at this juncture as a special example of advocacy against stigma and discrimination.

The hearing voices movement

Ron Coleman is one of several former patients who report that one of the most important steps towards recovery was to say: 'I am not Ron, the schizophrenic. I am Ron, the voice-hearer'. Everyone who chose this path had to let go of their identity as patients with schizophrenia in order to return to their lives. Their symptoms and difficulties might have been the same as before, but their identity had changed and along with that so had the opportunities for integrating their difficulties with real life. This has given them a huge reservoir of resources and also a great deal of health, which no one, including themselves, had expected. This experience and position is clearly displayed on one of Ron's T-shirts: 'Psychotic and proud'.

When we see Ron Coleman with another one of his T-shirts stating: 'I hear voices – and they don't like you', he is toying with our fears by suggesting that his voices may actually be talking to him about us, which could become dangerous. In actuality, his voices talk about him; and people he has met throughout his life speak to him, about himself, often about everyday matters, minor issues and nonsense – sometimes with humour. Even when we are physically close to him, we cannot hear them, but he can tell us about them. When he talks about the long goodbye from a woman who was with him for many years, as a voice after she had taken her own life, he can bring tears to the eyes of many psychiatrists attending a conference.

Ron is familiar with the wounds that propel his voices. Psychiatrists are astonished to hear that he has worked for a long time now as a successful businessman, teacher and activist in the UK, after many years as a patient in psychiatric hospitals (cf. pp 61). He and his family were astonished when he stopped hearing voices altogether. Another voice-hearer stated after 20 years of such experiences: 'I remember times when I, not unlike most other people, kept an inner dialogue going with myself. For twenty years now I've been discussing my decisions with my voices instead. I'm not sure whether I can relearn that other, silent, dialogue once again.' Ever since the term schizophrenia came into being – about 100 years ago – voice-hearing has become known as one of the cardinal symptoms of this condition. The belief in a biological model of brain disease in modern psychiatry has contributed to the development of a position that voice-hearing is merely used as a quantitatively relevant symptom, whose content is hardly examined. Whatever these voices are saying to people diagnosed with a schizophreniform psychosis is given little meaning, at the most it is seen as a way of predicting dangerousness. Usually even journalists deal with this subject only when they suspect a murderous intent is being caused by the voices.

Likewise, when crime fiction brings up the subject of voices it is with similar errors and the intention to hide the weakness of the story. Whenever the establishment of a motive becomes difficult, a voice might be implicated as having ordered an otherwise senseless crime. Propagating such erroneous information about the actual significance of voices can become risky for the people who are hearing them, by inducing fear of the voices and of the voice-hearers themselves. This is very unfortunate, since the world of voice-hearing is not dangerous at all, but rather a fascinating and compelling aspect of human experience.

Epidemiological studies have shown that today around 5% of the general population in the Western world hears voices at one time or another (Coleman and Smith 2005). For most of them, this occurs during periods of health, perhaps as part of a grief reaction, as a result of sleep-deprivation, during the period of awakening or following great exertion. Many experience these voices as helpful, or as pertaining to the spiritual sphere. Others are bothered by them, tormented and confused. One person in a hundred receives a diagnosis of schizophrenia, and many people so diagnosed experience certain changes in perception, for example a perpetual string of commenting voices, as a considerable burden. Even though their content might be banal and merely annoying, such voices can still have a considerable impact on the person's emotional and social life. Feelings of impotence and of being controlled by outside forces frequently characterize the relationship between voice-hearers and the kind of voices which deliver unwelcome and undeserved comments. Medication can often silence the voices and provide some relief, but does not always lead to the desired success. Isolation, stigmatization and discrimination are often debilitating consequences for people who hear voices.

When individuals who have experienced psychosis and psychiatric treatment demand greater involvement with these phenomena, it can lead to exciting developments. In 1987 the Dutch psychiatrist Marius Romme appeared on a TV talk-show with a woman whom he had not been able to help with her voices. They invited other people who heard voices to respond and received hundreds of calls from viewers. Many of them reported difficult experiences to do with their voices, but others managed to get along well with them, and quite a few even felt enriched by these experiences. More than 400 individuals participated in a conference organized soon thereafter (Romme and Escher 1993). Marius Romme and Sandra Escher interviewed subjects who heard voices without exhibiting any other mental idiosyncrasies, and others who had been diagnosed with depression or schizophrenia. They showed that the individual interpretations and coping strategies related to these voices determined what kind of a role voice-hearing would play in a person's life. In the meantime, other studies have revealed a multiplicity of diverse experiences of, and coping methods with, voice-hearing. Therapeutic strategies that assist in analyzing these experiences and optimizing coping-methods have been developed and are being used with considerable success.

People who hear voices have looked around and found each other (for example, on the internet, see www.intervoiceonline.org). Beginning in the Netherlands and the UK, a movement of voice-hearers has developed and excelled in both self-help and advocacy. Today there are local self-help groups and support networks for voice-hearers in many places, e.g. Manchester, London, Maastricht, Berlin, Adelaide, Vienna and Madison/Wisconsin, which are open to relatives and others who are interested. In such an environment it becomes possible to explicate and publicize the experiences of voice-hearers without discrimination. People with the experience of hearing voices are reclaiming their ownership of these experiences and their representation. For far too long these rather personal experiences have been usurped by psychiatrists, who were loathe to consider their meaning, and instead chose to see them as symptoms that needed to be eliminated.

The personal accounts of voice-hearers and an increasingly differentiated engagement with the phenomenon of voice-hearing among research psychologists and neuroscientists have opened up vistas into perceptual worlds that are not merely shaped by the great variety of voices, but also by an astounding number of interpretations and ways of addressing these phenomena. Voices do not always stay the same. Each voice-hearer perceives a different set of specific voices but the voices themselves can also become transformed. They reveal intentions, emotions and yield different interpretations. Voices can seem strange or quite familiar, they can be demanding, offended, annoying, whiny, lonesome, funny or even riotous. What they say might make good sense for everyday living, and their suggestions can urge caution or be helpful in some way. They can have meaning within a biographical or spiritual context, and exert a soothing effect. Voices can highlight problems, express conflicts, but they can also cause confusion and become threatening. They can take on an air of self-importance and even forbid the person hearing them to talk about them. It is essential to understand the extent and the kind of significance each voice has in order to cope with them successfully. Traumatic experiences can trigger hallucinatory perceptions and confronting these can be quite stressful, but it may also contribute to resolution and recovery.

The essential step towards liberation for many is to be able to talk about the voices, and thereby not be left alone with them. The experiences of many people in the hearing voices movement has shown that the initial confusion associated with the hearing of voices can be replaced by an acceptance of this concretely experienced phenomenon during a phase of 'organization', in which the relationship to the voices tends to improve. A phase of 'organization' is, in this context, a time to get more information, exchange experiences, find interesting partners for dialogue and clarify which explanatory models might be best suitable to help deal with these experiences and one's relationship to the voices. The decision whether a person wants to see the voices as a symptom of an illness that can be conquered, or as an inner voice, biographical information, messages from the unconscious, or a form of contact to another reality, opens different approaches for professional or self-help responses. Eventually, many voice-hearers reach a phase of stabilization where it becomes important to structure their life in a safe and meaningful manner, in order to solidify protective influences and coping strategies while fears and adverse effects progressively lose their impact.

Many people, like the members of the German hearing voices network founded by Hannelore Klafki, or Ron Coleman in Scotland and Stephanus Binder in Austria and many others all over the world, use their experience of hearing voices to make this phenomenon accessible, communicable and manageable. They inform, educate and conduct research. They provide information, help and advice to others who may be dealing with voices.

There is much to do and much to accomplish: the voices need to be taken seriously, the hearers need to take themselves seriously, and there is a need to overcome fears, isolation and the associated taboos. Hearing voices has been experienced and described differently in different historical and cultural contexts. Today we have the exciting opportunity of an emancipatory movement of voice-hearers that tries to appreciate the phenomenon of hearing voices in all its particularity and heterogeneity. A more sophisticated engagement with this exceptional way of perceiving makes it possible for voice-hearers to better integrate these experiences into their lives. Within the framework of a dialogue in which experts voice-hearers and members of the public have equal status, a domain of human perception becomes accessible that is also of interest to people who do not hear voices.

The question, 'Do you hear voices?' can become the beginning of a good conversation in a pub, rather than a feared inquiry in the process of establishing a psychiatric diagnosis. People who hear or have heard voices have much to say. And it isn't just the type and content of the voices themselves that arouses curiosity. The necessary examination of oneself that accompanies the experience of voice-hearing, the need to understand one's position in the world, to accept and to integrate both irritating and amazing perceptions, all of these promote an intellectual and emotional quality among voice-hearers that makes them rather desirable partners for conversation. The activities of the hearing voices networks and groups promote the kind of language that enables others to partake in the extraordinary perceptions of people who hear voices. To find a connection there opens up rather inspiring perspectives.

CHAPTER 6

Recovery – Implications for Scientific Responsibilities

Mike Slade's example of a debate it is necessary to have, regarding an intervention which is known to reduce symptoms, but which also fosters dependency and loss of hope, gives an indication of what kind of research is necessary if recovery outcomes are to be captured in a valid way ('research is better than rhetoric', Slade and Hayward 2007). He calls for the identification of the 'active ingredients' in recovery-focused mental health services, a task that would include finding out not only 'what they do' but also 'how' they do it. Fidelity Scales would then allow evaluation of just how successful services had been in promoting recovery. Regarding outcome measures that can capture recovery, he draws our attention to the fact that they would need to reflect personal preferences and that research design must make the best use of both quantitative and qualitative approaches as well as user-led approaches. Liberman and Kopelowicz (2005), in a clear demand for a research concept for recovery from schizophrenia and operational criteria for both the process of 'recovering' and 'recovery' as an outcome, argue for viewing process and outcome 'in apposition, not opposition'. Julie Repper and Rachel Perkins (2003) clearly state the obvious: 'Any services, or treatments, or interventions, or supports must be judged in these terms – how much do they allow us to lead the lives we wish to lead' and John Strauss's (2008) admonition regarding the question 'whether a field that systematically ignores a considerable amount of data can be considered an adequate science' is an attempt to encourage us to meet the methodological challenges of the research and theory of subjectivity. Of course, any relevant evidence-base in times of recovery-orientation would need to be multi-perspective and to be scientifically excellent in terms of multiple and mixed methods designs (Rose *et al.* 2006).

Whether recovery does need research in order to succeed or, as a civil rights movement should not be in need of scientific evidence, is debatable. Probably both perspectives are valid and fair. In any case, recovery-oriented research is auspicious and carries great scientific challenges and opportunities for hard work and much fun.

NEW DIRECTIONS

The chapter on 'Personal experience as evidence and as a basis for model development' could have featured Bill Anthony as well. In 2006, after many years of prominence in science as a world-famous expert and director of the Center for Psychiatric Rehabilitation

Recovery in Mental Health: Reshaping scientific and clinical responsibilities Michaela Amering and Margit Schmolke
Copyright © 2009 John Wiley & Sons, Ltd

at Boston University, he publicized his personal experience and the conclusions to which it had led him. In an article in the journal *Psychiatric Services* (Anthony, 2006) Anthony gave us a personal report about his own illness, multiple sclerosis (MS), and the assistance he has been receiving in connection with it. He describes the 'MS community' as exemplary with respect to instilling courage and hope and continually providing information and opportunities for exchange, and for never questioning a person's ultimate freedom of choice. At the same time he emphasizes the importance of professional helpers, other service users, and the pharmaceutical industry for underwriting research, conferences and publications. It is his wish that psychiatry will become just as successful in supporting those dealing with psychiatric conditions.

His words are very clear when he says that patients with MS face considerably less stigmatization and discrimination than those with psychiatric diagnoses. Unlike in the case of MS, he does not experience the medical profession, i.e. psychiatry, as acting with full respect and support for its patients. The 'person first' approach, he says has not been implemented in psychiatry. He sees psychiatry's efforts in the area of forced treatment as a serious obstacle, which undermines the trust between a helping profession and its supposed beneficiaries, and its relationship to the pharmaceutical industry. Also, he does not consider the fact that information for patients is called 'psychoeducation', which is conducive to obtaining helpful services and support. The kind of self-determination that is hardly in question for MS patients is for him an essential foundation for the encouraging experiences he has had in dealing with his illness. He maintains the vision that what is possible for MS should also be possible for severe psychiatric conditions. But he sees a great deal more work and transformation ahead if this vision is to be realized.

In their 2003 article, Bill Anthony and his colleagues Marianne Farkas and E Sally Rogers, outlined the requirements for scientific studies that aim to promote evidence-based supports in the age of recovery (Anthony *et al.* 2003). In addition to the important struggle to ensure that all interventions which are already backed by scientific evidence should be available to anyone who might benefit, future studies should be designed so that they can be measured against recovery-goals. In the following we present a short summary of their expectations, which are topical and applicable to the international field:

Outcomes emphasized in evidence-based practice research should include those that focus on recovery and that consumers believe are most critical

Most studies assess interventions according to how far they are able to reduce the number of days a person spends in hospital. They deal with symptoms, re-admissions, length and cost of inpatient stays and possibly also whether someone has been able to get a job. These types of outcome variables may not have much to do with the things that are important to people in achieving their goals and experiencing success. A voluntary hospital admission may be less relevant to people in recovery than the way they spend the majority of their days, where and how they live, and whether a person is meaningfully engaged and has friends. On the other hand, while a distinction between voluntary and involuntary hospitalizations may be crucial, it is hardly ever mentioned in outcome studies. Obviously, the traditional criteria are inadequate. Success in social roles, for instance, as an intimate partner, a family member, or among friends, in training or at work, and factors such as self-determination, self-efficacy and well-being, and the lessening of discrimination and the curtailment of harmful treatment effects, are variables that must become much more prominent.

Subjective outcomes and qualitative approaches should assume greater credibility and be used more in the context of evidence-based practice research

Since recovery paths can take rather divergent individual courses, any research that is based exclusively on groups of subjects and on statistical relationships can be of only limited value. Such studies must be supported by scientific methods that can take people's individual experiences into account and reveal certain unfolding processes. Quantitative procedures can only be used sensibly once qualitative methods have shed light on the way complex interventions make their impact and how transformation occurs.

Researchers should attempt to determine why currently published, evidence-based practice research has rarely demonstrated a positive impact on recovery related outcomes

It is a well-known fact that interventions whose impact on symptoms and hospital days has been clearly proven, may not have a scientifically measurable impact on recovery rates. This needs to change urgently, and we must find out how this might be possible. To achieve this, interventions, as well as scientific methods, must be improved. We cannot rely exclusively on randomized clinical studies, since there are important scientific concerns that require the use of more complex research methods and designs.

Evidence-based practice research should include more studies of the helper-consumer relationship, which appears to be an important component of recovery

There are strong indications that relationships play an important role in recovery. This applies equally to therapeutic and other supportive relationships. Concepts and methods with which to investigate therapeutic relationships are readily available. Recent work that has applied such methods in psychiatric research appears rather promising (Priebe and McCabe 2006). Much more needs to be done to achieve an evidence-base for further research and implementation.

Evidence-based practice research should attempt to separate out the programme models to research specific practices rather than programmes in general

Some psychosocial programmes have already shown that certain of their components are more effective than others. Nevertheless, these programmes are still being offered and evaluated in their entirety. The scientific work of 'breaking down' programmes into their components and identifying their effective elements, as well as the search for superior combinations of elements, is essential for broadening the evidence-base.

Evidence-based practice research should test its models for applicability in various cultural and contextual conditions

It has also been shown that many evidence-based programmes are only effective locally, and cannot be replicated with equal success in other cultures or environments, for example, urban vs. rural settings. Frequently, studies do not reveal for which circumstances interventions are designed and for which subgroups of clients they are deemed to be appropriate.

Evidence-based practice research should examine dimensions related to the field's underlying values

Apparently, the effectiveness of services does not merely depend on their specific elements, nor on the way they are organized. Their values and the image of humanity that undergirds them must play equally important parts. To examine these values and their effects systematically is another task of scientific research.

In summary, this means that specific approaches and experimental methods are necessary to ensure that psychiatric services which want to measure up to recovery parameters can satisfy the criteria of evidence-based practice. Whenever it is feasible to undertake the necessary efforts and to optimize the scientific know-how, the concepts of evidence-based medicine and recovery can go hand in hand.

THE INCREASINGLY ACTIVE ROLE OF UK USERS IN CLINICAL RESEARCH

Getting users involved in research collaborations and joint research projects between researchers with a lived experience of mental health problems and researchers without such experience in mental health, is a relatively new and exciting development. In other clinical areas, such as cancer, HIV/AIDS, and Alzheimer research, a collaboration between researchers and patients has also begun (for example, Dunbar 1991; Thornton 2002). Mental health service users are increasingly becoming involved in the evaluation of clinical interventions and in the development of research instruments, such as those assessing recovery. However, scientific reports and publications frequently fail to describe the extent and nature of the collaboration and during which phases of the research projects the users have been involved (for example, Telford and Faulkner 2004). For a first *Handbook of User Involvement in Mental Health Research* see Wallcraft, Schrank, Amering (currently in press, Wiley-Blackwell).

Mental health service users in the UK have proposed three levels of participation: consultative; collaborative; and user-led (Consumers in NHS Research Support Unit

2001). User-led research in mental health has been going on for some time and was actually a precursor to collaborative research between researchers with and researchers without first-hand experience.

1. In a consultation, user participation is rather minimal, i.e. consisting of an informal request to review a questionnaire, and often does not go beyond lip service on the part of the researchers.
2. Collaborative research attempts to integrate elements of user-oriented research into more traditional studies. Academic researchers are officially collaborating with users. In this fashion, participants and researchers with personal experience in psychiatry can have a substantial impact on various phases of a research project, for example, by formulating therapeutic goals or by recommending the use of certain outcome variables.
3. In user-led research, users control all phases of the research projects: design; sample selection; ethical guidelines; data collection; data analysis; preparing reports, and dissemination/publication of findings. The participants in such projects are users and ex-users of services and researchers at the same time, who are sharing their insights with other users who do not have a research background. Thus they have a dual identity as researchers and current or former service users. They are also called 'experts by experience' (Faulkner and Thomas 2002). Most of the multitude of smaller projects in user-led research are evaluations of clinical services and treatment methods from the perspectives of the users themselves, or investigations of subjective strategies employed by people living with psychiatric conditions. Until now, studies emerging from user-led research have hardly been accepted by the academic mainstream, and have been relegated to the 'grey' literature. Currently, interest in such studies, and their status, is on the rise. The Ministry of Health and several public funders of research in the UK have begun to demand that users be involved in research projects, even to the point where they are asked to take on a central role (Department of Health 1998; Royle and Oliver 2001).

The SURE model

SURE stands for Service User Research Enterprise. It is a research division of the Institute of Psychiatry in London and is an example and model for universities that employ service users in research positions and leadership capacities. SURE either conducts autonomous research projects or becomes responsible for sub-projects in large research enterprises, where the perspective of users on a certain research topic (for example, continuity of care) is being investigated as a complement to the perspectives of clinicians, relatives or administrators, which are obtained by clinical researchers. Members of SURE play an active role on official research boards at the Institute of Psychiatry.

Diana Rose is one of two directors of SURE (*www.iop.kcl.ac.uk/departments/?locator=300 8.8.08*). She had been diagnosed with 'bipolar affective disorder', and has a background in research on education, gender issues and the media; in the past she had to conceal the fact that she had a psychiatric disorder at her workplace. The stigma associated with the diagnosis made it impossible to be open with her colleagues. However, her efforts to hide her diagnosis were rarely successful. After a few years out of work, and once she had made contact with the user/survivor movement, Ms Rose decided to seek employment within the mental health field. This was at a time when user-led research was still in its infancy, and she encountered 'bafflement, if not hostility' (Rose 2003a). After pioneering user-focused research for seven years at a London-based charity, Dr Diana Rose today is Europe's first Senior Lecturer in User-led Research.

In her article, 'Having a diagnosis is a qualification for the job', Diana Rose says that the assessment by users of mental health services and clinical interventions – including those she received herself – is a central element of the work at SURE (Rose 2003a). Users bring a different perspective and, unlike professional clinicians, they are in a position to judge how services and treatments come across from the 'inside' (Rose 2003b).

Examples of research projects

Investigating the patients' perspective on electroconvulsive therapy

Rose *et al.* (2003) put together a literature review of studies that deal with the opinions of patients who have received electroconvulsive therapy. Twenty-six studies had been conducted by researchers in psychiatric settings and an additional nine studies were led by, or involved, current and/or former service recipients. Sixteen studies looked at the perceived benefits of the treatment, and seven studies identified criteria for an investigation of memory loss.

In 1995, the Royal College of Psychiatry issued a statement indicating that 80% of patients with depression who had been receiving electroconvulsive therapy responded positively; that any memory loss was clinically irrelevant, and that there was no long-term negative impact on memory or intellectual functioning. In contrast, the authors working with Rose found out that at least one third of the patients in these studies reported a significant memory loss following ECT and that routine neuropsychological tests do not capture the kind of memory loss that is being reported by these patients.

Two authors from this group had themselves received shock treatment and could use their personal experiences in the interpretation of those studies. The authors found that studies which reported high levels of satisfaction among patients were generally based on interviews conducted shortly after the treatments in the hospital, and that the interviewers were often the treating physicians. The authors tried to put themselves in the position of these research subjects and postulated that many of them would have wanted to curry favour with the doctor and therefore would have avoided making any complaints, and might even have expressed satisfaction in the hopes that the doctor would not trouble them any further.

These results show that the reactions of the patients to the ECT depended on the interviewing method. Studies run by users revealed a lower rate of subjective satisfaction when compared to the clinical studies. These divergent results can be attributed – according to the authors – to the fact that the clinical studies were conducted shortly after the treatments by medical investigators in clinical settings, and that the questionnaires had been brief, offering a rather limited repertoire of possible answers from which to choose.

Qualitative data from an expanded literature survey supported the above mentioned conclusions and showed that the views of patients about ECT are rather complex. The data revealed various ways in which patients considered the pro and cons of this intervention. The authors hypothesize that many patients do not simply decide for or against this treatment. Most clinical studies which were reviewed used narrow outlines to capture the answers and the attitudes of the patients. Furthermore, the authors criticize the fact that the conventional view of patient satisfaction and its measurement is far too simplistic.

The authors propose that future studies should include qualitative assessments of a representative sub-sample of patients who had received ECT. Furthermore, studies about treatment interventions should capture the complexity of subjective experiences, for example, by looking at a variety of outcome factors which are being considered by the patients. Factors that might influence effectiveness and satisfaction are particularly important. Furthermore, it is important to assess any loss of autobiographical memory, which has been described extensively, but hardly investigated in a systematic fashion.

This work was considered during the development of the new NICE guidelines (National Institute for Health and Clinical Excellence). NICE is the central UK agency that makes important decisions about psychiatric treatments and issues relevant guidelines.

Qualitative survey about the involvement of users in research projects

Trivedi and Wykes (2002) investigated the actual involvement of users in mental health research. The first author of this detailed and programmatic report is a user and associate of 'Share in Maudsley Black Action' group at the Maudsley Hospital in London. The second author is a professor of psychology at the Institute of Psychiatry in London, and a senior investigator at SURE. Both are co-authors of a study by Kavanagh *et al.* (2003) about the psycho-education of inpatients with respect to the use of psychotropic agents at the Maudsley Hospital. 'From passive subjects to equal partners' is an evaluation of the ways in which users took part in the study mentioned above.

To start with, Trivedi and Wykes describe the significance of collaborations between clinical scientists and users in mental health research from the perspective of the official psychiatric commissions in the UK. Here are some of the reasons given for such collaborations: 'users have the experience and skills to complement those of current researchers ... they know what it feels like to undergo treatments and their various side effects ... they will have a good idea about what research questions should be asked ... and how questions might be asked differently (Goodare and Lockward 1999); if the needs and views of users are reflected in research it is more likely to produce results that can be used to improve clinical practice' (Department of Health 2000).

Users who worked on the study to do with psycho-education offered a broader perspective on the conceptual design of the study. Parameters such as empowerment, self-esteem, and alliance with the clinical team were presented as primary outcome variables. Needless to say, aside from the advantages offered by the involvement of users in research projects, there were also certain costs to consider, such as the need for additional time and funding.

The authors list ten questions that should be considered during the actual development and implementation of collaborative research projects involving researchers with and without personal experiences as mental health service users.

1. What is the value of user involvement?
Does the involvement of users merely serve to obtain funds for the project by complying with the requirements of the funding agency, or is it based on a genuine belief in the value

of such collaborations? The concrete example was implemented by a clinical team that was convinced of the positive impact of a user-perspective on all aspects of the project.

2. How will users be involved in the research process?
The clinical team, with its theoretical point of view, desired a partnership and collaboration with users, including equal decision-making powers and control, but did not realize the extent of the time commitment and other challenges that such a collaboration would imply.

3. What projects might be suitable for user involvement?
The project presented here, with its subject of 'Educating inpatients about their medications: is it worth it?' was suitable for the involvement of users, since it had been initiated by patients themselves. The clinical research team saw it as an important opportunity to assess the effects of the intervention on the level of information, insight into problems/illness, and compliance with treatment among its subjects.

4. What proposal will be prepared for presentation to users?
The clinical research team should not present a fully formulated proposal to the user group at the beginning of a project. Users realized immediately that they were being shown a finalized proposal with all research questions, study design, and outcome variables having already been decided. Based on this, they responded with an outright refusal to get involved.

5. How will the initial approach be made to users?
Working within pre-existing relationships that have developed locally is the most productive avenue. Less direct contacts, i.e. through posters or advertisements in the media, could also be useful and potentially reach a larger group of users. The example study was able to build on the recommendation of the local user group 'Communicate' to involve users in this project.

6. How will users' responses be considered?
Clinical researchers are quite challenged by negative, emotional and passionate feedback that they get from users about the proposed project. If such feedback, based on personal and often painful experiences, is meant to have a real impact on the project, it needs to be taken seriously. As far as this project was concerned, serious concerns were raised about the proposed outcome variables of 'insight into the illness' and 'compliance' because many users associated these subjects and terms with the paternalistic, authoritarian and disempowering attitude of psychiatry they had been made to experience. 'Having insight into the illness' was often equated with 'agreeing with professionals' and 'being compliant' with 'doing what the psychiatrist ordered'. This prompted the leader of the clinical research team to hold group discussions that were hard work and not always pleasant. They did, nevertheless, serve an important purpose. A mutually respectful atmosphere developed between professionals and users and the professionals accepted the feedback constructively, with both sides continuing to work on the project in a collaborative fashion.

7. Will research partnerships with users be formalised?
An explicit agreement about the collaboration between the two sides is necessary, outlining, for example: at which phase of the project and to what extent users will be involved; how their payment will be handled; how the contribution of users will be reflected in

any reports, and any issues pertaining to confidentiality. This project used a contractual format that had been worked out by the user group 'Communicate' several years earlier. Even if this contract did not have a legal basis, it still served to protect the interests of the partners. In addition to the contract, the collaboration was formalized at an institutional level by including users as official members of the research team in the application to the research ethics committee.

8. How will the proposal be jointly assessed?

It is recommended that the research proposal be appraised jointly, using a series of questions (see below) and then revised accordingly before its implementation. In the example project such questions had not been formulated at the beginning, but came up during its implementation when it became apparent how the intervention (psycho-education about psychotropic drugs) was to be carried out. Assuaging the concerns of the users during the project was far from the best solution, but it turned out to be the best possible pragmatic compromise that could be found at that time.

Possible questions are:

How did the research come about and does it address users' priorities?
What is the purpose of the study and does it contribute to user empowerment?
For example, users in this study pointed out that the subject of empowerment (including strength, trust, authority, and power) had been completely ignored.
What outcomes should be assessed, and are they what users consider to be important?
The users in this study advocated for greater future collaboration with other user groups on developing methods that could measure empowerment as an outcome variable. In addition, the authors of the study feared that psycho-education about the use of psychotropic drugs might cause more problems to the mental health team by enhancing knowledge and empowerment among patients, and thereby reducing compliance and eliciting more questions about these drugs. However, these concerns turned out to be unfounded. In fact, the approach to, and the communication about, medication proceeded much more easily when greater clarity and information were being offered, and in fact certain myths about prescribing practices turned out to be unfounded. While this change in attitude among the team was not formally measured, it still illustrated to them that future studies should assess any secondary effects of an intervention on the team itself, beyond its direct effects on the patients.
Is the intervention 'user friendly' and is enough importance attached to delivery of the intervention?
One user-researcher was concerned that patients were being accused of not becoming sufficiently engaged in psycho-education whenever the intervention did not succeed, instead of the professionals making sure that it had been adequately explained. Several factors were relevant to the success of the psycho-educational intervention, such as the environment where it was being offered, the capacity of the facilitators who are carrying out the intervention, and the attitude of the inpatient team with respect to the patients who were participating. The importance of such 'non-specific' factors in all medical and psychological interventions was once again demonstrated.
Are the methodology and design of the study appropriate?
In this study, one of the user-researchers pointed out that different teams in the same hospital might have rather different opinions regarding psycho-educational programmes

about psychotropic drugs, which in turn might have considerable influence on the way patients respond to the interventions. This resulted in the addition of specific matching procedures, which enhanced the scientific methods of the study.

How will data be analysed and the results interpreted?

Interpreting data is subject to a great deal of variation and is never free of values. For example, clinical researchers are inclined to offer a positive 'half-full' interpretation, in order to increase their chances of publication or additional funding, while user-researchers are more prone to come up with a less positive, 'half-empty' interpretation. Working with different interpretations of the same data-set can lead to interesting new questions that had not been apparent at the onset of the study.

9. How will the project be written up?

Whenever users are part of a study, their contributions should be reflected in its documentation to make sure that their influence on the study is reflected in the publication of the findings. Their work should be appropriately credited, for example, via co-authorship. In the project discussed here, the user-researcher was initially reluctant to appear as a co-author, because the focus of the study had remained on insight into illness and compliance. However, since the impact of users on the study had turned out to be greater than expected, she decided not only to appear as a co-author of the published study, but to write a second article, outlining the process of user-involvement.

10. How will dissemination occur?

In general, study results are mainly published in peer-reviewed academic journals or presented at conferences. However, these reach only a relatively small sub-set of clinicians who might be interested in such research. The UK Department of Health and other funders have insisted on much greater dissemination. The Department of Health believes it to be especially important that this information reaches users, following the department's commitment to the importance of user demand when making decisions on implementation (Department of Health 1999). To publicize the results among participants of studies, members of the user organization in London have proposed their dissemination via a circular newsletter. Websites, conferences and discussions about the results in the context of user-networks and community groups could also be used for dissemination.

Critical views from both sides

Clinical researchers have raised objections regarding collaborative research projects with users along different lines (Rose 2003b). Examples include a considerably greater expenditure of time during all phases of the study as well as additional financial costs for the compensation of user-researchers; complicated discussions that are sometimes difficult because of their emotional aspects, at certain phases of the research process, in order to achieve consensus about controversial issues and goals, and finally, a sceptical attitude and a lack of trust on the part of many academic researchers towards user-involvement in research (for example, Tyrer 2002).

Users point out the status- and power-differential between professionals and users, not unlike the more general situation between junior and senior research team members (cf. Rose 2003b):

- Even if a user-researcher is equipped with all the required academic qualifications, he/she is not likely to achieve a professional career comparable to a researcher who is not identified as a user. Mental health problems can disrupt careers. Discrimination and stigmatization are still capable of preventing individuals with mental health problems from applying for research positions and actually obtaining them.
- There are differences in salary and status, which imply that even experienced user-researchers in collaborative projects are seen as 'junior' and thus inferior to others.
- It is rather problematic when the relationship between users and professionals becomes overshadowed by an implicit clinical doctor-patient relationship, such as when some team-members view the user-researchers through dual lenses, as a researcher on the one hand, and a patient on the other. This might indeed be an important issue in mental health research because there is a risk that the respect for the expert knowledge that patients have can be diminished because of their diagnoses.

As Diana Rose points out (2003a, p 1331): 'One's user status may be used to undermine one's opinions, as it is held that a person cannot be both logical and mad'.

In spite of all the criticism and doubts on both sides it can be assumed that the genuine contribution and active participation of users in research projects is seen as essential because the complexity of subjective experience can never be captured from just one side, i.e. from the professional vantage point. The unique contribution of people with a lived experience is not merely fruitful and enriching for clinical research, but has widespread benefits for the entire health care system. First of all, the users need specific training in research issues, but they also need encouragement from the scientific community to become actively involved in research projects. Qualified users – according to Rose (2004) – should then have the opportunity to advance in their professional careers and obtain a doctoral degree (such as a PhD), if they so desired, while users without such long-term research career goals could be trained and employed as interviewers or facilitators of focus groups or to do other tasks around research projects. A comprehensive presentation of background and principles underlying the concept of service user involvement in mental health research, including various examples and practical advice from eminent international experts, can now be found in the *Handbook of Service User Involvement in Mental Health Research* (Wallcraft, Schrank, Amering in press).

ASSESSING RECOVERY

Ruth Ralph and the Recovery Advisory Group

Ruth Ralph was a Senior Research Associate in the Health Policy Institute at the Muskie School of Public Service, University of Southern Maine. She has written extensively on recovery in mental health and is one of the most important experts on recovery conceptualization and research in the United States. She worked with a group of consumers to develop papers on consumer issues for the Surgeon General's Report on Mental Health (Ralph 2000a), and she was a principal investigator at one of the seven sites of the national evaluation of consumer-operated services.

In *Recovery in Mental Illness: Broadening our Understanding of Wellness* (2004) Ruth Ralph and Patrick Corrigan explore what recovery means from various perspectives.

The book discusses recovery as process, outcome, and natural occurrence, and examines evidence-based services as well as consumer-endorsed practices that may not be measurable by traditional quantitative methodologies. Researchers are invited to develop innovative approaches to studying the complex and exciting phenomenon of recovery.

Together with the Recovery Advisory Group, a group of pre-eminent consumer researchers, Ruth Ralph began the first large-scale effort to generate a suitable instrument. From 1998–1999 under the leadership of Ruth Ralph, the Recovery Advisory Group had monthly teleconferences in which they discussed their own and others' recovery experiences. In 1999 the group formulated a recovery model which reflects their reading of published and unpublished literature on recovery written by consumers/survivors as well as the experiences of the Advisory Group members themselves (Ralph *et al.* 1999). The recovery model served as an important conceptual basis for the development of currently available instruments.

The members of the Recovery Advisory Group are: Jean Risman, Kathryn Kidder MA, Jean Campbell PhD, Sylvia Caras PhD, Jeanne Dumont PhD, Dan Fisher MD, PhD, J Rock Johnson JD, Carrie Kaufmann PhD, Ed Knight PhD, Ann Lode, Darby Penny, Wilma Townsend, and Laura Van Tosh (http://www.mhsip.org/recovery 20.08.08).

The Recovery Advisory Group recovery model

One of the first results of this study was the realization that pathways of recovery are not linear. Participants from the Recovery Advisory Group discussed several stages of recovery through which individuals pass along the way towards well-being (Ralph *et al.* 1999):

- anguish (feeling at the lowest point of your life);
- awakening (turning point – is there something better?);
- insight (finding out more – becoming hopeful that you can get better);
- action plan (finding ways to get better);
- determined commitment to become well (knowing you must work hard, and promising you will work towards getting well);
- wellbeing/empowerment/recovery (accomplishing wellness and other achievements).

Not every person passes through all phases and also there are movements back and forth between these phases throughout the process of personal growth. These phases reflect a progression towards recovery and healing, as it is described in the literature, and in the discussions and personal experiences of researchers.

The model also indicates that recovery can be influenced by internal factors (within oneself) and external factors (interactions with others). Internal factors encompass cognitive, emotional, spiritual and physical domains, such as insight into oneself, 'self-talk' and growth. The external factors include a person's actions and reactions to external influences, and interactions with people and situations, such as activity, self-care, social relationships and social supports. The authors illustrate their model using grids and graphics to facilitate the understanding of the different stages and of the internal and external factors influencing the recovery process (Ralph 2004).

Many external influences cannot be controlled by an individual but still have a positive or negative impact on the recovery process. These could be health policies, decisions and actions on the part of the mental health system and individuals who are in charge of financing and implementing services. Furthermore, there are social factors to be taken into consideration such as financial support, housing and work, as well as the natural supports of family and friends and community – the latter including religious organizations and like-minded individuals in either an organized or an informal way. All these factors can have an impact on the process of recovery and transformation of individuals affected by a mental condition. External obstacles can be, for example, discrimination, prejudice, stigmatization, forced treatment, lack of information about treatment effectiveness, poverty, homelessness, joblessness, absence of restricted health insurance coverage, lack of support and lack of understanding among family and friends (Ralph *et al.* 1999).

The Recovery Model was meant to serve a scientific purpose and was also aimed at service users, clinicians, funders, and health policy-makers who were searching for definitions and studies that could shed light on the subject of recovery. Additionally, the concept was supposed to gain entry into the treatment methods of traditional mental health services that had not yet been recovery oriented.

Ruth Ralph and her colleagues have made an enormous effort to provide valuable literature reviews on various recovery concepts, models and study outcomes as well as measures and instruments with which to assess recovery as process and outcome (Ralph 2000b; Ralph and Kidder 2000; Ralph, Kidder and Phillips 2000).

Examples of published recovery instruments

The Recovery Assessment Scale RAS

This scale has proven to be psychometrically stable with respect to its reliability and validity (Corrigan *et al.* 1999). The analysis of nearly 2000 completed RAS-inventories showed dimensions similar to earlier reports in the literature by distinguishing among among five factors (Corrigan *et al.* 2004; Ralph, Kidder, Phillips 2000).

1. personal confidence and hope;
2. willingness to ask for help;
3. goal and success orientation;
4. reliance on others;
5. symptom coping.

These analyses have revealed that while these factors can be distinguished from each other, they are linked in a rather complex fashion. Hope seems to play a key role in all of these dimensions. Recovery seemed to be more difficult the more a person is dominated by symptoms, even though this correlation was less clear than the connection between recovery, self-esteem and empowerment.

In a validation study in Australia (McNaught *et al.* 2007) the above listed five factors were replicated and the reliability and validity of the RAS as a measure of recovery was supported. The RAS is offering a measure that succeeds in capturing information that is possibly unique, and of quite considerable interest to consumers and clinicians.

The Recovery Process Inventory RPI

Like the RAS the development of this 22-item questionnaire was also based on the published literature, but the RPI has also benefited from the input and discussions of focus-groups composed of service users, and professional service providers (Jerrell *et al.* 2006) The stated aim of this group went beyond merely assessing whether someone considers himself to be 'in recovery'; it sought also to determine to what extent services had contributed to the process of recovery.

The six factors that have been identified in this study as crucial to recovery confirm the picture that has emerged from earlier work: fear and hopelessness, links to others, confidence, mutuality of relationships, a safe and adequate housing situation, hope and self-care. As in other studies, no clear-cut associations between demographic and diagnostic factors and recovery have been noted.

The Recovery Attitudes Questionnaire RAQ

The RAQ was developed collaboratively by a group of students and scientists with and without personal experience of recovery (Borkin *et al.* 2000). The questionnaire aims to measure the attitude of subjects towards the assumption that recovery from severe mental illness is possible.

In the course of its validation and in other studies with a variety of subjects this questionnaire turned out to be psychometrically solid. The first results were surprising in an interesting way. Professional helpers and service users are most clearly convinced about the possibility of recovery, and students the least. Professional service providers see a clear connection between their work and the possibility of recovery and can hardly imagine that recovery might be possible without professional intervention. On the other hand, relatives are most convinced of the possibility of recovery without professional help. The aspects which are connected to trust and faith reveal cultural differences. African-American respondents considered faith and trust in god as more relevant than any of the other groups.

A 21- and a 7-item version of this questionnaire can be ordered from the authors at the University of Cincinnati (*borkinjr@email.uc.edu; steffenjj@email.uc.edu*).

The Stages of Recovery Instrumet (STORI)

The Australian researchers Retta Andresen, Peter Caputi and Laindsay Oades developed the Stages of Recovery Instrument (STORI) in order to assess the process of recovery in its various stages. This instrument was published in 2006. A preliminary five-stage model based on consumer accounts had been developed in an earlier study by the same authors (Andresen *et al.* 2003). These authors had advanced a model of recovery based on consumers' personal accounts of their experiences and identified four key *component processes* of recovery: (i) finding and maintaining hope; (ii) the re-establishment of a positive identity; (iii) finding meaning in life, and (iv) taking responsibility for one's life. These data as well as the consolidated findings of several qualitative studies suggest the following five *stages* of recovery:

1. *moratorium*: a time of withdrawal characterized by a profound sense of loss and hopelessness;
2. *awareness*: realization that not everything is lost, and that a fulfilling life is possible;
3. *preparation*: taking stock of strengths and weaknesses regarding recovery, and starting to work on developing recovery skills;
4. *rebuilding*: actively working towards a positive identity, setting meaningful goals and taking control of one's life;
5. *growth*: living a full and meaningful life, characterized by self-management of the illness, resilience and a positive sense of self. (Andresen *et al.* 2006).

This stage model of four component processes and five stages – 'a model of the personal experience of psychological recovery' – assumes the stages to be sequential with 'growth' as the outcome of the recovery process and the component processes representing the psychological state of the person as he or she progresses through the stages of recovery. The model is purposely flexible in terms of the time-frame and the means by which the person moves through this process. That means: 'that each person may find his or her own sources of hope and ways of finding meaning and building a positive identity'. The authors refer to the accounts of consumers about the complex and non-linear nature of recovery, with relapse possible at even the highest level of recovery. Importantly, relapses and set-backs in no way mean that someone has returned to an earlier stage, but on the contrary are possible sources of resilience.

According to the authors, the stage model of recovery, when validated, could be used in research into the promotion of recovery as well as research into the education and training of helpers, consumers and carers.

In order to test the model, the authors looked for existing measures of recovery which were based on qualitative work with consumers, had been published in peer-reviewed journals and consisted of self-rated measures suitable for quantitative analysis. Two instruments met these criteria and were examined regarding their suitability for testing the stage model of recovery: the Recovery Assessment Scale (RAS) (Corrigan *et al.* 1999), and the Mental Health Recovery Measure (MHRM) (Young and Ensing 1999). A postal survey was conducted of 94 volunteers from the Neuroscience Institute of Schizophrenia and Allied Disorders (NISAD) that keeps the Schizophrenia Research Register, a database of people with schizophrenia who are interested in taking part in research. The participants completed the STORI and measures of mental health, psychological well-being, hope, resilience and recovery.

Ten themes were identified for each of STORI's five stages, and a number of items were generated to reflect each theme. The authors agreed on ten items to represent each of the five stages, resulting in a 50-item measure with five sub-scales. For example, we find in Stage 1 "moratorium" items such as "no hope of recovery" or "loss of meaning in life", in Stage 3 "preparation" items such as "re-discovering personal value" or "building confidence", and in Stage 5 "growth" items such as "optimism about the future" or "different, but improved self".

Positive correlations between STORI-allocated stage and other recovery-related measures demonstrate its validity. Individual stage sub-scales were found to be internally consistent and inter-correlation measures between the sub-scales supported construct validity. Efforts to enhance STORI's power to discriminate between stages of the model are under way. It is exciting to watch this work, which aims to describe the complexity of a recovery experience through this stage model and to make the model available to prospective study designs and combinations with traditional measures without losing its individuality. We agree with the authors, who conclude that 'the results provide prelimi-nary empirical support for the STORI as a measure of the patient experience of recovery. (. . .) The model has already proven valuable in clinical training and may provide a useful heuristic for clinical work and a framework for research. A single, relatively short measure capturing this complex construct would prove invaluable' (Andresen *et al.* 2006, p 979). Naturally, the development of new instruments is not the whole story. For recovery to serve as a goal and orientation, scientific research in psychiatry must be transformed and expanded with regard to its emphasis and its methods. One notable development in terms of assessment is the emergence of instruments aimed to measure the degree to which psychosocial services have advanced in their transformation towards a recovery focus (see also chapter 7). The bibliographies of recovery-related instruments at www.power2u.org can provide information about this subject as well as many others.

RECOVERY AS A PROCESS

Turning points – living with contradictions

We decided to describe a study from Scandinavia in more detail, since the author is one of the first researchers to have presented results from qualitative interviews with people in recovery. He illustrates in a very refined manner various recovery processes as experi-enced and described by the study participants. These experiences reflect a highly complex process with ups and downs, phases of relapse and turning points towards recovery.

Alain Topor from Stockholm presented in 2001 a comprehensive and well differenti-ated study on the complex subject of 'recovery'. His aim was to collect empirically all those variables that had been experienced as valuable and helpful by individuals in their own recovery process. The first part of his paper provides a well grounded survey of all earlier research on recovery processes from serious psychiatric disorders and also con-siders the problem of chronicity in depth. He distinguishes between outcome studies that consider 'complete recovery' and 'social recovery'. Topor points out that the proportion of individuals who experience recovery within traditional outcome studies depends on certain relatively unexpected factors, such as the fluctuation of national and local unem-ployment figures, diagnostic criteria, and access to psychiatric services. The introduction of certain treatment interventions during recent years seems to have had a beneficial effect on relapse rates, but no notable impact on recovery rates (Topor 2001 p 25).

The second, empirical part of Topor's study is an analysis of in-depth qualitative interviews with sixteen participants who had been in treatment for many years because of a serious psychiatric condition. Nine of the participants reported schizophrenia as 'their' diagnosis, two reported having the diagnosis affective psychosis, two 'schizoid', one paranoid psychosis, one personality disorder and one borderline psychotic personality. Participants in this study had been out of hospital for two years or more and considered themselves as 'recovered' or as engaged in a recovery-process. The study was conducted within the context of the Nordic Recovery Research Group and seven of the interviews were carried out by the author.

Topor and his research team analysed the interviews using the qualitative method of Glaser and Strauss's 'grounded theory'. The divergent meanings and subjective experiences of symptoms, the relevance of social relationships for stability and the positive development of each individual were among the important findings of this study. Material conditions as a basis for participation in communal life, the underlying subjective theories of illness and the explanatory models of the participants for their personal recovery/life-path were also subject to detailed analyses.

Based on the statements of participants, it became clear that they had struggled with symptoms and whatever may be causing them throughout the entire duration of their illness. Frequently, what appeared to those around them as signs of illness, were failed attempts at coping with existential problems. An important factor for recovery was becoming engaged in and maintaining social relationships. Professional helpers from all fields, family members and other lay individuals were able to contribute substantially to their recovery, in particular by representing continuity in the face of the multiple facets of a person's life. Certain providers became involved with the entire person in their full complexity, rather than reducing them to a diagnosis and patient-role. But at the same time, these important individuals did not deny the actuality of the person's suffering. The material conditions which influenced the extent to which a person could resume fully fledged participation in society were another important factor for recovery-work.

Subjective explanatory models

The author had the impression in many cases that, during the interview, possibly for the first time, the participants realized that there were certain connections between their illness and their life circumstances. It appeared that the author and his team may have been the first people to whom the participants had spoken about these experiences. Some of the comments showed that this was indeed true in several instances.

Subjects offered different explanations which helped them understand and categorize their own recovery experiences. These attributions were based on certain subjective explanatory models, which Alain Topor categorized on a meta-level into a psychotherapeutic, medical, spiritual and interactional model. Frequently, these models did not appear in their pure form, but rather in a blended fashion. In what way the four models apply to the participants of the study is described as follows:

The psychotherapeutic model: Individuals who were involved in psychotherapeutic treatment were the ones who made the clearest connections to their biography and childhood experiences. Frequently, negative childhood experiences had led to increasing problems during adolescence and ultimately to a breakdown. Those individuals connected their recovery closely to their psychotherapy, which often lasted for a number of years. Individuals who did not participate in psychotherapy had similar explanations. They tended to use elements from the culture they live in as building blocks in order to arrive at sensible interpretations and to make useful connections. Even though certain mental health advocacy groups in Sweden consider psychodynamic thinking to be ineffective and without any explanatory value, it is nevertheless firmly anchored in Swedish culture outside of psychiatry.

The medical model: All study participants were taking neuroleptic drugs which, nevertheless, they viewed with considerable scepticism. While none of the interviewees used the medical model to explain the causes of their problems, many still regarded medication as an important element of their recovery. No one referred exclusively to the medical model. If anything, they predominantly referred to one or more of the other models. The general population of Sweden and its psychiatric profession gives full credence to medical explanatory models.

The spiritual model: Many biographies talked of spiritual experiences being a source of meaning and sense, but rarely used them as an explanation for their illness. Spiritual experiences had become an important element in their recovery for several participants. It appeared that spiritual experiences and affiliation with a religious group could help people to cope with life and could suggest a path to a community outside of the psychiatric realm. Swedish psychiatry rejects the spiritual explanatory model, and instead considers it as the tip of an iceberg of underlying symptoms. Someone who tends to favour spiritual interpretations is not seen by psychiatry as having recovered from their illness. On the other hand, spiritual models occupy a strong position in Swedish culture outside of the psychiatric domain, for instance within religious communities.

The interactional model: The interactional model is rooted in commonsensical thinking. All the life stories offered by the participants contained descriptions of interactions with other people which had triggered – at least partially – the onset of the illness, as well as descriptions of interactions that influenced the duration of their illness and the recovery-process in multiple ways. Many narratives emphasized everyday direct interactions with other individuals that became important. Participants felt that spending time with 'ordinary' people was a meaningful thing. This included members of the provider team who had a comparatively lesser status in the hierarchy of professionals. Swedish culture as well as psychiatry consider interactional explanations as lay opinions and anecdotes of little scientific value.

One example from the interviews illustrates a combination of all four models: A man stated that he had experienced traumatic events during his childhood (psychotherapeutic model), but connected his first psychotic crisis with tensions in his marriage and with excessive work at his job (interactional model). In giving explanations about his recovery, he mentioned his close contact with one family member and a doctor with whom he had a good relationship (interactional model). He also mentioned his faith (spiritual model) and was of the opinion that he had finally been prescribed 'the right medicine' (medical model).

Stepping out of an old role – 'role exits'

The recovery stories in this analysis showed clearly that whenever they spoke about their recovery experiences, the subjects were describing a profound process of inner transformation. Alain Topor established a connection between the basic process of change and the concept of 'role exits', which had been proposed by Fuchs-Ebaugh (1988). She examined the processes which people go through when they leave behind the identity of an old role and establish a new one in a different role. To this end, Fuchs-Ebaugh examined different groups of individuals, such as nuns who were leaving their convents, transsexuals who were undergoing gender reassignment surgery, alcoholics who were joining AA, and doctors, police officers and seafarers who were leaving their professions more or less voluntarily. She did not interview people diagnosed with a mental illness.

Topor recognized the parallels between the processes these types of individuals were going through and the processes the group he was studying were undergoing. Generally speaking, a person passes through several phases: from the original identity, through a phase of leaving this identity but still carrying the signs of that role as an ex-patient, ex-nun, ex-police officer, etc, then into the new identity, which is reached when there is a full identification with the new role. Each person takes several steps as an 'ex' in the direction of the new role (Topor 2001, p 172 ff):

Growing uncertainty: The first step is taken when the current role is being put into question. The person unconsciously displays behaviours which indicate a willingness to change. Any further development depends largely on the way the environment responds to these first changes.

The search for alternatives: Given a positive response, the person feels encouraged to believe that he/she has the freedom to choose. A change in behaviours appears at the conscious level and the person looks around for individuals or groups that could reinforce the desired change.

The turning point: Gradually, or all of a sudden, something occurs which will eventually appear as a turning point. From this time the new role is played openly and the person's sensation of cognitive dissonance is reduced. New inner and external resources are being mobilized. The feeling of 'hanging in the air' prevails until the new identity has become solidified.

The role of an 'ex': Now the person has to prove him/herself in the new identity before others who had known them in the earlier role. New relationships are established as well, and people come into the person's life who are not familiar with the person in the old role. Now the person will also encounter and recognize individuals who have left the same role, and others who are still attached to the old role.

Fuchs-Ebaugh (1988) emphasizes that such an exit from an old role rarely happens smoothly. Even if the person makes a transition into a socially desirably role, he/she must be prepared for difficulties with their new environment. Assuming a new role feels tenuous or implausible, transitory at best. It seems impossible to leave the former role once and for all, and this causes many difficulties for the person who is making such a transition. Remnants of the old identity still have an impact on current expectations. The person is caught in an ongoing dilemma: Not admitting the earlier identity might seem like a lie, but holding on to those earlier activities could pose a risk to the current situation and the new role.

Topor arrives at commonalities and differences between the people examined by Fuchs-Ebaugh and his subjects, with their experiences of psychiatry. Their experiences are often reduced to a diagnosis. Large portions of their lives are affected by the condition. Their social network shrinks to a minimum, consisting primarily of family members, the treatment team and other patients. The recovery-process involves a role change not only among the persons with the diagnosis, but also among their family members, who have been reduced to a 'concerned family' and who now must re-organize their lives and broaden their social circle once again in order to experience recovery themselves.

Critical 'turning points'

In the narratives provided by his subjects, Alain Topor discovered important turning points that push the course of the illness in a different direction at a certain moment in time. Most subjects reported a sequence of initial events that were spiralling downwards. Only when the person had hit bottom, could the critical transformative event occur which is needed to induce an upward movement towards a fundamental, and not merely a super-ficial, change of self-perception and identity. Study participants experience the moment of 'hitting rock-bottom' with a great deal of anxiety, fears of death and abandonment, intense doubt about life in general, and disorienting feelings of being totally untethered and empty. Topor describes the various phases before and after such a turning point that many subjects have gone through in the following manner:

A fragile normality – a turn for the worse
Such narratives generally start out with a more or less regulated life. At the same time, certain aspects of the personality or certain situations were often mentioned that had threatened the semblance of normality. Participants were nevertheless able to sustain this state for a while. The first psychotic break generally occurred as a result of heightened tensions and contradictions within the person, or it was triggered by external events, or by a combination of both (for example, parents divorcing, lack of attention, doubts about life in general). The breakdown resulted from a collapse of hitherto effective coping strategies. The illusion of normalcy that had been maintained so far, caved in and the individual became involved with public institutions, most often with psychiatry, for the first time. For some, the admission to a psychiatric hospital is followed by a turn towards the positive, but for most a downward spiral is set in motion.

The downward spiral – hitting rock bottom
The personal narratives reveal stories of individuals who were forced to give up every-thing in order to find themselves. At the lowest point in the downward spiral feelings of totally relinquishing any motivation or a sense of identity seemed to prevail. A premature attempt to rise up again was likely to fail because the dismantling of an 'alien identity' was not complete and the new identity still rested on a faulty and brittle foundation. A state of total hopelessness was the point of departure for a solid foundation that enabled the person to gain strength once again. Many recovery narratives described this place at the very bottom as a new starting point. One interviewee explained this as follows:

> *'One thing's for sure: something helped to calm me down after I had gone through that process, had become crazier and crazier – for years I just kept getting crazier. I've learned a lot from that. I've learned that you have to get a lot more crazy before you can climb back up again. And that idea doesn't scare me anymore' (Susanne, Topor 2001, p 185).*

From another very troubled biography: After many mental breakdowns and inpatient stays a young woman named Irene experienced an apparent stabilization (a relationship, training, employment) and thought that she had made it through. But the foundation of her new self was not solid. At the age of 18 a rapidly downward spiral began once again until she crashed completely, overwhelmed by feelings of doom and destruction along with psychotic experiences, drug consumption, a life-threatening infection and the impending loss of her child. Only at this point, at the very bottom, four years later, did she experience an upward turn towards the positive.

Sometimes there was more than one downward turn, until the person finally landed all the way down, at the 'true' bottom. At such moments of collapse, when nothing seemed possible anymore, an inpatient stay and therapeutic support was experienced as helpful or even as a blessing. The person stood there without any type of protection, the facade that had covered up the void until now, had collapsed. The gap between a role and an actual identity could no longer be bridged. When a person talks about having landed at this point in their recovery narratives, they often recall an overwhelming feeling of hopelessness. A woman describes her feelings and her yearnings for protection and safety in a hospital as follows:

> '... When I got to the point where I couldn't keep up the façade any longer, that's when I went into hospital. They gave me sick leave first time around, but I had already decided I wanted to be admitted. I wanted 24-hours care' (Susanne, ibid., p 187).
>
> 'I saw everything as being completely hopeless... I didn't have much faith that I could ever come out of it as a whole person... but I didn't have any choice either... Stopping therapy and going back to the way it was before wasn't a real option for me... because I had already moved on. I couldn't go back... so I felt, like, all I could do was keep going... to the bitter end' (Susanne, ibid., p 188).

Turning point(s) upwards

Some participants reported that there were several turning points for the better. There were quite a few different kinds. Such a point could come rather quickly, or after decades of psychiatric care. It could be brought about by one's own strength or by virtue of an inadvertent event, for instance if someone made a particular effort on behalf of the person or when a series of chance events led to positive changes.

Even though reaching a turning point in life is usually part of a process of achieving maturity, several participants in the study reported unexpected events or situations that forced them to make a decision. Such events did not have the expected negative results, but rather served as a push in the right direction; they worked as a kind of catalyst. Service users might have encountered similar situations or individuals earlier in their lives, but they hadn't had the same kind of meaningful catalytic effect on them earlier. Such changes, as they were being recounted in the biographical narratives, had to do with an actual encounter. But the external circumstances alone did not account for the change. The significance of the event could more often be ascribed to the internal state of the individual, his/her personality and their subjective biography. The person recognized the situation as *the* opportunity and assigned his/her own meaning to it. The encounter turned into a mutually engaging creative process.

A turning point does not have to be a dramatic event. The key factor is that it should trigger a different perception of the individual in terms of their own life, their symptoms and their life circumstances. The ascent from the very bottom occurred in small increments, which reinforced the power to make important decisions in life. Several recovery narratives are about the strategy of small steps. A man described this process as follows:

> '... But then I thought to myself: I have got to try to do this a little bit at a time. I have just got to try to loosen the knots inside a little at a time, take small steps, so maybe I can get somewhere, that's what I thought to myself ... And things have loosened up. And I did it a little at a time, like. I succeeded in loosening the knots, I mean' (Sven, ibid., p 189).

The way up

Topor describes the ascent to the top as not being a direct or linear path. Cosmetic changes that had only to do with material circumstances (i.e. a job, a place to live), but which did not influence the self-perception and the identity of the individual, only led to superficial and temporary changes. Over time such external changes carried the risk of merely reinforcing the original dichotomy 'facade versus the actual self' and thereby causing the person to lose the ground under their feet once again. Relapse was a recurring theme in these recovery narratives and the people explained this by suggesting to themselves that they must have tried too early to lead a normal life, without having really sensed they had a solid foundation. Two participants expressed this in the following way:

> 'And after a while I got a new psychosis. You could say it was my own fault. I had been doing too much for the user movement and got too involved and didn't get enough rest and so it got all mixed up. I overdid it and wore myself out ... I think I spent too little time on myself. So I'm much more careful about that today. Somehow I've kind of felt that there's a point to all these psychotic experiences. They're not completely meaningless ...'(Jan, ibid., p 190).
>
> 'Yes, I feel that part of me is gone forever... it's just gone, like, and in another way I think it's like a long drawn-out rebirthing' (Susanne, ibid., p 191).

Finally, Topor emphasizes that a turning point is a radical transformation of an attitude, a change from utter hopelessness to the notion that the situation might be amenable to change. In actuality, a turning point is only achieved after taking many small steps. He concludes that rising from the bottom to the top does not mean arriving once again at the point of departure. The regained or revealed self is not the same as before. Some participants described this process as a kind of rebirth. Topor views the reconstruction of inner connections as a central element in the recovery-process, a guiding red thread that ties together the various aspects of a person's life inside and out and that shapes it into a coherent whole.

The central point: complexity

The analysis of these interviews reveals an overarching category, which Alain Topor calls 'complexity'. Its particular characteristic is the understanding that several things can happen at once, not that merely either one thing or another happens. This applies to each individual in recovery and to the people around them, as well as to the places where they are and to whatever it is that triggers and promotes recovery. The idea of complexity includes the possibility of being insane and rational, ill and healthy at the same time. These analytic categories contain contradictions. Alain Topor made a crucial and important point about these recovery-narratives when he suggested that a resolution of these contradictions was not the primary aim, rather one must find a way of living with them. Which means being able to experience life and oneself without too much pain along the way, and having the ability to deal with these kinds of contradictions.

According to Topor, the recovery-process seems to consist of events and coincidences that happen precisely when the individual is capable of using them for their own purpose and thereby emerging from the one-dimensional identity of a psychiatric patient towards a more complex understanding of oneself. It should be possible to increase the chances of such coincidences occurring, but they cannot be planned. One way might be to eliminate the element of isolation which is imposed on people who deviate from the norms set by society and by its institutions. It would be of paramount importance to offer such people a variety of possibilities and interventions which more closely reflect the plurality and diversity of human needs.

Findings from four countries

An article by Davidson *et al*. (2005c), which includes recovery-experts from Italy, Norway, Sweden and the USA, presents the results of an international study on the varying processes of recovery. The interdisciplinary team was composed of researchers from the fields of psychiatry, psychology, social work and occupational therapy. The study was based on complex qualitative interviews with individuals who had long-standing psychiatric conditions. Their diagnoses included schizophrenia, major depression with psychotic features and paranoid psychosis. Participants had a variety of experiences of both general, everyday life and of using mental health services. All participants had been admitted to psychiatric settings ranging from in-patient care in hospitals to respite care provided by 24-hour community centres, some for extended periods. One participant spent many years homeless on the streets. The interviewees considered themselves as 'recovered' or reported that they were in the process of recovery. At the time of the study they had not been hospitalized for two years.

Twelve participants from centres in the above mentioned four countries completed in-depth interviews and other qualitative measures. The interviews were transcribed and translated into English. The researchers used consensus-groups to identify key themes, which emerged in the following areas: 1) how the individual deals with his or her difficulties; 2) the role of material resources; 3) the various roles of formal and informal health systems; 4) the roles, and absence, of significant others, and 5) the roles of social and cultural factors. The authors began their article with a quote from a young man who had been diagnosed with schizophrenia:

> 'At the bowling alley it doesn't matter if you're mentally ill, if you're a foreigner, an asthmatic, a dyslexic... In a bowling match everyone's a bowler.

*It's the number of strikes that counts, nothing else' (Davidson et al. 2005c,
p 178).*

By using this quote the research team emphasized a frequently overlooked aspect of
recovery, namely how people spend their time every day of their lives. The example
from the bowling alley shows, as many others do too, that recovery refers also, or
even mainly, to the way a person with psychotic experiences spends their day-to-day
life. Obviously, such a life takes place largely away from psychiatric institutions and
services, for instance in communal settings such as bowling alleys.

In the following we will summarize the main findings from the analysis of these
interviews.

How the person deals with his or her problems:

Most persons go through a long process which gradually reveals to them that the illness
has brought something new into their life, which they have to confront, lest it dominate
and destroy their entire life. Many were not prepared for this challenge, did not know
anything about mental illnesses or had misconceptions about them. Several elements had
to be present if they were to cope in a constructive fashion. Above all, there had to be
hope for the possibility of a different and better life. Carol, a study participant from the
USA, described it in this way:

*'Hope of knowing that everything that is, that I go through, would not continue
the rest of my life, that there would be an end of it; and just knowing that I
knew that, I could keep going' (ibid. p 184).*

Other factors were the wish to get better; having faith in oneself and having the ability
to move forward and to take on the difficult task of rebuilding oneself step by step, and
at the same time be able to bear the fact that outsiders might see all of your efforts
as trivial and negligible. For the participants themselves each of these little steps was a
major accomplishment, requiring patience and steadfastness. Other important conclusions
were the need to become focused on the present, planning the next required steps and
setting reachable short-term goals (for example, getting up in the morning, writing down
a recipe, signing up for a course). Such things must be taken care of by the person
and cannot be taken over by others, even if they mean well. Such small steps enable
individuals to gradually rebuild their capacities, competencies and talents and thereby
see themselves as more worthwhile.

It was very important to learn, with the help of information, psychotherapy, self-help
materials, the internet, or through one's own 'experimentation', to distinguish between
those aspects of one's experience that were tied to the illness (for example, difficulties
remembering) and those that belonged to everyday life. In order to once again lead a
normal life, it was important to do normal things, such as going to school, finding work,
making friends, having intimate relationships, participating in social and leisure activities,
and to accept that there is such a thing as a 'normal' life outside of the illness with its
own ups and downs, and its own joys and disappointments.

The role of material resources:

It was helpful for a person to have a private and safe place where they could carry out the above mentioned activities, and where they could spend time by themselves and replenish their strengths. A place to which they could retreat was especially helpful when a person experienced active hallucinations. Unfortunately, just this kind of private, personal space may be lost due to psychosis (for example, the person has become homeless) or has yet to be achieved as part of becoming independent. Living at home with family, in a supportive residence, a shared apartment or a psychiatric institution often means lacking such a space for retreat as it has been described by a participant.

> 'I spend a lot of time on my own because I have an enormous need to unwind and chill out. To recharge my batteries ... when I'm around people I get so worked up that I need time to calm down, so that when I spend time with people I like to retire early because I need several hours of peace and quiet on my own before I can go to bed' (ibid. p 188).

Participating in important and everyday activities, such as starting a training programme, getting a cup of coffee or seeing a movie, were helpful in that they lent structure to otherwise empty time. And it was also helpful to experience meaningful activities, and to feel joy and pleasure – all these things contributed to a positive sense of self-worth and belonging. Carol (USA) explained:

> 'Having joy is one way to stay out of depression' (ibid. p 189).

Not everyone could engage in such activities, especially if they were short of funds. Being financially dependent on the state or on a poorly paid job meant having only limited access to these positive resources. The self-worth of participants was compromised if they had to accept the status of being 'permanently disabled' in order to receive a disability pension, or were employed below their qualifications.

Roles of formal or informal health systems:

Participants considered those mental health professionals as being the most helpful, who had the ability to listen and to follow, rather than lead, and who allowed the person to make his or her own decisions, along with any mistakes that might be part of that. It was also experienced as helpful when the professionals genuinely cared about them and when they communicated the attitude and expectation, that the consumers were capable of doing many things themselves towards their own recovery. Such a therapeutic attitude makes people feel accepted; they sense a respect for their own desires and decisions. Unfortunately, such therapeutic positions were encountered only infrequently, as illustrated by the statement of interviewee Kari from Norway:

> 'When you are allowed to make mistakes as you go along, without being corrected all the time, then you realize that what you are doing is not such a good idea' (ibid. p 191).

It still appears to arouse resistance among professionals when a patient seeks affirmation, and wants to be recognized and accepted as a person and as someone who has something to offer. Most of their training still emphasizes problems and deficits rather than the capacities and successes of the patients.

Communicating with peers, whom the participants encountered in a great variety of psychiatric and psychosocial services, was of great importance. While the relationships in formal health services are of a rather hierarchical nature, the informal, private environment of the participants was filled with mutual support and encouragement. Whenever they could help others and assume an important role in their lives, this had an especially positive impact on their self-worth. Jan, a participant from Sweden:

> 'By helping others, you're not totally worthless. Like, it's a natural, human characteristic that if you're able to help others then you're worth something ... It's essential to life for people to feel necessary. ... Giving something to someone else makes you worth something yourself' (ibid. p 193).

The meaning and the absence of significant others:

Davidson et al. (2005c) found the reasons for the fact that individuals with psychotic experiences tend to support each other and help others, which in turn enhances their sense of belonging, in several of the interviewees: participants often felt isolated and lonely, and had few friends or acquaintances outside of their family or their peers in psychiatric services. The feeling of basic abandonment was qualitatively different from just feeling a bit alone for a spell, as Tisha, a participant from the USA, describes:

> 'To wake up and to feel nothing. Just, you know, I can walk endlessly forever and not, not know where I'm going or what I'm doing. I just feel like I wake up and there's nothing there ... When I'm alone a lot I have flashbacks' (ibid. p 194).

In certain instances, family members or friends could lessen this sense of being abandoned or they could respond to the person's need for acceptance or attention; other interviewees assigned these functions to God or some hallucinated other (such as voices). A few had pets which took over this function.

The roles of social and cultural factors:

The authors could not identify any significant social or cultural differences concerning the recovery-process as described by the interviewees. In other words, there were no fundamental differences between these four countries in terms of the individual needs to deal with psychoses and the associated limitations, and the need to compensate for and overcome such limitations. The authors attribute the lack of fundamental differences to the fact that Anglo-Saxon or Western European cultural characteristics are found in each of the four countries and thus influence the nature of mental illness across these cultures. The only differences they did find were in the actual environment that played a role in recovery, i.e. the social and cultural factors operating in that environment. Different experiences were reported depending on the availability of certain services and opportunities. Participants in Italy spent more time talking about their work situations, while Swedes focused on their activities in clubhouses and user-organizations. North-American interviewees mentioned their participation in advocacy organizations more often.

Participants from all four countries found it important to speak about their experiences of their illness and their inclusion or exclusion from community. Experiences of stigmatization and rejection by their own families were considered especially troubling and destructive for their own lives and for their prospects of recovery. In contrast, the following factors played an important part in the recovery-process: the experience of having one's rights respected; being listened to and taken seriously (for example, with respect to taking medication); being informed about one's rights; rebuilding a positive social identity; finding meaningful work; having experiences of success; establishing new contacts, and ultimately, finding the way back to a normal life in society.

The authors conclude that the interviews showed the lives of the participants moving back and forth, at various points in time, and to varying degrees, between health and psychosis. Accordingly, the categories of "sick" and "well", or "ill" and "normal" may not be as clear cut or categorical as they appear to be in the clinical literature. These narratives lie closer to the consumer end of the spectrum on recovery, emphasizing more the process than the outcome.

Identity and recovery in personal accounts of mental illness

Including recovery as a topic of research into personal accounts is a new and promising scientific path. Jennifer Wisdom from Columbia University and her colleagues (2008) examined 'identity-related themes' in published self-narratives of family members and individuals with serious mental illness. The authors chose 45 personal accounts from people with severe mental illness and family members which were published in two prominent research journals (*Schizophrenia Bulletin* and *Psychiatric Services*) in the years between 1998 and 2003 and analyzed them qualitatively.

The personal account writers wrote about the negative effects of mental illness on their perception of themselves and their family members which needed to be overcome, or at least managed, for recovery to become possible. Writers described, in the order of prominence:

a) a loss of self;
b) the duality of (ill/well) selves;
c) perceptions of normality;
d) specific concerns about parenting and identity, and
e) hope and reconciliation.

Loss of self

The researchers point out that in this phase, writers often described the onset of mental illness as "taking away a person's sense of self". For many writers, this resulted in the loss of their previously held identity. Prominent themes at this stage were lack of hope and focus on symptoms and illnesses. According to the authors, these writers seemed to have internalized longstanding patterns of belief and negative expectations regarding prognoses for serious mental illnesses. This was illustrated by several examples (Wisdom *et al.* 2008):

Example from Ben-Dor (2001):

> '*My son was already long gone, dying bit by bit over the 16 years of his battle with schizophrenia . . . I had never had a real chance to say goodbye to David. He had disappeared into his illness so slowly, imperceptibly*' *(ibid., p 491)*.

Example from Hartmann (2002):

> '*. . . For me [depression] has always been more than a disease: it has taken my self-esteem, confidence, and pride, heaved them into a swamp of worth-lessness, confusion, and frequently, utter hopelessness*' *(ibid., p 491)*.

The duality of (ill/well) selves

In this section, the authors worked out that other writers described themselves 'in terms of dichotomies that maintained perceptions of their real, authentic selves, separating those from the alternative selves that were present during a bad episode'. The alternate selves were regarded as part of who they were, but were separated as parts 'that they did not much like or were ashamed to show the world'. Simultaneously, it was possible for these individuals to retain a sense of their authentic identities as well as 'a sense of hope for rebuilding'. This is clearly illustrated in the quotations from the writers below (Wisdom *et al.* 2008, p 491).

Example from Williams (1998):

> '*Someone answering to my name was once a terrified, angry person who was showing up in emergency rooms nearly every night and throwing up into a basin, or was being looked for regularly by the police when threat-ening suicide. . . . But that wasn't the real me. That's not who I want to be. Nor are the other people who are seen through the pathology of borderline personality disorder showing their real selves*' *(ibid., p 491)*.

Example from Goldowsky (2003):

> '*My sociologist friend reminded me that we are not only mental patients, we are also writers, doctors, fishermen, husbands, wives, and children. For so many of us, mental problems are really just a fragment of our being. But sometimes societal pressures make our condition a self-fulfilling prophecy*' *(ibid., p 492)*.

Striving for normalcy

The study found out, that for many writers it was a primary goal to be 'normal' and to lead a 'normal life'. Having a mental illness made them feel 'abnormal'. They had the strong desire to become normal, and some had a sense of hopelessness that 'although they may be able to "act normal", they would never truly be normal'. The authors found different definitions of being normal, some people defined themselves as not normal solely because they had a mental illness. One person who had recently been diagnosed with bipolar affective disorder reported that 'everyone treated him differently because of his mental illness' (Wisdom *et al.* 2008, p 492):

Example from Parker (2001):

> *'Whether it was stigma from my peers, stigma perpetuated by the profession-*
> *als "helping" me, or the self-stigma I experienced, any chance at having a*
> *semblance of a normal life seemed lost' (ibid., p 492).*

Using a quotation from a mother whose son committed suicide, the authors illustrate the "identity dilemmas" in which individuals struggling with mental health problems are often involved. The authors describe this dilemma clearly and powerfully: "To behave in ways other than what are perceived to be correct, risks losing others' perceptions of one's valuable self, and interferes with one's ability to belong. What then, does a person with severe mental illness do when it is not possible to behave correctly at all times? These are some of the most difficult tasks associated with healing, recovering, and establishing an identity that encompasses these past experiences while supporting personal hope and growth" (Wisdom *et al.* 2008, p 492).

Specific concerns about parenting and identity

In some of the writers' accounts the authors could see that it was particularly painful, in connection with their sense of identity, to make decisions about whether or not to become parents. Those individuals who made the difficult choice not to have children often felt regret or felt unfulfilled. Those who felt unable or unwilling to take the risk of having children experienced themselves as having fewer role and identity options (ibid., p 492).

Example from Perkins (2003):

> *'Feeling doubtful was my constant state of mind when I considered issues*
> *of pregnancy and parenthood. . . . My mother tried to soothe my pain and*
> *told me I was still a loving person and that not giving birth to my own child*
> *didn't make me any less of a woman. She said I shouldn't need a baby to*
> *feel complete and that I was deserving and worthy of a loving husband.*
> *However well intentioned she might have been, I interpreted her words as*
> *meaning that I absolutely wouldn't ever be able to have a stable life with*
> *children and that the sooner I accepted that fact, the better off I would be.*
> *I was left feeling even more patronized and unworthy' (ibid., p 492).*

Hope and reconciliation

The authors discovered that some writers maintained a sense of hope despite the challenges related to their changing senses of self and identity. The individuals maintained the hope that they would continue to make progress in 'reclaiming their old selves or in developing new identities'. Some of the writers indicated hope 'that the "essence" of self would return', and one woman struggled with reconciling the 'thought-voices' that were part of herself (Wisdom *et al.* 2008, p 493), as illustrated in the following quotations:

Example from Greenblat (2000):

> *'I wonder sometimes, as I grow even healthier, if the voices will fade away completely. Will I miss them? Having lived with them for so many years, I wonder if it will feel empty or lonely without them. Thought-voices are part of who I am, and what makes me unique. With what will I replace them? I believe I will find other ways to be unique. Can I do it? I believe so. I am willing to try' (ibid., p 493).*

Example from Hartmann (2002):

> *'Hope, sometimes even blind hope, must somehow be grasped. It is best grasped not by a lone sentry of the night, but within true community: a place to go, to feel worthy, to nourish a self-respect: a job, a friend, a neighbour, a lover. This is the true lifeblood, and it is this that incessant mental disease steals' (ibid., p 493).*

The authors of the study come to the conclusion that the narratives they analyzed confirm the central role of identity transformations, both positive and negative, taking place in the recovery process in the context of mental illness. They point out that challenges to individuals' sense of self and sense of self-worth were significant. Furthermore, they emphasize that much work needs to be done to include 'positive voices of recovery' in published personal accounts of mental illness. Because of the importance of hope in the literature on recovery, they believe it is important to recognize and remedy the relative absence of hope in personal accounts of recovery. The lack of hope indirectly reflects ongoing community beliefs that include low expectations and little likelihood of success for those with mental illnesses. Therefore, hope could be an important catalyst in the recovery-process for patients with mental illnesses, their relatives and clinicians.

The researchers' conclusions also contain a call for the publication of more personal accounts that focus on strengths-based, patient-centred stories, rather than on deficits. Messages of hope, strength, and encouragement are greatly needed, and clinicians could assist in providing these messages: 'A positive life is possible for patients suffering from mental illness, and recovery narratives have the potential to convey this message' (ibid., p 494).

Recovery as lived in everyday practice

Marit Borg and Larry Davidson (2008) carried out a qualitative research study in which they explored how individuals with severe mental illnesses experience the illness and its consequences within the context of their daily lives, and how they overcome these challenges and other barriers to find their place, a sense of meaning, and a valued social role as members of their community. In this study, narrative phenomenological methods were used, based on interviews with individuals in recovery. Refering to their research results, the authors conclude that conceptualizing recovery in severe mental illness within the context of everyday life may offer the opportunity to understand mental health problems as an integrated part of people's lives. This way, recovery unfolds within the context of 'normal' environments and activities. Consequently, the authors recommend to clinicians that everyday life expertise should be included on the practitioners' agenda.

This study was intended to 'contribute to an increasing knowledge-base that attempts to explore, understand, and address severe mental health problems within a person's everyday life'. Such attempts should arise from a profound curiosity about the person, who continues to exist behind, beneath, or beside a severe mental illness and about how the problems and challenges that are associated with the illness are experienced and addressed by this person within the context of his or her everyday life' (Borg and Davidson 2008, p 130) acknowledging the impact of little things in a person's life, such as meals, birthdays, or recreation; experiences and events which might otherwise be overlooked in studies that focus merely on illness and impairment (Davidson et al. 2006). Daily life is considered by the authors as the place for people's acts and interactions with other persons. With Gullestad (1989) the authors refer, firstly, to organizational and functional aspects of daily life such as concrete organizations of tasks and activities. A second dimension is the 'experienced daily life'. Phenomenologists such as Husserl (1970) have described this as the 'Lebenswelt' (life world), intending to convey what is important to the person beyond recorded facts or events.

Assuming a dynamic process of individual, material and social issues and that the person is an active agent, Borg and Davidson (2008) come to the conclusion that once we realize the importance of this sphere of everyday life and its various components, our major challenge as researchers and clinicians would lie in 'making explicit, capturing, and recognizing the simplicity as well as the complexity of daily life among individuals with severe mental illnesses' (p 131).

Seven women and six men were interview partners in phenomenological-approach, in-depth qualitative interviews about their experiences, material and social situations, actions and choices. The study included participants who a) had a permanent place to live; b) considered themselves as being in recovery or having recovered from severe mental illness; c) were coping satisfactorily with their lives, and d) who had improved their lives with the help of mental health services and/or from other sources. The participants had various histories, and various experiences with different types of services and support systems and lived in varied social situations. Their ages ranged from 26 to 54 years, two were married, two were engaged, nine were single, two had children, six had higher education, and two had ordinary jobs and an income, while the others were receiving disability payments but were all working part-time. Several had, or had had, financial problems that were considered as a hindrance to living a meaningful life in the community. In terms of clinical diagnoses, ten participants had been treated for schizophrenia, one for reactive psychosis, one for manic depression, and one for paranoia. The time since the onset of illness ranged from under ten to over 35 years.

The research process included a reference group of five individuals with recovery-experiences who were involved in project design, interview content, inclusion criteria, and ongoing discussions during the analysis phase. The authors evaluated the contribution of the reference group as highly important because its input of first-hand knowledge and expertise resulted in a more comprehensive understanding of lived experience and its context.

Thematic and step-wise analyses identified four major themes: 1) Being normal, 2) Just doing it, 3) Making life easier, and 4) Being good to yourself.

Being normal

Normality had a very concrete and practical meaning in the participants' stories, as in 'spending time in ordinary environments with ordinary people'. Daily life activities that are usually taken for granted, when experienced as difficult become embarrassing, troublesome, and annoying. One participant described her struggles with daily life activities, such as shopping, cleaning, paying bills:

> 'Ah, I would describe it [recovery] probably as functioning as normal, in terms of ... I work and that takes a big, big chunk of my time and energy, probably too much. I am married, and that's a big chunk that, yeah a very central part. I think the normal things of hanging on and doing those things we have to do, like shopping and cleaning and paying bills and having resources to keep living' (Borg and Davidson 2008, p 132).

It can be a struggle to manage the consequences of mental illness in a way that allows you to maintain life in a normal setting, as illustrated by the example of Nina, who 'tired easily, but she found her ability to cope nonetheless to be quite gratifying'. To take over responsibility for 'all kinds of practical things' is a struggle and frightening for her at times. But she wouldn't like to live her life in any other way and 'felt pleasure and pride in being independent and accepted the worries associated with this'.

'Being normal' also meant 'being situated in ordinary social settings and environments, and fulfilling ordinary roles, such as being with parents, siblings, or spouses and children'. For many participants family life represented a sense of continuity and stability and offered regular contact and activities. Visiting and helping each other in practical ways was part of family life. It was not necessarily the person with mental health problems who received support. Giving and taking in more general terms was emphasized and this mutual interchange seemed to be based more on traditional family patterns than illness-related roles. Taking your share of daily responsibilities, especially in relation to other people, even at times of crisis is often possible and can be essential.

Having a job in an ordinary setting as opposed to a sheltered occupation was experienced as valuable and meaningful, and as giving people a chance to spend at least part of their time in situations that both provide and expect a normality that is shared with others.

In summary, 'being normal' is signified on the one hand by 'stepping out of the problematic areas of their lives' (for example, psychiatric settings) and on the other hand 'to be just an ordinary person carrying out ordinary activities' and thus 'being one of the (normal) crowd as opposed to being a mental patient among other mental patients'.

Just doing it

Being in recovery can 'require the person to do something concrete in order to improve his or her situation', for example:

> *'I identify with the Nike slogan: 'Just do it!' Just do it! It's about having to do it. Yeah, really... I probably think about the things that I don't think it is, and that about when someone else decides for me... When I read about recovery written as goal-driven... that can only be written by practitioners because how many of us get up in the morning and say: How am I going towards my goals today? That is not something that you do' (Borg and Davidson 2008, p 134).*

'Continuing to believe in their capacity to recover' people find sources of hope, pathways towards a better life. As was suggested in the quotation above, the practicalities of recovery can be summed up as 'just doing it' in the sense of 'being creative in dealing with your problems, looking again and again for new solutions, and discovering what works for you' (Borg and Davidson 2008, p 134).

The participants reported positive expectations of others towards them which were experienced as helpful, for example, a husband who does not accept his wife staying in bed all day and a 'family who had never given up and who continued to expect her to get well and despite her distress, expected her to get up every morning to take care of the house and her children'.

For some participants, 'accepting that they had mental health problems meant accepting limitations in their lives, not being able to take part in as much as they used to or would have liked to do'. 'Just doing it' can mean finding pleasure in managing small tasks and 'little things' and carrying on in spite of the times when you are worrying about becoming ill again.

Making life easier

Other people – as well as coping strategies and certain situations – were experienced as helpful in terms of 'making life easier'. Mental health professionals who were available, who recognized the need for assistance or support in all kinds of practical matters, and who did not give the impression of primarily being interested in symptoms and problems were highly valued. Having service systems available also made life easier, for example, for Martin, who experienced a sense of security in a special hospital ward:

> *'Yes, I've used one ward at the hospital as an asylum, collaborate with them when problems get worse. I've got a deal when I can go there without all kinds of bureaucracies. I can just call and then go there' (Borg and Davidson 2008, p 135).*

Another aspect of life that was seen as being helpful was having adequate material and instrumental resources, for instance, having a home you could feel safe in and take pleasure in. The participants described their home as a place where they could relax and find peace, which they decorated and furnished in their own way, and which was a safe place and a 'platform from where they could enter into the larger community and encounter and form relationships with the community, for example, going for a walk in the park, going to work, to church, going to swim or bicycle, or to meet friends'.

Finding out what makes life easier is not always easy but it is often a big help to people on their journey to recovery.

Being good to yourself

Participants mentioned a variety of situations that 'created good feelings, gave peace for a shorter or longer period of time, or gave pleasant memories' and talked about 'spoiling yourself, giving yourself a treat, and taking care of your body'. One participant described it in her own words:

> 'I feel I get so much back for the good experiences, and I can take them up again if I feel down and low, then I can think about the good moments. I find good experiences so important. You get much more out of them than things and that kind . . . ' (Borg and Davidson 2008, p 137).

Other examples of 'being good to yourself' were building up and maintaining vital bodily processes and preventing illness by taking vitamins and supplemental nourishment; a solitary activity, for example, watching TV alone, meditation, listening to music; meeting friends, and travelling with friends. Concentrating on a healthy life-style meant physical exercise, healthy food and a sensible diet.

In the narratives in this study, the wish to give back, to share their experiences through writing or talks, and to offer advice and practical help to others was a prominent theme. This is interesting because usually patients and clients have been viewed as being on the receiving end of relationships with others, and rarely have had the opportunity to give back. 'Being good to yourself' may also involve being good to others.

In summary, the authors propose that this study has the following four implications for practice (Borg and Davidson, 2008 p 138f):

1. Recovery is inevitably a social process as well as an integrated part of the person's daily life. It is these small bits of life that are often experienced as being of critical importance during an individual's recovery-process.
2. People experiencing severe mental illness do not report a life-history characterized by having lost their overall ability to function. Rather they describe a life full of interests, skills, and expertise which they had acquired before the onset of illness, and which remained useful to them in their recovery.
3. Ordinary environments and activities emerged as the most effective places for recovery, in contrast to mental health service settings. In these ordinary places the participants could keep their position and role as a family member, a friend or a neighbour, as opposed to becoming only a "mental patient".
4. Rehabilitation and treatment programmes should elicit, listen to, and appreciate 'both the dramas and the trivialities of everyday life, as well as the individual's own expertise in managing these tasks'. Quite apart from the assessment of suffering and difficulties,

and from applying traditional interventions such as medication and psychotherapy, it may have an equally therapeutic function to support a person in his/her practical, material, instrumental, and social life areas, and environmental accommodations.

Qualitative research as one royal road

The detailed and informative review article of Davidson *et al*. (2008), entitled 'Using qualitative research to inform mental health policy', gives examples of different ways in which qualitative methods have informed mental health policy. The authors, who come from the USA, Canada, Sweden and Norway, emphasize the increasing importance of promoting recovery in mental health policy so that it will lead, it is hoped, to the transformation of mental health systems in the future. The authors argue that since the individuals' own first-hand perspectives play a central role in the recovery-process, qualitative methods will become increasingly useful in psychiatric research, 'as psychiatry shifts away from symptom reduction to enabling people to live satisfying, hopeful, and meaningful lives in the community' (Davidson *et al*. 2008, p 137).

The authors highlight the following arguments in favour of qualitative methods:

- Qualitative methods have reached 'a sufficient degree of maturity and rigour' to inspire quantitative researchers who start asking what qualitative research can do for them. Likewise, practitioners are eager for clinically relevant research and policy-makers are searching for useful data.
- The 'recent shift to recovery as the overarching aim of mental health care' creates a policy environment that might be highly receptive to qualitative studies of the lives of persons with serious mental illnesses.

The authors identified three initial uses of qualitative methods:

a) The first use was to generate hypotheses to be tested by other, often quantitative, means. The example used to illustrate this little contested use of qualitative methods concerns early findings about the now well recognized problem of the access to health care for service users who live in the community. This problem had already been picked up in initial studies of de-institutionalization, which explored concerns about the real-life experiences of people in transition between long-stay hospitals and the community (Davidson *et al*. 1996).

b) Qualitative research could be aimed at exploring the subjective experience and everyday lives of people with mental illnesses, in the tradition of the pioneering work of Sue Estroff (1989) and John Strauss (1989 a and b). In 2008 these two researchers impressively remind us that it is questionable 'whether a field that systematically ignores a considerable amount of data can be considered an adequate science' (Strauss 2008).

Davidson *et al. (2008)* refer to the groundbreaking work of the Yale Longitudinal Study (Strauss *et al*. 1985) in establishing the 'principle of the non-linearity of course' and essential new insights into the complexity of the interaction between the environment and the individual – discoveries with major implications for policy-makers and systems of care. The same authors also refer to qualitative studies in Scandinavia which had a similar impact for clinical practice in a different, but similarly important area. The discovery of how important it was to 'break the rules' (Borg and Kristiansen, 2003) in Scandinavia, which means stepping outside the traditional roles and therapeutic boundaries of the therapist-client relationship, brought about important discussions and adaptations to the rules of and the opportunities for therapeutic relationships. (See also the section on recovery-oriented professional helpers in chapter 7).

Davidson *et al*. (2008) highlight another very large qualitative study which aimed to change policy to do with the reform of psychiatric practice in the direction of promoting recovery based provider performances. The study was the 'What Helps and What Hinders Recovery Project' (Onken, Dumont and Ridgway *et al*. 2002). The study not only produced clear descriptions of elements of the mental health system which promote recovery, for example, having valued choices and the support of peers, but also of those that hinder recovery-processes, for example, stigmatization and abuse of power. In a second phase of the study a set of items were generated and tested which served as recovery performance indicators, and a 42-Item Consumer Self-Report Survey and a 19-Item Administrative Data Set were produced (Dumont, Ridgway, Onken *et al*. 2006).

c) Qualitative research could be used to understand recovery and the active role of the individual with the disorder in order 'to define and delineate what is meant by the term recovery in relation to serious mental illness and to identify and describe the various ways in which the person with the disorder can play an active role in his or her recovery' (Davidson *et al*. 2008, p 141). In Davidson's (2003) own qualitative studies on people in recovery, who are trying to live their everyday lives, it emerged, for example, that people invest a considerable amount of their available energy on efforts 'to look or pass for normal' and on efforts 'to restore order, meaning, a sense of routine, and normality to their everyday lives'.

CHAPTER 7

Recovery – Implications for Clinical Responsibilities

While much of recovery is lived outside clinical settings there clearly are important responsibilities for clinicians in supporting and assisting people with mental health problems in their efforts towards making full use of their health and resilience, and achieving their goals in life. For services and mental health workers recovery-orientation not only means fighting for a system that is able to offer everyone evidence-based interventions – currently only available to a small proportion of people with severe mental illness (Anthony, Rogers and Farkas 2003) – it also means accepting that what is essential for one person's recovery will not necessarily work for the majority of patients. Sometimes it is the very specific and individual approaches that are the most effective.

Patient self-determination, individual choice of flexible ways of support and opportunities, interventions aimed at promoting empowerment and hope, and assistance in situations of calculated risk are the new indicators of the quality of services. In contrast to a deficit model of mental illness, recovery-orientation includes a focus on health promotion, individual strengths, and resilience. A shift from demoralizing prognostic scepticism towards a rational and optimistic attitude towards recovery, and broadening treatment goals beyond symptom reduction and stabilization require specific skills and new forms of co-operation between practitioners and service users, between mental health workers of different backgrounds, and between psychiatry and the public. New rules for services, for example, user involvement and person-centred care, as well as new tools for clinical collaborations, for example, shared decision-making and psychiatric advance directives, are being complemented by new proposals regarding more ethically consistent anti-discrimination and involuntary treatment legislation and participatory approaches to evidence-based medicine as well as evidence-based policy (Rose *et al.* 2006).

The following chapter will cover new forms of communications between mental helth workers, users and carers and collaborations between professionals with and without a lived experience of mental health problems and treatments. Models of sharing expertise and developing alternatives will be presented in brief overviews of exciting international developments. Data and initiatives on recovery-oriented relationships between users of services and professional helpers as well as examples of recovery-oriented programmes, services and system transformation initiatives will highlight relevant and actual changes in how clinical responsibilities take shape in an era of recovery.

SHARING

Trialogue

'Trialogue' (Amering *et al.* 2002) or 'psychosis seminar' (Bock and Priebe 2005) are both terms which are used to describe an innovative development which has long been exclusive to the German-speaking countries. In trialogue groups, users, carers and mental health workers meet regularly to have an open discussion that is located on 'neutral terrain' – outside any therapeutic, familial or institutional context – with the aim of communicating about, and discussing the experiences and consequences of, mental health problems and ways to deal with them. The groups also function as a basis and starting point for trialogic activities at different levels (for example, serving on quality control boards) and different topics (for example, a work group on religion and psychosis) and activities (for example, a trialogic day in the training of police officers with regard to interacting with people with mental health problems). In German-speaking countries, trialogues are regularly attended by approximately 5,000 people. Trialogues are inexpensive, a great number of people seem to benefit from participation, and the movement has certainly brought about concepts and language different from the still widely prevalent narrow discourse of the medical model of mental health and illness. It is a new and exciting form of communication, an opportunity to gain new insights and knowledge, a chance to interact beyond role stereotypes, and a training ground for working together on an equal basis. Participants learn to accept each other as 'experts by experience' and 'experts by training'. In other words, they learn skills that are well suited to recovery-oriented work as well as to the involvement of users in therapeutic and service development decisions (Slade *et al.* 2008). The scientific evaluation of trialogues with regard to process and possible outcomes poses conceptual and methodological challenges and is in its fledgling stages.

Open Dialogue

In an open dialogue (OD) family-and-network approach, patients with psychosis are treated almost exclusively in their homes. The patient's social network is involved right from the start, within 24 hours of the first contact with the patient. The same team has responsibility for the entire treatment process, even if the setting changes. The main aim is to generate dialogue with the family and to construct a language, a way of talking about the experiences that occur when there are psychotic symptoms. In Finnish Western Lapland, in a historical comparison, five-year follow-ups of two groups of first-episode patients with non-affective psychosis were compared. One group had been treated using the OD approach, the other one had been treated before the introduction of the OD approach. Amongst the group who had been treated using the fully developed OD approach, the mean duration of untreated psychosis was found to have declined and they had both fewer hospital days and fewer treatment meetings. No significant differences between the two groups emerged in the five-year treatment outcomes, with 82% of Open Dialogue clients having no residual psychotic symptoms. Eighty-six per cent of the OD-treated group had returned to their studies or a full-time job, only 14% were on disability allowance. Seventeen per cent had relapsed during the first two years and

19% during the next three years. Twenty nine per cent had used neuroleptic medication in some phase of the treatment (Seikkula *et al.* 2006).

'Open Dialogue' is a network-based, language approach to psychiatric care which has a clinical and scientific tradition in Finland; it is associated internationally with the name and work of Jakku Seikkula from the University of Jyvaiskyla. Gregory Bateson's work and Bakhtin's dialogical principles are the most important foundation stones of Open Dialogue. Two levels of analysis can be described (Seikkula and Olson 2003), namely poetics, which includes the three principles of 'tolerance of uncertainty', 'dialogism', and 'polyphony in social networks' and which work to generate a therapeutic dialogue, and micropolitics, the institutional practices that support this way of working and are part of the Finnish need-adapted treatment (Alanen 1997).

From a Bakhtinian perspective, 'understanding requires an active process of talking and listening. Dialogue is a precondition for positive change in any form of therapy. Using the perspectives of dialogism and neurobiological development, we analyze the basic elements of dialogue, seeking to understand why dialogue becomes a healing experience in a network meeting. From the perspective of therapist as dialogical partner, we examine actions that support dialogue in conversation, shared emotional experience, creation of community, and creation of new shared language. We describe how feelings of love, manifesting powerful mutual emotional attunement in the conversation, signal moments of therapeutic change' (Seikkula and Trimble 2005).

Shared vision

The Care Services Improvement Partnership (CSIP) of the National Institute for Mental Health in England has recently conducted a draft guidance for consultation on 'Finding a shared vision of how people's mental health problems should be understood'. It aims to:

- 'identify a shared vision of how people's mental health problems should be understood that is recognized equally by different provider groups and by service users and their carers;
- raise awareness of the wide variety of different approaches to assessing mental health problems and well-being and,
- to build mutual understanding of these different approaches as resources for drawing together, through a shared process between service users, carers and service providers, ways of understanding a mental health problem that reflect the particular and often very different strengths and needs of individual service users' (www.dh.gov.uk/en/Consultations/Liveconsultations/DH_080913; 20.08.08).

The shared vision, in the words of a service user, is about 'having a say in how our problems are understood' instead of being 'assessed to death' or viewing the whole process as 'all Greek to me'. It involves three key elements:

- 'active participation of the service user concerned in a shared understanding with service providers and their carers, in a process of assessment that,
- draws together different provider perspectives in a well-integrated way, to produce,

- a person-centred assessment that builds on the strengths and resiliencies of the individual service user, as well as identifying his or her needs and difficulties, as a basis for recovery and for developing the skills of self-management',

which are supposed to reflect and build on best practice, with contributions from service user, carer, and a number of different provider perspectives. The shared vision is *evidence-based* in that 'it builds on a range of diagnostic assessments reflecting different areas of professional and other expertise', and *values-based* (Woodbridge and Fulford 2004) in that it balances positive (strengths and resiliencies) as well as negative (needs and difficulties) aspects of an individual's mental health problems in the process of person-centred assessment (www.dh.gov.uk/en/Consultations/ Liveconsultations/DH_080913; 20.08.08).

Sharing Voices Bradford

Sharing Voices Bradford is a ground-breaking UK project in terms of:

- a community development approach to community care, as well as
- an action-research project

which aims to explore 'how a critical perspective in mental health can be put into practice' (Henderson *et al.* 2007).

Individuals with mental health difficulties played a central role in this project which aims:

- 'to liaise with statutory service providers to improve the range and quality of services to people in Bradford from BME (black and minority ethnic) communities;
- to develop capacity within communities and support voluntary sector and self-help activity in mental health and well-being;
- to stimulate wider debate locally and nationally about the nature of mental health, diversity and ethnicity.'

People were engaged in peer groups, some were single faith and others were gender groups, for example there was a group for Muslim women. Some groups, for example a music group, were mixed. These groups of volunteers were 'sharing voices' and over a three-year period:

- 'enabled people from diverse communities to set up groups where they could address shared experiences of distress in their own way;
- supported individuals to develop their social, spiritual and economic potential;
- developed partnerships and support networks that increased capacity in the statutory, voluntary and community sectors and widened access to support for people from BME communities;
- increased BME participation in service design and delivery and other local issues, in statutory and voluntary forums;

- signposted people who needed resources to the statutory and voluntary sectors;
- advocated choice and citizenship in dialogue and debate on non-medical understandings of distress' (Henderson *et al.* 2007, p 40).

The results of the participatory action-research project apply to issues of relevance in contexts beyond Bradford:

- 'Community development at Sharing Voices involves a combination of safe spaces and networks which extend ever outwards, linking the mental health field with sports, leisure, arts and other local organizations. Understanding of mental ill-health is increased and stigma reduced as organizations become more inclusive. The networks have also led to an increase in social capital and community cohesion.
- The research evidence on the value of peer support and mutual aid in promoting recovery from mental ill-health is strong and further supported at Sharing Voices.
- By tapping into the specialised knowledge of experts by experience of and BME communities, stigma is tackled more effectively and the benefits for the individuals involved, their communities and the NHS can be considerable (Henderson *et al.* 2007, p 40).
- Primary care trusts can opt to be ambitious ('radical') or more cautious, but they need to manage the expectations of their staff and communities accordingly.' (Henderson *et al.* 2007, p 40).

On the basis of the Sharing Voices Bradford experience and research results, and other examples, Henderson *et al.* (2007) make suggestions about how to strengthen the links between community development and community care. One of the things they suggest is the evaluation and collection of the success stories of such approaches and 'champions', looking beyond 'Westernised' assumptions about communities and mental health, and connecting 'community care issues more powerfully to the promotion of social justice and the tackling of social exclusion'.

ALTERNATIVES

Recovery demands all our best efforts in terms of human rights, patients' rights, scientific and clinical responsibility, and service, in the interest of those who might become patients and those who are. We learn from those who are using services, those who have used services (ex-users), and those who define themselves through overcoming harmful experiences even in the support system (survivors). Co-operation between people with and without lived experience of mental health services has been successful but needs more support. Support is also needed for those who work on the development of alternatives outside the traditional system. The ideas and concepts which are broadly covered by the umbrella term and/or the concept of 'alternatives', have a lot to offer and we briefly present a few examples here.

Alternative Conferences

'Since 1985, the Community Support Programmes (CSP) has supported the annual national Alternatives Conferences organized by and for consumers (also referred to as ex-patients or survivors) of mental health services. The purpose of these conferences is to provide a forum for consumers from all over the nation to meet, exchange information and ideas, and provide and receive technical assistance on peer support and peer-operated services along with other relevant topics, such as self-help, protection and advocacy issues, empowerment and recovery. The conferences also provide information on best practices in mental health and support services. The knowledge gained through attending these conferences helps consumers advocate for effective treatments and services, and improve service systems. Starting in 1992, the Consumer Technical Assistance Centers have rotated the hosting of the Alternatives conference.' (www.mentalhealth.samhsa.gv: 20.8.08)

Alternatives Conferences rotate between different cities in the U.S.A. The titles of the last several Alternatives Conferences give a good impression of what is being presented there; there is always an amazing list of speakers and a very special atmosphere:

Freedom to Remember. Freedom to Choose. Freedom to Dream. (2001)
Strengthening Networks and Taking Action Together. (2002)
Achieving the Promise of Recovery: New Freedom, New Power, New Hope. (2004)
Arizona Leading the Transformation to Recovery. (2005)
Blazing the Trail to Recovery through Transformation. (2006)
Spanning the Recovery Movement: Consumer Control and Choice. (2007)
Creating Community through Active Citizenship. (2008):
(www.power2u.org; 20.08.08)

'Alternatives beyond psychiatry'

- 'What helps me if I go mad?
- How can I find trustworthy help for a relative or a friend in need?
- How can I protect myself from coercive treatment?
- As a family member or friend, how can I help?
- What should I do if I can no longer bear to work in the mental health field?
- What are the alternatives to psychiatry?
- How can I get involved in creating alternatives?
- Assuming psychiatry would be abolished, what do you propose instead?'

Those are some of the questions which are addressed by the 61 authors – (ex-)users and survivors of psychiatry, medical practitioners, therapists, lawyers, social scientists, psychiatrists and relatives from all continents, who contributed to *Alternatives Beyond Psychiatry*, edited by Peter Stastny and Peter Lehmann, and published in 2007 by Peter Lehmann Publishing in USA (Eugene), UK (Shrewsbury) and also in Germany (Berlin).

The book contains contributions from: Volkmar Aderhold, Laurie Ahern, Birgitta Alakare, Karyn Baker, Ulrich Bartmann, Agnes Beier, Regina Bellion, Wilma Boevink, Pat Bracken, Stefan Bräunling, Ludger Bruckmann, Giuseppe Bucalo, Dorothea S Buck-Zerchin, Sarah Carr, Tina Coldham, Bhargavi Davar, Anne Marie DiGiacomo,

Constance Dollwet, Jeanne Dumont, Merinda Epstein, Sandra Escher, Jim Gottstein, Chris Hansen, Geoff Hardy, Petra Hartmann, Alfred Hausotter, Michael Herrick, Guy Holmes, Andrew Hughes, Theodor Itten, Maths Jesperson, Kristine Jones, Hannelore Klafki, Miriam Krücke, Peter Lehmann, Bruce E. Levine, Harold A Maio, Rufus May, Shery Mead, Kate Millett, Maryse Mitchell-Brody, David Oaks, Peter Rippmann, Marius Romme, Marc Rufer, Gisela Sartori, Erich Schützendorf, Jaakko Seikkula, Andy Smith, Zoran Solomun, Peter Stastny, Chris Stevenson, Dan Taylor, Philip Thomas, Jan Wallcraft, David Webb, Uta Wehde, Scott Welsch, Salma Yasmeen, Laura Ziegler and Ursula Zingler.

Translations by Christine Holzhausen, Katy E. McNally and Mary Murphy (www.peter-lehmann-publishing.com; 20.8.08).

The International Network Toward Alternatives and Recovery - INTAR

'The International Network Toward Alternatives and Recovery' is an international summit of world renowned survivor leaders, psychiatrists, psychologists, family members, and other mental health professionals who meet annually to counter the belief that people with diagnoses such as schizophrenia or bipolar disorder can never completely recover.

'INTAR believes that the dignity and autonomy of the person in crisis are of the utmost importance, that full recovery from distressing/altered mental states is possible, and that these two convictions should shape the social response. For these reasons, we find established psychiatry and public mental health systems in which many of us work, seek (or have been forced to seek) treatment (for ourselves or our loved ones) and do research, to be deficient. Instead, we seek, and some of us provide, alternative settings where people in crisis can find the care, connectedness, respect, and interventions they need and elect to use. Our backgrounds range widely, from peer/user organizing to biomedicine and psychoanalytic training to Eastern meditative disciplines to family advocacy to academic research. But we are, each of us, committed to building safe spaces and positive relationships, wherein the ordeal presented by extreme states of mind can be met with proven tools and seasoned presence. This includes people who have been through it before and know how to offer the steadfast support needed. As an international network, we undertake to document the effectiveness of such alternatives, to refine and expand their use, and to make them more accessible to people who need them' (www.intar.org: 20.8.08).

RECOVERY-FACTORS IN THERAPEUTIC RELATIONSHIPS AND PSYCHIATRIC SERVICES

Recovery-oriented professionals

In 2004, Marit Borg and Kristjana Kristiansen published an article entitled *Recovery-oriented professionals: helping relationships in mental health services*. Both researchers are affiliated to the Department of Social Work and Health Science, Faculty of Social Sciences and Technology Management at the Norwegian University of Science and

Technology in Oslo. They looked at factors involved in the relationships between service providers and users that seemed helpful from the perspective of the users. The authors conducted a qualitative study based on interviews with 15 service users, who had been or were still suffering from serious psychiatric conditions. They also wanted to find out whether any of the factors were discussed by service providers and users as part of their therapeutic relationship and whether such discussion was experienced as helpful.

Research projects and literature about personal accounts of recovery from serious psychiatric conditions are still quite rare. The few reports that have been published show that therapeutic relationships seem to play a key role in facilitating recovery. In this Norwegian study, the researchers addressed the question whether a person was being seen as a fellow human being with insight and expertise, or, in contrast, as someone with a chronic illness who needed to be cared for, maybe forever. Studies about this subject are pretty important for professional service providers, but are quite rare and difficult to access. That is why we are presenting the results of this study here in greater detail.

The empirical material for this project came from a larger study which investigated a broad array of factors that might be helpful in the recovery from mental illness (Topor 2001; Borg and Topor 2003). The study presented here aimed at understanding the characteristics of helpful relationships in psychiatric services, especially the kinds of relationships where recovery-oriented service providers work most effectively with service users.

The 15 interviewees had been diagnosed with schizophrenia, schizoid personality, paranoid psychosis, affective psychosis, personality disorder, and borderline psychotic personality. This study included people who: a) considered themselves as having recovered or being in recovery from severe mental illness; b) were coping well in their lives; c) had improved their lives with the help of mental health services and/or other sources, and d) had not received inpatient psychiatric care during the past two years.

The interviews began with an open question: "What was helpful in your process of recovery?" The researchers were particularly interested in the way the participants dealt with challenging situations in life, including their experiences with mental health professionals, provider agencies, and other sources of support. They wanted to learn more about the person's own role in recovery, as well as the impact of other social supports and contextual variables. The aspects that the participants considered particularly important for their recovery were investigated further with additional questions, in order to capture the variability of personal experiences. The transcripts of the audio-recordings were sent to the participants for editorial changes and consent. Subsequently, the research team reviewed the transcribed interviews and took note of recurrent topics which seemed relevant for recovery. Summaries were developed inductively and discussed among the entire research team.

Group-level analyses of the summaries were used to identify specific recovery-related themes. These included the active role of the person; the support and influence of others; events; environmental factors, and the understanding and meanings underlying the experience of mental illness and recovery.

The interviewees reported several positive and negative experiences and challenges along the road towards recovery. Their stories were punctuated by times of fear, loneliness, hopelessness, anxiety, and inexplicable pain. The stories revealed both the individual behind the diagnosis and also the human being in his/her role as a professional helper. Below we list the main topics that the researchers found.

The human distinction: discovering fellow humanity

The participants experienced the following elements as most helpful in their relationships to the professionals: empathy, respect, and a general person-to-person investment. This included careful listening on the part of the professionals, showing an interest in the priorities of the participants, and being open to discussing more than just problems. Participants did not particularly value the traditional ways of displaying professional competence, such as intervention programmes or methods, but instead appreciated the willingness of professionals to share power and promote an atmosphere of trust, in which the professional provider and the service user could collaborate on the therapeutic agenda. Several participants emphasized regular contact and collaboration with supportive professionals as vital to their recovery. Overall, helpful relationships seemed to be characterized by the following elements:

The apparently small things and 'being seen': The participants emphasized the importance of "being seen" in their relationships with their helpers and offered concrete personal stories. For example, a mental health care provider asked how a person's mother was doing; a staff member in a day-centre shared stories about her dog, and one nurse presented a user with a rose, as an acknowledgement of the fact that she had stayed in her new job for over a month. These apparently small acts, which often just consisted of a few words, were nevertheless experienced as having a profoundly positive value to the participants in their daily struggles.

Being ill and well at the same time: The interviewees valued those professionals and services who permitted them to be ill and well at the same time. The professionals were ready to share both the positive and the less favourable experiences of a fellow human being's totality, both the times of suffering as well as the hopeful opportunities.

Genuine interest, continuity, and safety: Some participants reported that finding and getting to know a provider who showed genuine interest in them was an important turning point in their lives. Others considered those professionals as helpful, who could bear with them, staying the course with them over several years. Others told about one particular provider who represented the essential thread of continuity and safety that they needed at certain difficult times.

On the other hand, a few participants said professionals had only a minor influence on their recovery. For them, recovery had to do with other helpful factors, such as faith in god, having a job and adequate funds, or even having a pet dog as a companion and provider of comfort.

Available everyday helpers

Helpers who were truly dedicated were experienced as particularly useful, since they were available for the large and small challenges of daily life, especially in times of crisis, i.e. when the participants heard tormenting voices, experienced extreme anxiety or found it difficult to carry out the practical tasks of everyday living. During such times, professionals who were open to the individual person's own priorities were seen as helpful in the sense of simply being there when required and helping in doing whatever was necessary.

Finding time and just being there: 'Being available' had mostly to do with the element of time. The main contribution of a helper was to be available for a little chat, to do something together, or to offer support in various ways. It seemed important that the provider found time to "just be there" and also had the sensitivity to understand the person's unique and most pressing needs. Many participants expressed deep gratitude towards providers who could set aside their professional role for a moment and do something unexpected. Providers who offered their own unpaid time beyond their "professional time" were experienced as surprising and extraordinary. One participant expressed this as follows:

> '*Last time Ragna (a community nurse) called me, I wasn't able to answer even a single question properly, so I was . . . so miserable and useless, feeling so bad, and she noticed while we were on the phone, that I wasn't well at all. And she came and visited me, 3–4 times a month, on her own time and just came here.*' (Borg and Kristiansen 2004, p 497)

Sense of humour, good talks, helping in practical things: One participant appreciated the team's sense of humour and that she could speak to them about things other than her troubles. The same person also had other people with whom she could get in touch, like her doctor, a community nurse and a volunteer. Good conversations, visiting a café, knowing each other for a long time, getting help in practical things, as well as dealing with her pain and hearing voices – all this was important to her.

Psychotherapist's patience and endurance: Another participant especially appreciated the patience, tenacity and continuous availability of her psychotherapist. Even though he changed his place of work three times during her treatment, he never interrupted the therapy, nor did he refer her to another colleague. He took her along on his professional journey, and gave her priority, which resulted in six years of working together. This long relationship with the therapist was important for the woman, because of its continuity and the fact that they kept getting to know each other better. She expressed this as follows:

> '*What really matters is that you have not many, but a few good helpers over time. Someone who can keep it up, who's there . . . That's what I feel is the most important my therapist has done for me . . . that he stuck with me all these years.*' (*Borg and Kristiansen 2004, p 498*)

Experiencing what is 'therapeutic'

Some of the interviewees mentioned psychotherapy as being helpful in their recovery-process. How exactly this was being experienced as helpful and what the psychotherapy was about, presented itself in a number of ways.

Psychotherapist as saviour: Some felt that psychotherapy was a turning point in their life. To find someone who is helpful was often compared to finding a 'saviour' who can start a process in which an individual feels safe and secure enough to talk about inner feelings as well as the chaotic circumstances of their daily lives. Such helpers were described as almost divine and seemed to have a strong influence on the life of the subjects.

Psychotherapist as ordinary person: Other psychotherapists were described in mundane rather than godlike ways, for instant as pleasant partners for conversation. Encountering someone like that did not seem to be a turning point in their lives, but rather a supportive relationship, maybe just for a certain time and with less significance over the long term.

Hope and courage to move on: Professional helpers were especially valued at the times when hope and courage to move on could emerge during the course of the therapeutic relationship. Providing a certain kind of stability and continuity was important in times when no one else in the person's life could offer that.

Therapeutic partnership and equality: Attention was being paid more to the person than to the professional as psychiatric expert. Emphasizing a human relationship is important, since it is the essence of a therapeutic relationship that it is actually a partnership defined by equality. Professionals who practised standard procedures and who prioritized their own professional agenda over that of the person seeking help, were often described as 'cold' or 'not really interested in me and my situation'.

Breaking the rules

Unexpected, surprising actions: Participants frequently mentioned unexpected and surprising actions or gestures on the part of providers whom they experienced as 'good' helpers. They were talking about those little things that had a lot of meaning for them. This included behaviours that were seen as being at the very edge of what is typically considered 'professional conduct'. For example, a community nurse loaned one of her clients some money over the weekend because she would not be getting her welfare cheque until Monday. Another provider accepted a present from a female client and thereby had given her the opportunity to offer something to someone else. Such 'good helpers' were described in warm and friendly terms, participants talking about kindness, patience, a sense of humour, wanting to help, giving time, or even just acting in ordinary ways.

Friendship-like relationships: Some participants had the feeling that they could talk about anything with their community nurses, and trusted that they would always be of help. Such a friendship-like relationship gave one of the women the sense that she could give presents to her community nurse (such as poems that she had written, magazines and music cassettes), and that they would be accepted. By feeling she could be herself in relation to the helpers she had contact with, she became someone more than 'a patient with mental problems', she experienced herself as an equal human being of equal value.

Giving and receiving presents: Exchanging gifts is a common feature of ordinary human relationships. It speaks of mutual respect and appreciation. Normally, giving presents between professionals and 'patients' is not allowed, or at the very least, discouraged. Such an exchange is usually not part of a paid, helping relationship. It is assumed that gifts might lead to an unhealthy dependency of the patient or could be a threat to the therapeutic alliance. The authors of the study suggest that the fact that such rules are being broken in daily practice should be openly discussed.

Making demands: The helpful professionals were not merely described as nice and pleasant. It is not enough to be nice, even though it definitely helps sometimes. To be a supportive helper also means to make demands. Not having the same opinion, or responding clearly when the provider has a demand, is generally experienced as helpful. Two participants, for example, were asked to attend group therapy or a day programme instead of just hanging around all day. At first they rejected this. What made them change their minds was the support they received from more than one provider whom they trusted and who helped them to understand that it was really necessary for them to attend such an activity, especially given the situation they were in at the moment. As long as a few 'good' or trusted professionals were around, they managed to deal better with certain therapeutic programmes which at first they had experienced as senseless or difficult.

'Good chemistry': Expressions such as 'good chemistry' or 'we just got on with each other' were frequently used to describe helpful professionals. It seemed that in this kind of partnership, offering simple and concrete services works best. Help was given in a collaborative relationship, where there was opportunity for negotiation.

Going beyond the professional role: The participants clearly demonstrated through their stories and examples that just the knowledge that providers had about mental illness, professional guidelines, and therapeutic treatment programmes, was quite inadequate and insufficient to support recovery. The high value they bestowed upon those helpers who went beyond their professional role is an interesting and rather striking paradox, which raises the question as to what professionalism really is and should be.

In summary, the factors which were experienced as helpful for the recovery of service users clearly implied the need for a transformation of the professional role. An orientation towards recovery meant that professionals had to transform their thinking to the point where they no longer saw themselves as experts on the lives of others, but rather could assume a position of support for their clients' own ways of dealing with their problems and struggles. If we are to have positive mental health services, those services have to accommodate the needs and preferences of users, instead of forcing them into pre-formed institutional structures. Professionals who showed the courage to deal with the richness and unpredictability of life in general, were held in great esteem. Such an approach also needed to include the ability to offer one's capabilities and professional experiences in the context of a collaborative partnership rather than as part of a hierarchically structured therapeutic relationship.

Human qualities seem to be more important than academic titles, professional background or concrete therapeutic modalities and techniques. Whenever providers and service users were ready and able to show their human sides and dared to be themselves, the therapeutic relationship was experienced as more beneficial. Showing oneself to each other makes collaboration and mutuality possible, which the participants considered to be important, if not essential, for the recovery-process. Mutuality seems to arise from the acknowledged and shared strengths, weaknesses, possibilities and limitations on *both* sides.

Recovery is a concrete and practical process that involves activities shared with several providers, whereby the individual can regain and maintain control over his/her own life and can develop and experiment with competencies and new information. Recovery is seen as an active process by the users, and not as something that is being done by the professionals for a "passive and sick" person. The task of professional helpers is to discover the capacities for recovery in each person who is seeking help, to provide support and encouragement, and to stand by them along the way.

The understanding of "severe psychiatric disorder" has to be modified. Instead of using an illness-based approach, which is based, for example, on the diagnostic criteria for schizophrenia, it is essential to implement a person-centred approach. This means that the roles and competencies of mental health service providers should be developed towards more open perspectives so that they are enabled to find out what actually helps each individual and what might be a hindrance to his/her recovery.

The authors of this study point out that believing in the prospects for recovery and having hope for a better life seem to be essential. In contrast to the pessimism existing in many professional textbooks and cultures, the participants of this study did not see themselves as passive victims of a chronic illness. 'Hopefulness' and 'a positive expectation towards the future' are mentioned as important factors in outcome research, but have been rather poorly defined and given little attention by psychiatric researchers yet (Schrank *et al.* 2008). According to Borg and Kristiansen, many participants were helped by having hope for a better life to deal with their everyday problems, especially during times of crisis. Accordingly, the providers who were seen as helpful in this study gave priority to building a positive relationship with the person seeking help, and emphasized optimism and a focus on inner resources. In contrast, helpers who were mainly interested in symptoms and deficits were experienced as providing little hope for the future.

Recovery Self Assessment (RSA)

The Recovery Self Assessment (RSA) was developed by Maria O'Connell and co-workers at Yale University to assess perceptions of the degree to which programmes implement recovery-oriented practices. Nine hundred and sixty-seven participants (directors, providers, people in recovery, and significant others) from 78 mental health and addiction programmes in Connecticut, U.S.A completed the instrument for an evaluation (O'Connell *et al.* 2005) with a factor analysis revealing the following five factors:

Factor 1: *Life-goals*
Contains 11 items that reflect perceptions of the extent to which staff help with the development and pursuit of individually defined life-goals such as employment and education.
Factor 2: *Involvement*
Contains eight items reflecting perceptions of the extent to which people in recovery are involved in the development and provision of programmes/services, staff training, and advisory board/management meetings.
Factor 3: *Diversity of treatment options*
Contains six items that indicate perceptions of the extent to which an agency provides linkages to peer mentors and support, a variety of treatment options, and assistance with becoming involved in non-mental health activities.
Factor 4: *Choice*
Contains six items measuring perceptions of the extent to which service users have access

to their treatment records, staff refrain from using coercive measures to influence choice, and the choices of service users are respected by staff.

Factor 5: *Individually-tailored services*

Contains five items that reflect perceptions of the extent to which services are tailored to individual needs, cultures, and interests, and focus on building community connections.

Data analyses of the RSA summary score showed that service providers had significantly lower ratings than people in recovery. On the individual factors, service providers had significantly lower scores than directors on *life-goals*. Providers also had significantly lower scores than people in recovery and family members/significant others/advocates on *Involvement* and *Individually-tailored services*. Finally, there were no significant differences between the various categories of respondents on *Choice* or *Diversity of treatment options*.

For the authors it was encouraging that the highest rated items were those related to services focusing on helping people explore their own goals and interests beyond symptom management. However, agencies were rated lowest on items regarding the involvement of service users in service design, management and provision. The authors found this result consistent with the literature, indicating that one of the most difficult barriers for 'practitioners in recovery' is being accepted as equal members of agency staff.

That people in recovery had consistently higher ratings than providers is surprising. These higher ratings have been explained by the authors 'as possible selection bias due to the fact that agency directors and providers hand-selected the respondents', and as reflecting 'common difficulties that occur in conducting service user satisfaction surveys' (O'Connell *et al.* 2005, p 383). The authors point out another problem of service user surveys, saying that people 'only know that to which they have been exposed' and 'if someone is not familiar with alternatives, it is easier to be satisfied with what he/she has' (p 383). The authors suggest a solution to this problem: an ideal administration of the RSA would be the application of the instrument across sites, programme participants, and staff, maintaining anonymity of respondents, and assessing the majority of the programme participants/staff.

What needs to be done in the future, according to the authors, is to examine scores on the RSA in relation to other recovery-oriented constructs such as quality of life, satisfaction with services, and empowerment. Furthermore, the authors suggest that future research should also examine the degree to which the subjective perceptions of recovery-oriented practices are consistent with the actual implementation of the practices and more objective measures of fidelity (such as data available in chart reviews, policies, and procedures).

Measuring recovery-orientation in a hospital setting

The authors Salyers, Tsai and Stultz from Indiana University, USA (Salyers *et al.* 2007) state that there is growing emphasis on the need to examine the process of delivering recovery-oriented services as a necessary complement to measuring recovery-outcomes.

According to the authors, programmes that are recovery-oriented promote partnerships with consumers, emphasize consumer choice, and instil hope. The authors refer to elements of a recovery-orientation which include: the recognition that people with mental illness have the same wants and needs as everyone else (Anthony 2004); priority being given to consumer choice in all aspects of treatment, housing, employment, and medication (Drake *et al.* 2003); and a focus on consumer strengths (Rapp and Wintersteen 1989). The authors point out that it can be made clearer by saying what recovery is not, for example programmes solely devoted to medication adherence and stabilisation, or programmes that take a paternalistic or coercive approach and discourage consumer autonomy.

The authors wanted to examine the psychometric properties of the 36-item provider version of the Recovery Self Assessment (RSA) (Conell *et al.* 2005) in a sample of 302 hospital workers from a State Hospital in Indiana. In addition they used the Life Orientation Test-Revised (Scheier, Carver and Bridges 1994) which assesses personal optimism, and an adapted version of the Consumer Optimism scale (Grusky, Tierney and Spanish 1989). As a comparison group, the authors included a smaller sample of community mental health providers (N = 182), working on the hypothesis that the recovery-orientation of community providers would be higher than that of state hospital providers. The staff members of the state hospital included attendants, nurses, psychiatrists, psychologists, rehabilitation therapists, social workers, and other mental health professionals with a majority being white and female.

The following results can be reported:

- The RSA demonstrated good to excellent internal consistency, test-retest reliability, and adequate convergent and discriminant validity.
- Staff members who had higher levels of personal optimism were more likely to view consumers as having more potential and to view their agency as more recovery-oriented. A positive view of consumers was positively correlated with a positive view of their agency overall.
- The RSA discriminated between state hospital and community providers. As expected, the community providers scored significantly higher than state hospital providers on consumer expectations, and all five sub-scales of the perceptions of agency recovery. With moderate to large effect sizes, the community providers demonstrated greater recovery attitudes. The authors expected that the community sample would be much more 'recovery-oriented', primarily because the population served by staff members in the state hospital consisted of consumers in greatest need.
- Interestingly, while other differences were moderate to large in effect, the absolute score of hospital staff was not strikingly low, with mean scores on RSA factors ranging from 3.1 to 3.4, on consumer optimism at 2.8 and personal optimism at 3.5, all on a 5-point scale. Some level of social desirability cannot, of course, be ruled out.

The provider version of the RSA can be considered as a potentially useful scale to assess the recovery-orientation of services including hospitals. However, including consumer and significant other ratings as well – as originally foreseen for the use of the RSA - would provide a fuller account of recovery-orientation.

Recovery Knowledge Inventory (RKI)

After the development of the Recovery Self-Assessment (RSA) (O'Connell *et al*. 2005), a tool that can be used to evaluate the recovery-orientation of mental health services from a variety of perspectives, the RKI represents a second contribution to the process of operationalizing recovery. The RKI describes the development and implementation of a knowledge and attitude regarding recovery-oriented practices among providers of mental health services. Bedregal, O'Connell and Davidson (2006) from Yale University developed and administered the Recovery Knowledge Inventory (RKI) throughout the state of Connecticut, USA.

While the authors express welcoming words towards the emerging recovery concept in the mental health system they also express some concerns. They welcome the concept of recovery 'as it has taken over thirty years for the original recovery research of Strauss, Carpenter, Harding, Ciompi and others, to cross over from psychiatric rehabilitation into the broader clinical arena where it can influence all of psychiatric practice' (Bedregal *et al*. 2006, p 97). On the other side, they are concerned that recovery 'as practice, or at least rhetoric *about* practice, may quickly be outstripping the field's evidence-base' (ibid., p 97). They express fear that through the rapid dissemination of the recovery-concept, the many different definitions suggested, and the even more varied approaches to recovery-oriented practice, researchers and practitioners may be at risk of losing the unique opportunity to move psychiatric practice into an entirely new direction, namely into 'recovery-oriented systems of care' (ibid., p 96). The authors hope that one strategy that might be effective in rescuing recovery from this fate is to operationalize the characteristics of recovery-oriented care in as clear and specific a manner as possible.

The researchers provide, with the RKI, a description of the items and the preliminary psychometric properties of the instrument. Furthermore, they illustrate its utility 'as a needs assessment for tailoring staff training to better prepare them to offer recovery-oriented care' (ibid., p 97). The instrument was developed as part of a statewide initiative in Connecticut to make all behavioural health services more recovery-oriented (cf pp 227). A central component of this process was training on the principles, values, and practice of recovery-oriented care.

In order to integrate the various meanings and to create a tool for assessing the nature of recovery-oriented care, recovery was broadly conceptualized as involving a 'redefinition of one's illness as only one aspect of a multi-dimensional sense of self capable of identifying, choosing, and pursuing personally meaningful goals and aspirations beyond or despite continuing to suffer the effect and side effects of mental illness' (Bedregal *et al*. 2006, p 97). The following issues were identified as integral to the provision of recovery-oriented care:

- consumer directedness;
- the individual nature of recovery;
- cultural competence;
- self-determination;
- strengths-based care;
- choice and risk-taking,
- illness and symptom management;
- incorporation of illness into sense of self;

- involvement in meaningful activities;
- overcoming stigma;
- redefining self;
- hope, and
- the non-linear nature of the recovery process.

For measuring providers' knowledge and attitudes towards the different recovery domains, a 36-item instrument was developed after empirical considerations and discussion with various stake-holders. Completed assessments of 144 staff members from nine different agencies were analyzed and produced the following underlying dimensions:

Factor I: *Roles and responsibilities in recovery*
Includes seven items regarding risk-taking, decision-making, and the various and respective roles and responsibilities of people in recovery and mental health providers. For example, people with mental illness/substance abuse should not be burdened with the responsibilities of everyday life.

Factor II: *Non-linearity of the recovery-process*
Includes six items regarding the role of illness and symptom management and the non-linear nature of recovery, for example, recovery is characterized by a person making gradual steps forward without major steps back.

Factor III: *The roles of self-definition and peers in recovery*
Includes five items regarding the person's activities in defining an identity for him or herself, and a life that goes beyond that of 'mental patient' or 'addict'; also included are the valuable roles that peers can play in this process, for example, the pursuit of hobbies and leisure activities is important for recovery.

Factor IV: *Expectations regarding recovery*
Includes two items regarding expectations, for example, not everyone is capable of actively participating in the recovery-process.

Major results regarding training needs include:
'Staff members' obtained the highest mean scores on Factor III, *The roles of self-definition and peers in recovery*, which means that providers appreciated the need for the person in recovery to develop a positive identity beyond that of 'mental patient' or 'addict', and the importance of having the assistance of peers in this process.

The next to highest mean score was on Factor I, *Roles and responsibilities in recovery*, indicating that staff showed good understanding of the importance of differentiating the roles and responsibilities of each party (provider and client) in the treatment and rehabilitation process.

Staff's third highest mean score was on Factor IV, *Expectations regarding recovery*, which means that staff had less knowledge of how to develop realistic yet hopeful expectations of their clients with respect to their participation in their own recovery and in their lives in general.

The lowest scores were found in Factor II, *Non-linearity of the recovery process*, indicating that staff had least knowledge about the nature of the recovery-process, including its non-linear nature. This means they had little grasp of the idea that illness and symptom management not only precede recovery but can also be part of it (for example, a person does not necessarily need to be free from illness and symptoms to be in recovery). And it also means they had little awareness of the multiple pathways by which people could recover that went beyond formal treatments and rehabilitation settings (Bedregal *et al.* 2006, p 101).

In summary, the authors highlight the potentially important implications for training by identifying aspects of recovery-orientation with which providers are both more and less familiar with the aim of increasing staff knowledge, attitudes and beliefs and enhancing competence.

Developing Recovery Enhancing Environments Measure (DREEM)

Originally developed by Patricia Ridgeway (Campbell-Orde 2005) the DREEM has been edited for UK use by Allott and Higginson (www.recoverydevon.co.uk; 20.08.08) and used in a small but very apt collaboration between service users and staff in a residential rehabilitation service in Devon (Dinniss *et al.* 2007; www.recoverydevon.co.uk 20.08.08). DREEM allows an assessment of the importance of recovery elements as well as of the effectiveness with which a service is supporting these elements and can be used to highlight similarities and differences between users' and staff's assessments to identify the weaknesses, strength and needs of a service situation where change is wanted in the direction of recovery-orientation. While little is known yet about its psychometric properties, feasibility and face validity are quite satisfactory.

INITIATIVES OF THE WORLD PSYCHIATRIC ASSOCIATION

Psychiatry for the Person

The World Psychiatric Association (WPA), which has more than 130 member countries from all continents, has conceived an important programme which declares the person within his or her bio-psycho-socio-cultural context as its central focus. We welcome this perspective, since it affords a central role not only to aspects of illness but also to the positive elements of health in every person, and thereby aims to encompass the powers of recovery and resilience in clinical practice and research.

The WPA Institutional Programme on Psychiatry for the Person: From Clinical Care to Public Health has been developed under the chairmanship of Juan E Mezzich, the president of the WPA from 2005–2008. The programme was introduced in September 2005 at the General Assembly of the WPA in Cairo and fully endorsed by its member societies. The co-ordinating committee and the various project groups are staffed internationally and the project is planned several years ahead. 'Given the early programmatic achievements and responses received from throughout WPA and initial contacts with external organizations (World Federation for Mental Health, World Medical Association, World Federation for Neurology, etc.) it is becoming clear that Psychiatry for the Person (and eventually a Medicine for the Person) has to be seen as a long-term initiative aimed at innovatively refocusing the objectives of the psychiatric and medical fields in consonance with their fundamental soul' (Mezzich 2007b, p 1).

The following section summarizes key themes and activities of the programme (Mezzich 2005b, 2007a). The principal goal of the programme is to ensure that the whole person who seeks help within his/her context is regarded as the central focus of treatment and health promotion, at an individual as well as a community level. Science and humanism should optimize attention to the ill and the positive health aspects of the person who consults the mental health services, should seek to integrate all relevant health and social services, and also to advance related health policies. This programme encourages science and humanism to promote:

- a psychiatry of the person (of the totality of the person's health, both ill and positive aspects);
- a psychiatry by the person (with clinicians extending themselves as full human beings with high ethical aspirations and not merely as healing technicians);
- a psychiatry for the person (assisting the fulfilment of the person's health aspirations and life project and not merely disease management), and
- a psychiatry with the person (in respectful and empowering relationship with the person who consults rather than imposing treatments on a passive carrier of diseases) (Mezzich 2007b).

The Institutional Programme on a Psychiatry for the Person (IPPP) has developed four projects in the following areas: Conceptual Component, Clinical Diagnosis Component, Clinical Care Component, and Public Health Component (Mezzich 2005b).

The *Conceptual Component* aims to explore the historical, conceptual and ethical foundations of a Psychiatry for the Person in comparison to other perspectives, for example, a psychiatry that focuses exclusively on mental disorders and their symptoms. Participants come from the WPA sections on the History of Psychiatry and Philosophy and Humanities in Psychiatry and from other parts of the WPA, such as the Ethics Committee. International experts in these areas also participate.

The *Clinical Diagnosis Component* has to do with the ongoing WPA project on the International Classification and Diagnostic Systems (ICDS) which is contributing a) to the development of ICD-11 of the WHO and b) delineating a new person-centred integrative diagnostic model. This new diagnostic model will combine standardized and idiographic aspects in order to incorporate illness-related variables, as well as positive aspects of a person's health, into the interaction with clinicians, patients and their families. The clinically complex problem of co-morbidity is given special attention in this process, as the area of caring for people with co-morbidity would benefit particularly from a person-centred approach. The participants in this project are the WPA Section on Classification and Diagnosis, along with other WPA Sections, in collaboration with the WHO and other national and regional classification groups.

The *Clinical Care Component* includes the development of training curricula and continuing education modules within the framework of a multidisciplinary clinical training programme, which is based on contextualized and person-oriented clinical care. Promoting the doctor-patient relationship is at the centre of these activities as is the inclusion of the patient's family in the diagnostic and treatment process. Methods that are being used to attain these ends are small group learning and intense supervision of medical students and postgraduate trainees among others. Another project included in this component is the drawing up of Guidelines for Person-centred Clinical Care. Health promotion should be an integral part of clinical care. Input from psychiatrists across the world is being sought, via workshops at various regional congresses. Networks to enhance and monitor implementation and follow-up will also be organized. Participants in this component are the WPA section on Education in Psychiatry, several WPA sections related to clinical care and consumer and family organizations.

The *Public Health Component* is engaged in evaluation and epidemiological approaches which encompass illness- and health-related variables and the whole person of each individual within community settings. The project includes the development of public health initiatives which aim to promote mental health among the general population and to support the implementation of person- and community-oriented health services which take into consideration all the relevant socio-cultural factors. This component covers community mental health services; new challenges to communities such as catastrophic events and violence; by-products and consequences of globalization; efforts towards enhancing social supports; communication skills, and positive health. Participants in this project are the WPA sections on Epidemiology and Public Health, and Public Policy and Psychiatry, and colleagues from the WHO, experts from international psychiatric associations, and representatives of consumer and family organizations.

These various components of the WPA have already begun work and the ethics guidelines of the WPA will be followed throughout the entire project. It is expected that various results and products will be generated in the course of the programme, including: publications (a book series, scientific journal articles, brochures, CDs, etc.); instruments (such as the Person-Centred Integrative Diagnosis); manuals for clinical practice; statements and guidelines pertaining to health policies; teaching programmes and continuing education modules; symposia and workshops at WPA congresses and other conferences; research projects and surveys, and a collaborative network for implementation and evaluation.

A Person-centred Integrative Diagnosis

Another example of the World Psychiatric Association's projects are the activities of the scientific section on Classification and Diagnosis, which is making a substantial effort in collaboration with the WHO and national psychiatric associations towards developing the foundations for future diagnostic systems (Mezzich and Üstün 2002; WPA 2003; APAL 2004; Banzato *et al*. 2005).

The WPA section on Classification and Diagnosis, has become involved with the WHO in the development of the ICD-11. Beyond this, the section has assumed a leading role in the development of an innovative integrative diagnostic model consistent with the concept of a Psychiatry for the Person. The aim of such a Person-centred Integrative Diagnosis (PID) is a 'diagnosis of the person, by the person, for the person and with the person' (Mezzich and Salloum 2007, p 1).

'This broader and deeper notion of diagnosis goes beyond the more restricted concepts of nosological and differential diagnoses. The proposed Person-centred Integrative Diagnostic model, involving both a formulation and a process, employs all relevant descriptive tools (categorization, dimensions, and narratives), in a possibly multilevel structure, engages the interactive participation of clinicians, patients, and families, and intends to provide the informational basis for person-centred integration of health care.' (Mezzich and Salloum 2007, p 1)

The building blocks for such a diagnostic system have been assembled over a ten-year-long international work-project of the WPA, led by Juan Mezzich and the Classification section. The International Guidelines for Diagnostic Assessment (IGDA) which came out of this project were published in a special issue of the *British Journal of Psychiatry* (WPA 2003). They provide a framework and contain the essential components for diagnostic assessment. Depending on the institutional context and the diagnostic requirements, clinicians can modify the content and focus, in an individualized and flexible manner. *The International Guidelines for Diagnostic Assessments* (IGDA) have since been picked up by a number of South American psychiatric associations and adapted to local cultural conditions. *The Latin-American Guide for Psychiatric Diagnosis* has been published in several Latin-American countries (APAL 2004). Thereby, a widespread use in psychiatric services for Spanish-speaking populations has become feasible.

Just as the overarching programme of a Psychiatry for the Person in general, and the Person-Centred Integrative Diagnosis (PID) in particular, have illustrated, the central element of these efforts is a turning away from the reductionist notion of the patient as bearer of symptoms and the clinician as distanced provider of services, towards an encounter between two entirely real individuals. Therefore, we would like to quote Helen Glover. What she says demonstrates the essential importance of the whole person for the recovery process:

> 'The most important thing in a person's recovery is the person himself or herself. A recovery space cannot be realised without the person. Everything else is negotiable' (Glover 2005, p 1).

RECOVERY AND PSYCHOPHARMACOLOGY

New goals and new roles for psychopharmacologists

In an article published in 2000, Douglas L Noordsy, William C Torrey, Shery Mead, Mary Brunette, Daniel Potenza and Mary Ellen Copeland outlined which attitudes and competencies psychopharmacologists must acquire in order to assume meaningful roles within the recovery model: 'Recovery-oriented psychopharmacology: redefining the goals of antipsychotic treatment'. Their definition, delineation and description of possible psychopharmacological interventions as part of a medical as well as a rehabilitative model are a good example of the extent to which an adaptation to the new challenges of recovery by prescribing physicians can influence the practice of professional providers.

About the authors

Noordsy, Torrey, Brunette and Potenza are psychiatrists in Dartmouth, New Hampshire (USA). Shery Mead and Mary Ellen Copeland are non-medical professionals with their own experiences of a serious psychiatric disorder (cf. pp 83).

Mary Ellen Copeland's story and her work have already been reported, in the chapter about the Wellness Recovery Action Plan (WRAP). Shery Mead is co-author of their *Manual on Wellness Recovery and Peer Support*. She is an independent consultant and trainer in the area of 'peer-run' mental health services. 'Peer-run' means that a service is led by one or more individuals whose expertise importantly also comes from the fact that they have experienced a serious psychiatric disorder. Shery Mead worked for many years as the director of such services in New Hampshire. Many of her lectures and training programmes address the issue of alternative crisis support methods and the ways in which a service system can be transformed in order to meaningfully incorporate peer-run programmes. She is particularly interested in non-pathologizing ways of dealing with traumatic experiences and the development of research methods for the evaluation of peer-run programmes. Her website provides information about her personal story, her publications and the point in her life when she put the patient role behind her and dedicated herself to the establishment of user-organizations (www.mentalhealthpeers.com)

The basic idea

Noordsy *et al.* (2000) begin their article with a description of biological psychiatry's successes concerning psychopharmacological treatment. They point out that psychiatrists often experience their role as restricted to the biological part of treatment, while other disciplines are left to deal with rehabilitation and self-help. Nevertheless, psychiatrists still take on responsibilities in those areas, by making direct referrals, co-ordinating the overall treatment plan, and thereby integrating the recovery-oriented services that have sprung up outside of psychiatry. The authors suggest that because of the many fragmented services that are being offered, a considerable distance has developed between treating a person with psychosis according to the medical, the rehabilitative and the recovery model. This distance will need to be bridged. They recommend that psychopharmacologists integrate the principles of all three models, depending on the individual situation, and assume a variety of roles – according to the predominant model being used to treat a particular person at a particular point in time. To understand what kind of competencies within psychopharmacological treatment need to be applied, the authors describe the three models and their theoretical concepts, as well as their consequences for medical interventions.

The medical model

The medical model is based on the assumption that psychoses are brain diseases. This implies that the diagnostic assessments involve:

- identifying symptoms;
- taking a history of illness;
- identifying physiological abnormalities;
- generating a diagnosis using standardized diagnostic criteria;
- documenting disabilities.

Treatment follows this theoretical basis in a biological direction, determined by the diagnosis. There are guidelines and recommendations for the treatment of psychoses of the schizophrenia-type that doctors are expected to follow. The aim of treatment is essentially a reduction of symptoms without causing unwanted side effects. The research attempts to identify underlying causes in order to optimize treatment. The authors draw a parallel with Parkinson's Disease, where the identification of a causal factor – a dopamine-deficit – has led to a treatment of the causes by substituting dopamine. They also point out that even an accurate definition of the cause, as in the case of Parkinson's Disease, has not led to optimal treatments.

Therefore, a doctor's role, according to the medical model, consists of making an accurate diagnosis while ruling out other conditions that might cause similar combinations of symptoms. The diagnosis is the basis for prescribing medication that should reduce all symptoms associated with this particular diagnosis. Additional diagnoses might also be made, such as 'depression', which might also be treated with medication. In addition to this psychopharmacological intervention, psychiatrists need to co-ordinate their treatment with other medical or non-medical providers, something which it is not always easy to do.

The rehabilitation model

According to Noordsy *et al.* (2000), rehabilitation is traditionally an intervention that aims to improve the social functioning of a person with an illness beyond what can be accomplished with medication. The basis for such interventions is the assumption that psychoses are the cause of functional deficits, for which there are no curative treatments. Rehabilitative interventions are tied to resources and attempt to strengthen the capacities of the person that can help them overcome these deficits. They are based on diagnostic assessments about

- strengths;
- historic interests and abilities;
- physiological capacities, and
- functional capacity.

Evidence-based interventions are available in the areas of vocational rehabilitation, social skills training, social network development and life-style changes such as diet and exercise. Rehabilitation aims to optimize functioning and social integration. Rehabilitation research deals with the development of effective methods for promoting optimal functioning. In analogy to other areas of medicine, the authors point to cardiac rehabilitation, which is organized according to a similar methodology.

The demands that the rehab model makes on prescribing physicians are manifold and begin from the fact that psychiatrists are frequently responsible for appropriate and well-timed referrals to rehab services. This means that psychiatrists need to have current knowledge about locally available services. However, a referral does not put an end to the responsibility for the success of rehab interventions. There is a definite need for a close collaboration between the rehab team and the prescribing physicians. Medication has to be adjusted in a manner that facilitates optimal everyday functioning within the rehab service. This relates particularly to 'negative symptoms' and cognitive disturbances.

While acute treatment aims primarily at a reduction of positive symptoms, it is negative symptoms which mainly influence the results of rehabilitation. The prescribing physicians need to be regularly informed about their clients' concentration, tolerance of stress, energy levels, etc. in the rehab setting. On the other hand, rehab staff need to be informed about planned or necessary changes in medication, since these could affect the capacities of the patients in their day to day functioning at the rehab facility. Ideally, the prescribing physicians should be able to witness the functioning of their patients in vivo, i.e. at work, in the rehab setting and in their homes, to assess their successes and difficulties, and to find out how psychopharmacological treatment might promote a better adjustment.

Unfortunately, this ideal situation, as it is described here, rarely occurs in actuality. The fragmentation of mental health services in the USA and Europe often creates a situation where, instead of regular collaboration between the various service providers, they work in a disjointed and uncoordinated fashion. This means not only that opportunities for enhancing the effectiveness of interventions are being squandered, but also that they might actually be working at cross purposes.

The recovery-model

The authors acknowledge that the recovery-model has been developed from within the user movement and not from the professional realm. Frequently, the motivation to develop recovery-models originated from great dissatisfaction with professional services. The authors are nevertheless proposing that the recovery-model should not be viewed as antagonistic to the traditional models, but instead as complementary. Work within a recovery-model starts from the assumption that individuals with psychoses are more likely to define themselves anew in social roles and relationships, rather than through their disabilities. This means that 'personally relevant consequences of illness', 'consumer's ownership of life and illness', 'sick roles', and 'institutionalism' need to be assessed by consumers and professionals. Treatment in the context of the recovery-model consists of a consumer-driven change process, in which clinicians can serve as consultants and facilitators. It involves mutual-help and self-help interventions that can encourage growth and consider possibilities, hopes, and dreams. Service providers must be prepared to learn alongside service users and to be open to new experiences. And they need to believe in the potential of the users to achieve a meaningful life in place of the patient role. This means that important judgments must be openly and honestly expressed. 'Motivational interviewing' is proposed as a useful method for achieving clarity about certain limitations that might be encountered along the way towards goals and desired changes. The aim of the recovery-model is a meaningful life. This requires a focus on wellness instead of illness and a shift from patient role to meaningful life roles.

Noordsy *et al.* (2000) propose that the paradigm shift in cancer treatment and the approach to alcohol dependency, with their focus on mutual support, can be seen as prototypical recovery-models. The authors present results from a review of consumer literature on recovery and a series of focus groups, and conclude that:

1) promoting hopefulness;
2) developing skills and knowledge to take personal responsibility for health, and

3) 'supporting efforts to get on with life beyond illness' are central elements of successful work in the recovery-model.

They outline how these three areas should inform the role of the psychopharmacologist. Concretely, this means that consumers are to be given clear information about the prospects for their condition as well as access to scientific data that have frequently shown that recovery is possible. Service providers must steer clear of accepting limitations and poor prognoses as given, because by so doing they can stand in the way of patients' goals. Doctors must also realize the power-differential that characterizes their relationship to patients, and be prepared to accept change in the direction of responsibility being assumed on both sides. Quite a bit of work is necessary to establish the practice of shared decision-making. This does not only mean taking patients' suggestions about medication regimens seriously, it also means actively identifying areas where patients can assume control, even in times when they are struggling with limitations. Collaborative crisis-plans or advance directives for future situations when autonomous decision-making might be curtailed, are just as important as ongoing work aimed at enabling responsible risk-taking.

In order for psychopharmacologists to fulfill their important roles, they must go beyond merely acquiring the capacities relevant to each of these models; they must also be charged with making sure that the various treatment approaches can be integrated into a flexible and individualized overall treatment concept.

Pat Deegan's concept of 'Personal Medicine'

Pat Deegan (2005b), highly regarded as a pioneer in the consumer movement and icon of the recovery movement, (see also pp 71) who has personal experience of the diagnosis of schizophrenia and who is a distinguished clinical psychologist and teacher, begins her publication on personal medicine with the statement: 'People with psychiatric disabilities are resilient' (p 29). What a start! In saying this, Deegan refers to the more optimistic results of longitudinal studies about people diagnosed with schizophrenia and other severe psychiatric disorders, where recovery has been noted among up to two thirds of participants. Resilience and recovery are connected, being that they are two aspects of a multi-faceted phenomenon (see also pp 25). Deegan's main thesis is that the capacity for resilience does not cease when someone has been diagnosed with a serious psychiatric condition. On the contrary, those who are struggling towards their recovery should be considered as particularly resilient.

The author welcomes the notion that the concept of recovery and resilience can prompt clinicians to redirect their attention from illness-related processes towards the service user as a whole person, with his/her own life-circumstances. The focus should be more on the sources of health than on the origins of illness, in other words on 'salutogenesis' (Antonovsky 1979). This change of perspective would help clinicians learn how to inquire about clients self-assessed health resources and how to identify those qualities and strategies that are seen as health-promoting from the perspective of the clients.

Deegan's study on personal medicine was funded by the University of Kansas. Its results are currently being disseminated across the USA in continuing education programmes for users and staff of user-run organizations, as well as for mental health service providers. Deegan wanted to investigate the question: 'How do people with psychiatric conditions show their capacity for resilience in everyday life?' She was particularly interested in this question with respect to the taking or not taking of medication. Her personal experience with recovery and her concerns about the overuse of neuroleptics motivated her to conduct the study summarized here.

Implementation of the study

Deegan and her research team chose a qualitative method which they found especially suitable for an understanding of resilience. In the course of a participatory action-research design, study participants became involved in the interpretation and use of the data. A group of 29 individuals in the State of Kansas were interviewed, ten men and 19 women between the ages of 20 and 69. They had diagnoses such as schizophrenia, bipolar disorder, major depressive disorder, and personality disorder. Nearly half of them also had a history of substance abuse. All the participants except three were taking psychotropic drugs at the time of the interview, and everyone had participated in outpatient psychiatric treatment at one point or another for an average of fifteen years.

The participants were informed about the study, which included participation in semi-structured interviews, and were reimbursed for their efforts. They were asked how they came to use psychiatric services, and about their experiences with psychotropic drugs. Finally, they were asked to consider which was the most important element of their experiences, in the context of any useful aspects of taking medication, that service providers should know. The interviews took place in the homes of the participants, in public libraries, or in user-run programmes. Pat Deegan introduced herself personally in her dual role as a psychologist/researcher, and a former psychiatric patient who had herself, at one time, also taken medication in her recovery from schizophrenia. She wanted to communicate two things. First, she wanted participants to know that she was a nationally known lecturer and author on topics related to recovery from psychiatric disorders (her name was already known to some of the research participants). And second, she wanted her self-disclosure to help to create a more trusting atmosphere for the interviews. This she felt would be much more likely if people understood that the study was being run by and for people with psychiatric disorders. The transcribed interviews were analyzed according to the phenomenological method of Amedeo Giorgi (1997), which led to a contextual understanding of the participants' experiences. The results were discussed several times in a focus group which included research participants with a psychiatric diagnosis. The discussions centred on the usefulness, accessibility, and relevance of the findings from the service users point of view.

Results

The most interesting finding was that many answers to the question about taking psychotropic drugs included individual, non-pharmacological strategies, namely 'personal medicine'. Many autonomous self-help activities served the purpose of reducing psychiatric symptoms and avoided unwanted consequences (i.e. hospital admissions), while having a beneficial effect on mood, outlook, thought, behaviours, and overall sense of well-being. The participants reported that they generally did not speak with their providers about their personal medicine, and that those providers had never initiated any questions about these strengths. Taking medication only made sense to the participants when it could reasonably be fitted in with the array of their own individual strategies. Medication was not taken when it interfered with their personal medicine and thus resulted in a diminished quality of life.

Personal medicine

Personal medicine was discovered by the participants within the context of their everyday lives. For example, one participant (Joe), who had been diagnosed with bipolar disorder, found that solving mathematical problems was a more effective way to stabilize his mood than taking medication. He expressed this in his own words:

> '*I think there are a lot of other things that are medication, that are not really considered medication. There's things that you can do that changes what your body does. And it may not be medicine . . . I still think that one of the best mood stabilizers there is in life – maybe not for everyone but for me – is math. That stimulates your intellectual process.*' (Deegan 2005b, p 32)

All 29 participants mentioned different forms of personal medicine that they used in addition to, or instead of, taking psychiatric medication. Two main categories of personal medicine were identified: a) activities that gave meaning and purpose to life, and b) specific self-care strategies.

a) *Personal medicine as meaning and purpose in life:* This type of personal medicine includes positively valued social roles and activities which gave the individual a sense of direction, meaning and purpose, enhanced their self-worth and helped them persevere through difficult times. A woman participant who had been diagnosed and treated for schizophrenia since childhood discovered that singing in a group helped her avoid hospitalizations and medication over a period of five years. She was the principal singer of the group.

Personal medicine did not necessarily replace psychotropic drugs. Frequently, both were used successfully together. A woman of 29 years of age, who had been diagnosed with major depression with psychotic features, continued taking her medication, while also using personal medicine that included being a good mother and serving her community as a volunteer. Also, work was reported to be powerful personal medicine. For one participant, working full-time made life hectic but also filled her life with meaning, decreased her depression, and helped her stay out of hospital.

Personal medicine was not necessarily free of stress either. One young woman (Tamika), with a diagnosis of major depression with psychotic features, distinguished between stress and 'good stress'. She reported that the stress involved with attending the university was bearable since it had a *purpose*:

> *'(Going to university)... is stressful but it's a kind of good stress. I mean there's a purpose to it. A good purpose. And I think that's why I still do it. It keeps me from thinking about other things and going to other sources [street drugs] to relieve my stress'* (ibid., p 32).

b) *Personal medicine as self-care strategies:* Self-care strategies helped the participants to improve wellness and reduce psychiatric symptoms, or to limit undesired consequences. Nearly half of the participants mentioned that helping others in formal or informal ways had a mutually beneficial effect, for example for Thomas:

> *'I found by helping others, I found out how to live for myself'* (ibid., p 33).

Many activities helped to strengthen a person's well-being: keeping busy; physical exercise; engaging in advocacy; spending time with loved ones; sex; going fishing; solving math problems; shopping; changes in diet; having a good cry; spending time with 'normal' people; being alone; being in nature; making phone calls; going for a car ride; taking a day off; pushing oneself to achieve; collecting dolls, and exposure to sunlight. Even though many of these activities were quite ordinary and familiar, they helped participants by ameliorating different kinds of distress such as anxiety, confusion, lack of concentration, depression, insomnia, worries, suspicion, troublesome voice-hearing and racing thoughts.

Disclosure of personal medicine to healthcare providers

A large proportion of the participants reported that they did not speak to their psychiatrists about their personal medicine. A 42-year-old woman with severe depression still had difficulties falling asleep and struggled with depressed moods. At night she often watched horror movies and found that she could fall asleep better and felt less depressed – at least for a while – when she kept watching certain violent scenes. She was afraid to tell her psychiatrist about this, since she feared his disapproval. Another participant used alcohol, street-drugs and tobacco for self-soothing, but avoided talking about this to his doctor. Interestingly, even 'positive' wellness strategies that would probably meet with approval were not discussed voluntarily. Only four of the 29 interviewees reported that mental health care practitioners inquired about personal medicine activities.

Non-adherence: when psychiatric medicine interferes with personal medicine

Whenever psychotropic drugs interfered too much with the activities or the effects of personal medicine that were meaningful for the participants, several of them discontinued the medication. One woman (Nancy) felt, for example, that caring for her children was the most important part of her life. Her illness, diagnosed as a psychotic depression, interfered as much in carrying out the tasks of being a good mother, as did certain kinds of medication. She lacked all motivation to care for her children, and had to put them into day care, as she needed excessive sleep due to a certain drug. Then she found a practitioner who suggested a different drug that was able to strengthen her personal medicine of being a mother.

> *'She's a nurse practitioner... She wants you to be the best person you can be so she tries to get medication for that. Not something that's just going to, as I call it, zombify you out and get rid of the symptoms. She wants to get rid of the symptoms but also wants you to live.'* (ibid., p 33)

According to certain statements in the interviews, some clinicians interpreted the personal strengths and self-identified health resources of the participants as part of their psychopathology. For example, a single mother of three with a diagnosis of bipolar disorder valued her energy and stamina as positive, while her psychiatrist considered the same attributes as evidence of hypomania and prescribed a neuroleptic. It was not surprising that this woman (Kim) did not take the prescribed medication, which was supposed to 'treat' the very things she considered to be strengths.

> *'I don't really see it as mania. I see it as part of me. I just see that as an extension of me when I am full of energy. I am able to do things... this is the me that I know but then there's somebody else calling it a disease, a problem. Well for me, this problem has got me through a lot!'* (ibid., p 33)

Discussion of the results

Deegan does not consider herself a neutral observer. Her own background as a person who has taken psychotropic drugs as part of her recovery-experience, influenced the study design, the way participants were recruited, the data analysis and the composition of the focus group. She welcomed critical feedback from focus-group participants, who all had psychiatric diagnoses. According to Deegan, other qualitative researchers might have come up with different but equally valid interpretations of the data, which would also have contributed to a greater understanding of the complex phenomena related to resilience and personal medicine. However, she believes the participants would probably not have opened up as much to a more distanced interviewer or clinician. Regarding the representative nature of the findings, Deegan assumes that patient groups in other countries or with different issues, such as chronic physical illnesses, might offer similar responses about personal medicine and recovery. She hopes that future studies can shed more light on the way clinicians and patients might apply the concept of personal medicine in order to improve clinical outcomes and enable a more effective prescription of pharmaceuticals.

Participants in the focus groups, all of whom had experience with psychotropic drugs, considered the strategies of personal medicine as very valuable for their own recovery. From their perspective, should recovery be simply ascribed to the effects of psychotropics, this would rob people of the ability to make autonomous decisions. In such a case, the individual would merely be reduced to 'swallowing pills faithfully'. They believed that recovery means changing your life and not your biochemistry. Their recovery is hard work and requires much personal dedication, willpower, vision, hope, strength, courage, imagination, commitment, and resilience. The concept of personal medicine helped them to speak about their daily experiences and they felt empowered by the ways they worked to improve their lives.

Deegan wants to reach many peer support groups run by and for people with psychiatric disabilities and their families. She hopes that people can share and teach recovery-strategies in these groups. This way, people could be taught to identify their personal medicine and to create 'power statements' in order to convey the importance of personal medicine to their health care practitioners. An example of such a power statement could be: 'Singing lifts me up and gives my life meaning ... Singing is powerful medicine for me. I want to work with you to find a medication and dosage that does not interfere with my singing' (ibid., p 34). Deegan refers to a similar concept developed by general practitioners in Scandinavia (Malterud and Hollnagel 1999; Hollnagel and Malterud 1995), where patients are invited to share their experiences and the resources they discovered with their doctors. In the case of personal medicine, the information would be initiated by the patient instead of being elicited by the practitioner.

Resilience and personal medicine can be found in the lives of many people with psychiatric diagnoses, and Deegan refers, for example, to the work of Strauss *et al.* (1987) and Roe *et al.* (2004). The reasons why psychiatrists do not inquire about their patients' strengths and self-help strategies, and why service users generally do not mention them, are connected, according to Deegan, to the training of doctors and other clinicians, where a deficit-oriented model is still prevailing. This deficit-orientation goes so far that John Strauss (1989, p 182) – eminent researcher and proponent of the recovery-concept – offered an example from one of his many interviews during which a woman with a diagnosis of schizophrenia asked him: 'Why don't you ever ask what I do to help myself?'

Deegan demands that clinicians routinely inquire about any self-help activities among their clients which they may already be practising, and mentions Rapp's strengths approach: 'The strengths model then is about providing a new perception. It allows us to see possibilities rather than problems, options rather than constraints, wellness rather than sickness' (Rapp 1998, p 24). Deegan highlights other studies – for example, of patients with asthma – which revealed that the taking of medication became problematic when important personal attributes and activities of the patients were interpreted as symptoms of the illness, and medication was recommended to treat these (for example, Rogers *et al.* 1998; Britten *et al.* 2004; Scherman and Lowhagen 2004).

In summing up, Deegan states that medication adherence might increase if clinicians regularly ask clients about their personal medicine before prescribing and if they work with the patient to establish the goal of pharmaceuticals in supporting or enhancing personal medicine. When this is done, medication can be experienced as supportive and not as inhibiting the recovery-process. Ideally, treatment with psychotropic medication should enhance personal medicine.

'Personal medicine reminds us that there are many ways to change our body's chemistry and that, within the task of recovery, pill medicine must complement and support personal medicine, or the things that give one's life purpose and meaning' (Deegan 2007 p 65).

A programme to support shared decision-making

DVDs with three-minute recovery-stories in which people talk about how personal medicine supported their recovery are a core feature of a software programme designed to assist a process of shared decision-making concerning the use of psychiatric medication (Deegan *et al.* 2008). The use of a peer-staffed Decision Support Center (DSC) in a medication clinic is one of three tiers of a 'Recovery-Based Programme for Supporting Clients through Decisional Uncertainty Regarding the Use of Psychiatric Medicine' (Deegan 2007) developed by Pat Deegan, (see also pp 71) which is currently being disseminated and scientifically evaluated.

Deegan's own lived experience of using psychiatric medication ranges from 'compliance' and progress in the eyes of the psychiatrist, which led to the tragic realization that 'I lost years of my life in this netherworld, and although I was treatment compliant and was maintained in the community, I was not recovering', to an extremely different experience, namely that of 'using medication as part of my journey of recovery' (Deegan 2007 p 63). For such a change to happen much has to be learned by both client and psychiatrist (Deegan 2007; Deegan and Drake 2006). Deegan (2007) explores the complexities of decision-processes in the context of whether or not to use medication in the recovery-process. It is her belief that overcoming the oversimplification and dehumanizing quality of 'compliance versus non-compliance', acknowledging that rejection of medication can sometimes be a sign of resilience and hope rather than a symptom of illness, acknowledging that respect and interest for the 'authentic struggle involved in learning to use psychiatric medications in the recovery process' (Deegan 2007 p 63), and understanding that there are many sources of 'decisional conflicts', are important issues on the way towards a successful therapeutic alliance.

Deegan conceptualizes shared decision-making as:

- 'a person centred alternative to traditional notions of medical compliance' (Deegan 2007, p 62);
- an ethical imperative;
- consistent with the tradition of building therapeutic alliances;
- a superior approach to medical paternalism and insistence on compliance (Deegan *et al.* 2008);
- founded on the premise of two experts who 'must share information in order to arrive at the best treatment decisions possible and bridge the scientific and the personal knowledge domains through this process';
- an emancipatory praxis breaking silence and enhancing dialogue (Deegan 2007, p 64).

To support people through decisional conflicts and assist them in shared decision-making processes Deegan (2007 p 67) developed her programme around three principles:

1. 'The goal of using psychiatric medication is recovery';
2. 'Psychiatric medication must serve personal medicine and the overarching goal of recovery';
3. 'The goal of the treatment team (in relation to medication) is to support clients through decisional conflicts to achieve optimal use of personal medicine and psychiatric medicine in the recovery process'.

All three of which apply to the three tiers of the programme:

1. a peer-to-peer workshop;
2. a peer-run decision support centre;
3. training of case management staff.

One decision support centre that was set up in a typical medication clinic has been evaluated after one year of having been used by 189 consumers, 622 times. A randomized controlled trial is currently under way (Deegan *et al.* 2008). Apart from a welcoming environment with healthy snacks and all sorts of information, an internet-based software programme with which clients can create a one-page computer-generated report was offered. The report includes their assessments of problems, concerns and goals, and highlights decisional uncertainties, which might be due, for example, to side effects. Different formats and peer assistance allow people with low literacy and a lack of computer skills to use the programme. The one-page report can be printed out and is forwarded to the practitioner. It serves not only as a basis for interaction in the sense of shared decision-making but also allows easy access to specific further support, such as information and decision aids, which the client might have asked for.

Results of the pilot project (Deegan *et al.* 2008) clearly suggest that this ground-breaking programme for the amplification of clients' voice helps to enrich dialogue and deepen shared understanding as well as helping to bring to light concerns that might otherwise go unexpressed or misunderstood, concerns that can lead to an effective refocusing of support.

SYSTEM TRANSFORMATION

The United States Department of Health and Human Sciences in its Federal Action Agenda clearly states that for a recovery-oriented mental health system 'reform is not enough' and that 'transformation is not accomplished through change on the margin but, instead, through profound changes in kind and in degree' and is supposed to 'change the very form and function of the mental health service delivery system to better meet the needs of the individuals and families it is designed to serve'. (http://www .samhsa.gov/Federalactionagenda/NFC_EXECSUM.aspx#link_group_1; 20.08.08)

Hopper's (2007) assessment concerning the politics of recovery that 'after nearly a decade of work, wholesale system transformation is still pending' (p 872) is in part a reflection of his observation that 'operational specificity was unwisely sacrificed in the interest of more efficiently spreading the good news' (p 873). As far as efforts towards real change in terms of a capabilities-informed agenda are concerned, he does expect 'abrasive relations with traditional decision-making processes' (p 877).

In a similar down-to-earth assessment Meehan *et al.* (2007), speaking from an Australian perspective, assume that 'it is possible that transition to recovery-oriented services, if implemented in practice (rather than in rhetoric), will be as radical as the transition from institutional to community care' (p 181).

Recovery-oriented services

At the rather sanguine end of the spectrum of people considering system transformation, Wesley Sowers (2005) for the American Association of Community Psychiatrists states that the promotion of recovery has been 'recognized as an organizational principle for the transformation of behavioural health services', and that this 'represents a major cultural shift in service delivery' with:

- paternalistic, illness-oriented perspectives replaced by collaborative, autonomy-enhancing approaches;
- the myth of chronicity and dependence replaced by a message of hope and personal growth, empowerment and choice;
- a context of collaborative relationships between service providers and people who use services.

As a model that might allow the system to grow and change in this way, the recovery-model offers valuable advice for the 'extremely challenging task' which requires 'vigilance, dedication, skill, patience, humility and a great deal of hard work', and 'open mindedness and willingness to accept help'. This last essential capacity would, according to a recovery-model, lead to 'the assistance of people in recovery as partners in this process' (Sowers 2005, p 760).

The guidelines for recovery-oriented services (ROS) have been developed through clinical consensus, literature review and stakeholder consultation and address systems, in a process of transformation towards recovery-orientation in regard of quality improvement and management. For the three domains and several elements of each domain, recovery-enhancing characteristics are defined and supported with available evidence.

- Administration (mission and vision: strategic plan, organizational resources; training: continuing education, continuous quality improvement, outcome assessment);
- Treatment (an array of services, advance directives, cultural competence, planning processes; integration of addiction and mental health, coercive treatment, seclusion and restraint);
- Supports (advocacy and mutual support, access facilitating processes, family services, employment and education, housing).

Example indicators for each element provide direction as well as opportunities for evaluation. For example, indicators for the element of continuous quality improvement (CQI) in the domain of administration are:

A) 'Process in place to ensure that consumers are included in CQI activities as equal partners with professionals.
B) Agency budget will reflect compensation for consumer involvement in CQI activities.'
(Sowers 2005, p 763)

The model of the American Association of Community Psychiatrists (Sowers 2005) was one of the first to have been taken up by German-speaking colleagues at the University of Zurich, where Bridler and Lötscher are in the process of developing an assessment instrument for the recovery-orientation of psychiatric institutions (personal communication).

Recovery-oriented mental health programmes

Marianne Farkas and Bill Anthony are prominent rehabilitation researchers in the field of mental health and directors of Boston University's Center for Psychiatric Rehabilitation. For several decades they have been among the leading researchers in this field worldwide and they are among the most highly respected researchers in the area of determining scientific standard in this field (see also pp 153). They also have a decisive influence on many important developments in the mental health arena and belong to those established professionals who have endorsed the recovery-concept from its beginnings. In the era of evidence-based psychiatry, they have been pioneers in defining a recovery-orientation for services.

In several publications, including books and professional journals, and as members of state and federal advisory committees, Anthony and Farkas have applied their scientific backgrounds and developed ideas and proposals that captured the recovery-concept in a meaningful way and promoted its application in research and services. Several of their publications have been co-authored with activists with lived experience, for instance, in 2005 with Judi Chamberlin from the National Empowerment Center (Farkas, Gagne, Anthony, Chamberlin 2005).

The authors describe in clear language the kind of substantive changes that a recovery-orientation would imply for psychiatric services after almost an entire century during which the treatment and rehabilitation of people with 'severe and persistent mental illness' focused on relapse prevention and stabilization. Over recent years, long-term psychiatric treatment has aimed primarily at a reduction in the frequency and duration of hospitalizations, or, if possible, their elimination altogether. This meant that scientific research, correspondingly, followed the same goals. Recovery-concepts did not feature in this context. This does not mean that no one – neither patients, professionals nor relatives – had been working towards recovery in those years. But it does mean that the goals of treatment had never been formulated according to recovery-principles, and services had never been evaluated as to the percentage of people who were being helped in their recovery. Psychiatric services were never organized to implement recovery-concepts.

Currently, things are in a considerable state of flux. Many service organizations and individual practitioners want to work according to a recovery-orientation concept. ROMHP is the acronym for Recovery Oriented Mental Health Programmes. Farkas *et al.* (2005) point out that the term 'programme' can be used in a variety of ways, but usually indicates a service, for instance a psychosocial treatment facility, that offers several components, i.e. individual and group therapies, day treatment, vocational rehabilitation, and much else. Such a service or programme defines for itself what it is or desires to be, how it functions, and what its mission might be. It formulates guidelines and informs its customers about them. Staff are recruited and trained accordingly. Quality assurance and evaluation are also oriented according to the mission and the goals of the programme. The way programmes define themselves and how they formulate and monitor their mission and goals, determines whether they are recovery-oriented or not.

Increasingly, researchers such as Farkas *et al.* (2005) have expressed the opinion that it is not sufficient to assess the impact of one component of a programme or another, such as medication or a day treatment programme, but that the basic attitude of the programme staff, their mission statement, self-definition and their values must be captured by any research endeavour. There are some indications that these values, which are at the core of these services, have a greater impact than any one component of the programme, or than answering the question how much of this or that can have what kind of effect. Most likely, what we are calling the recovery-orientation of a service is largely contained in these basic values. Farkas, Gagne, Anthony and Chamberlin (2005) refer to earlier publications in order to define and describe four key values that they see as indispensable ingredients of recovery-orientation. These four key values are: person orientation; person involvement; self-determination/choice, and growth potential.

Person orientation: Person orientation implies that the services are primarily defined according to the needs of an individual, with all his/her strengths, talents, interests, and limitations. This is in stark contrast to the focus on an individual as a 'case', along with the signs and symptoms of an illness, and a diagnosis which determine the services to be delivered. Many recovery-concepts and plans place a major emphasis on the way people are being approached. Davidson and Strauss (1992), Pat Deegan (2005a) and many others have pointed out that people are always more than just patients and that it serves them well to be seen as whole human beings. They should not merely be viewed and understood in their patient-role, but rather in their many life-roles along with their possibilities and limitations. Deegan underlines explicitly that professional service providers who are denying such a holistic view to the people they encounter as patients, are causing them harm.

Person involvement: Services are concentrating on the right to a partnership in all relationships pertaining to recovery. This means that the people who are supposed to be assisted by those services have the right to have input in the planning, organization and evaluation of those services. Rehabilitation research teaches us that people are more likely to be successful when they have been meaningfully involved in the organization and evaluation of their services. User involvement is increasingly seen as a benchmark for quality in organization, planning and evaluation (see also p 21).

Self-determination/choice: The service places an emphasis on the rights of all people to make individual decisions and choices in all aspects of their recovery. This includes, among others, treatment goals, choice of supports that should assist in reaching these goals, and determining when and whether to make use of services. The literature has repeatedly cautioned that compliance, i.e. simply going along with interventions suggested by professionals, should not be overestimated. It might very well be that such compliance could weaken a person who found himself dependent on the decisions of others.

Growth potential: Services are focused on the inherent potential for recovery of every person – irrespective of whether he/she is currently overwhelmed by the illness or disability, is struggling with adversity or living with disadvantages. It cannot be stated too often: hope is an essential ingredient of any recovery-orientation. Concentrating on the potential of every person to grow, implies a dedication to sustain hope on the part of the professional service providers as well as on the part of the recipients. For the services this means that they need to assess themselves according to the amount of hope and belief in possibilities that is being offered. This might require a fundamental change in the way services are being offered.

What does this mean for the organization, administration and staffing of services?

Mission: The mission of service provision is no longer to assure people, in the traditional way, that they will receive comprehensive services with optimal continuity of treatment, but rather the mission now is to help people in a way that enables them to be satisfied with their lives and to live successfully in their communities under circumstances of their own choosing. The guiding principles emerge from discussions with clients and are accessible at any time to everyone.

Policies: Even today, many services users are still being offered programmes with strings attached, as for instance when they are told that they have to attend one or other of the structured day-programme in order to gain access to certain types of housing. Recovery-oriented services would have to make it possible for everyone to determine which kind of support they would be using at what point in time and to what extent. Guidelines need to be presented in language that can be understood by everyone, by, for example, using 'person first' language that doesn't use a diagnosis as an attribute, i.e. calling someone a 'schizophrenic person', but instead talks about a 'person with a certain diagnosis, problem, disability, who is in recovery, etc'.

Procedures: General information packages should be replaced by a stepwise procedure that uses individualized methods of communicating. Clients should receive only the kind of information they want and they should receive it in a manner with which they are comfortable. The information should primarily be about the kinds of things the programme can offer and those that it cannot. The expectations of the programme should be presented as explicitly as the options available to clients so that clients can provide feedback and become involved in the structure of the programme. In particular the information should include guidelines about the way medical records can be accessed: 'clients should be able to gain access to their records at any time'. Beyond this, clients should also have the opportunity to comment about their records and to amend them. Strengths, talents and interests should be documented as well as difficulties and problematic areas.

Quality Assurance: Instead of programmes having to use officially mandated outcome assessments – even if they have little relevance for clients – results should be measured according to criteria identified by the clientele. Services should use quality assurance teams that represent all groups – workers, users, and relatives, as well as other interested public parties.

Physical Setting: Something that has come up consistently, ever since the first European studies on client satisfaction were conducted by Farkas and her colleagues also needs to be addressed, namely the problem of restrooms. Restrooms and other public facilities should be equally accessible to everyone. Signs indicating 'staff' and 'clients' do not make sense, but rather proclaim the inappropriate distinction between 'us, the healthy ones' and 'you, who are ill', which runs counter to person orientation. Clients should be able to become successfully involved in creating a pleasant environment.

Network of services: Programmes should not only be connected to other professional services, but also to the community at large. Otherwise, a segregated world might emerge, with leisure activities, religious services and training all taking place within mental health settings, which would thwart personal growth and integration.

Staffing: Traditionally, personnel choices occur according to criteria composed of relevant professional qualifications and years of experience. Recovery-oriented programmes must be careful to find staff who have knowledge about recovery and who have the values and capabilities which will enable them to work according to the principles of recovery. Therapeutic relationships play an important role in determining the success or failure of recovery-efforts. The capacity to sustain hope, the belief in the potential for further growth, and a non-discriminatory attitude towards clients are essential characteristics of staff in recovery-oriented services. It has also proven to be helpful when at least some of the staff comes with knowledge gained from personal experiences of psychiatric crises, quite apart from any professional competencies they may have.

Training: A significant component of traditional training is likely to be preparing mental health staff to deal with problems. They learn how to respond to relapses, deal with a lack of compliance, and manage risk. Mental health workers are generally not prepared to deal with successes and with the inherent potential of their clientele. They are not especially familiar with the ways of relating deteriorations and crises to an overall life-trajectory. Consequently, training programmes must be changed accordingly. This requires communication and interaction with people/experts who have overcome illness and disability and who are living examples of recovery.

Supervision: Recovery-values are also new for supervision and the administration of programmes. Career ladders and the potential for advancement should reflect the knowledge of staff about recovery-values and their competencies in supporting people throughout the recovery-process. This also includes the ability to facilitate well-informed decision-making and to accept such decisions of clients, even if one would not have chosen in the same way.

The authors stress that, on the one hand, such a recovery-oriented form of practice might contribute to a more successful realization of already existing aims in evidence-based mental health services. And on the other hand, additional goals that are more directly linked to recovery might emerge. These could include enhancing self-esteem, empowerment, and well-being. A clear outline of the recovery-orientation within a service agency would enable potential customers and other interested parties to evaluate the service. It would also help administrators to determine their strengths and weaknesses in the area of recovery-orientation. Researchers might be able to specifically investigate the implications of the recovery-concept for evidence-based mental health services.

A Recovery-Process Model

The example provided by the Ohio Department of Mental Health (Townsend *et al.* 1999) of a system-wide reorientation towards recovery has been met with great interest internationally and was also used by the National Institute for Mental Health in England as the basis of their 'Emerging Best Practices in Mental Health Recovery' plan in 2004.

The Institute proposed several meanings of recovery. These include a restoration of health, experiencing a recovery-process, and the achievement of an acceptable quality of life and satisfaction with that life in spite of persisting disabilities or an ongoing illness. They emphasize the significance of recovery as an individual process of combating the negative consequences of a mental illness or disorder, even if it still persists. Recovery is whatever people experience when they become empowered to lead a meaningful life, along with a positive feeling of belonging in their communities. This assessment has to come from the users themselves.

The concept of four phases begins with a state where a person lacks autonomy and needs help ('dependent'), but is unaware of what exactly is going on. In this first, *'dependent/unaware'* phase, it is frequently not apparent what the person's problems and needs actually are, there is no clear conception of what has to be accomplished, and no motivation to change anything. During this time there is a great demand for patience from the environment and the support systems. There is also a big challenge not to proceed in a resigned and devaluing manner, but rather to spend a lot of time conveying information – often in many brief interactions – and to enhance awareness.

People who have learned to rely on the service system and have become somewhat familiar with their psychiatric conditions, but have not yet developed trust in their own capacities, are entering the second phase, *'dependent/aware'* during which they live with an awareness of their dependency. This can be a result of institutionalization. The providers tend to take care of things for the users, rather than working with them. Patients suffer from stigmatization and social exclusion. Self-worth and self-efficacy are minimal. Life is marked by unfulfilled dreams and desires.

During the third phase, *'independent/aware'*, people are – once again – able to resume responsibility for themselves and their actions. They realize that they have to contribute to their own well-being and find ways to obtain support. Certain life-styles are identified as risky and people pay more attention to their own health during this phase. At this time people also develop the capacity to tell their own story and show interest in helping others. Relationships are now increasingly based on mutuality. Some people assume tasks and leadership roles in advocacy and other social spheres. Relying on the mental health system becomes less and less important and loses its attraction. At this point the service system needs to encourage clients to become engaged in outside activities and support their independence.

The fourth phase, *'interdependent/aware'*, means to live one's life and to be in charge, finding supports whenever, and in the way, one needs them. Health-promoting interventions, such as psychotherapy and pharmacological aides, can continue without people staying involved in the mental health system. Their careers are elsewhere. If they do stay involved in the system, they serve in active roles, for example as paid co-workers or volunteers. Mental health providers can be supportive when clients are leaving the patient-role behind. However, it must be clear that one can always come back in case of need during crises, or for other kinds of support.

Naturally, people do not fit neatly into such cubbyholes, but it is helpful to think about which phase is currently relevant. It is also obvious that some people pass through some of these phases more than once.

The significance of each of the four phases for clients, clinicians and community support is being considered in great detail. Each of the nine core areas of service are being dealt with separately: clinical treatment; family support; self-help; work and meaningful activities; power and control; stigma; participation in community life; access to resources, and training. This comprehensive matrix is the foundation of professional work. It provides a profile for the demands and activities of providers. Staff qualifications, competencies, basic and continuing education, and supervision are derived from it.

Essential capabilities

The definition of essential capabilities plays a core role in basic and continuing education and human resource development in all domains of health care and social services. They convey clearly which minimal requirements and basic competencies are expected from staff in recovery-oriented services. The National Institute for Mental Health in England's (NIMHE) ten essential capabilities relate to the following domains:

1. working in partnership;
2. respecting diversity;
3. practising ethically;
4. challenging inequality;
5. promoting recovery;
6. identifying people's needs and strengths;
7. providing service user centred care;
8. making a difference;
9. promoting safety and positive risk-taking;
10. personal development and learning.

Each of these is aimed at promoting a new culture in psychiatric services and thera-peutic relationships. Both content and form of communication and organization need to express and promote the existence of hope. The values and aims of the individual, and their strengths, must be at the centre of all efforts. The right to full participation and self-determination, as well as protection from discrimination must move to the centre of all efforts to promote recovery. All services need to aim towards a development beyond the limitations of the patient-role and towards a self-determined, meaningful life.

The 2008 policy paper published by the Sainsbury Centre for Mental Health, 'Making Recovery a Reality' (www.scmh.org.uk), is a great example of international language and an emerging consensus on recovery. In addition to the essential capabilities high-lighted above, various other UK and international experiences and formulations such as STORI from Australia (page 166); META from Arizona (www.recoveryinnovations.org 08.08.08); WRAP (page 83), and Davidson *et al.*'s (2006) top ten concerns, among others are integrated.

'A common purpose: recovery in future mental health services', a 2008 joint position paper by the Care Services Improvement Partnership (CSIP), the Social Perspectives Network (SPN), the Royal College of Psychiatrists (RCPsych) and the Social Care Institute for Excellence (SCIE) provides an overview of recovery-concepts and developments, including international and UK-based model examples (www.scie.org.uk/publications/positionpapers/pp08.asp 20.08.08).

Ramon *et al.* (2007) draw our attention also to the special UK situation, with its emphasis on social inclusion (www.socialinclusion.org.uk 20.08.08), and to the impact of the work of Repper and Perkins (2003) on the wealth of expert experience and the opportunities of hope-inspiring relationships. Reporting on Australia as well as on the UK, they conclude that: 'In the UK, the policy change – again drawing on service user perspectives – has perhaps been stronger and clearer, but the task of implementation largely lies ahead' (Ramon *et al.* 2007 p 119). For Australia, the Collaborative Recovery Model (Oades *et al.* 2005) provided training all over the country, but 'training clinicians has not ensured the routine implementation of recovery-based practice, with significant difficulties with the transfer of training' (Slade *et al.* 2008 p 132). Hope lies in the growing impact of the consumer movement (Ramon *et al.* 2007) and in the progress of research into recovery and the recovery competencies of the mental health workforces (Slade *et al.* 2008).

Practice guidelines for recovery-oriented behavioural health care

Connecticut's recovery initiative aimed from the start for statewide transformation 'warranting an entirely new approach to the design and delivery of care' in several interrelated steps:

- 'developing core values and principles based on the input of people in recovery;
- establishing a conceptual and policy framework based on this vision of recovery;
- building workforce competencies and skills through training, education, and consultation;
- changing programmes and service structures;
- aligning fiscal and administrative policies in support of recovery;
- monitoring, evaluating, and adjusting these efforts'(Davidson *et al.* 2007, p 24).

The involvement of 'people in recovery' as well as a recovery definition in line with a disability/civil rights model rather than a medical model – 'a process of restoring a meaningful sense of belonging to one's community and positive sense of identity apart from one's condition while rebuilding a life despite or within the limitations imposed by that condition' – set the scene for 'operationalizing recovery' (Davidson *et al.* 2007 p 26). Connecticut's recovery-oriented practices and supports for nine basic components of recovery are:

1. Being supported by others;
2. Renewing hope and commitment;
3. Engaging in meaningful activities;
4. Redefining self;
5. Incorporating illness;
6. Overcoming stigma;
7. Assuming control;
8. Managing symptoms;
9. Becoming empowered and exercising citizenship. (Davidson *et al.* 2005)

These have been formulated in detail with regard to:

- the person in recovery ('To me, recovery means....');
- the direct support provider ('I can support people in their recovery by ....');
- the manager/administrator ('I can lead an organization that supports recovery by ....).

For the practice guidelines for recovery-oriented behavioural health care (www.ct. gov/dmhas/LIB/dmhas/publications/practiceguidelines.pdf) the following eight domains of recovery-oriented services have been identified:

A. Primacy of participation;
B. Promoting access and engagement;
C. Ensuring continuity of care;
D. Employing strengths-based assessment;
E. Offering individualized recovery planning;
F. Functioning as a recovery guide;
G. Community mapping and development;
H. Identifying and addressing barriers to recovery.

The specifics of each domain are explained and this is followed by concrete action steps and guidelines. The practical implications are imparted through various instructive examples, following the didactic example of: 'You will know that you are placing primacy on the participation of people in recovery when .... :' (answers A1-A14, for example, A1 '... people in recovery are routinely invited to share their stories with current service recipients and/or to provide training to staff', and A2 '.... people in recovery comprise a significant proportion of representatives to an agency's board of directors, advisory board, or other steering committees and work groups').

For all domains instructions are given in the way illustrated by the following example: 'What you will hear from people in recovery when you are placing primacy on their participation:' for example, *'I knew I was in recovery when I could help somebody else that was in the same awful place that I used to be. But I think about where I am today: healthy, and drug free, and being a real Grandma. And getting back in the workplace as a peer provider makes me feel good; makes me understand that I can do this. I can really do this. And if I could do this, anybody can do this. Folks get hope when they look at me.'*

Another example of this system of standards and guidelines goes as follows: 'You will know that you are functioning as a Recovery Guide when .... :' (answers F1-F16), for example, F7 '... people are allowed to express their feelings, including anger and dissatisfaction, without having these reactions attributed to symptoms or relapse.' You will hear from people who realize that you are functioning as a recovery guide statements like: *'When he asked me: "So how can I best be of help!" I thought, "Oh great, I've really got a green one. You are supposed to be the professional – you tell me!" But I get it now. I need to decide what I need to move ahead in my recovery. And I needed to know it was OK to ask people for that. That was the key!'*

The Recovery Self Assessment tool RSA (O'Connell *et al.* 2005; see page 201–203) and the Recovery Knowledge Inventory RKI (Bedregal *et al.* 2006; see page 203–205) were widely and enthusiastically used to allow services and people engaged in the process at different levels to identify practices that either help or hinder recovery, as well as the extent of the variety of attitudes and knowledge (Davidson *et al.* 2007).

Commissioner Kirk Jr's policy on recovery included, in addition to the Recovery Education and Training Institute, the development of Centers of Excellence and Exemplary Programmes. The importance of peer-run programmes was particularly emphasized.

After several years of great success, Yale University recovery experts Davidson, Tondora and O'Connell, along with Commissioner Thomas Kirk Jr and Peter Rockholz of the Connecticut Department of Mental Health and Addiction Services and Arthur C Evans, former Deputy Commissioner (Davidson *et al.* 2007) still consider themselves to be at an early stage in the transformation process and offer lessons to do with two major issues:

1. 'It is key that people in recovery lead the way' and it is important and not always easy to avoid the grave yet common mistake of assuming that one can do recovery 'to and for people'.
2. Transformation is initiated through 'changing and realigning current policies, practices, procedures, services and supports to be oriented toward and effective in, promoting recovery'. Recovery-orientation is neither add-on nor is it waiting in an if and when sort of way for the resources to be in place. Instead, recovery happens through the integration of various system initiatives, for example, evidence-based practice or cultural competence, and the re-orientation of those system initiatives to support recovery.

Peer support and consumer-driven transformation

If the US Department of Health and Human Services is right in that a 'revolution' is required in mental health service delivery, the revolution will be about 'reconceptualizing the role of the person who has serious illness'. This assessment by Peebles *et al.* (2007) is meant as an encouragement for people to take on, in addition to the tasks associated with their own personal recovery, the tasks associated with the role of offering support, role modelling, mentoring, and other services to their peers. In this way, says Peebles, they will lead their peers towards presenting and discussing peer support and the initiatives of the Georgia Peer Specialist Programme regarding this essential innovation.

Solomon (2004) has defined peer support as 'social emotional support, frequently coupled with instrumental support, that is mutually offered or provided by people having a mental health condition to others sharing a similar mental health condition to bring about a desired social or personal change' (Solomon 2004, p 393). Such peer support can be either voluntary or financially compensated, and it can be provided in six different categories of services:

1. self-help groups;
2. internet support groups;
3. peer delivered services;
4. peer run or operated services;
5. peer partnerships;
6. peer employees.

Peebles *et al.* (2007), concentrate on a definition that talks about 'involving one or more people who have a history of mental illness and have experienced significant improve-ments in their psychiatric conditions offering services and/or supports to other people with serious mental illness who are considered to be not as far along in their own per-sonal recovery process' (Davidson *et al.* 2006c). This is more in line with the concept of 'peer provider' or 'consumer provider' (Chinman 2006) and implies a helping relation-ship with a certain asymmetry somewhere between a classical 'one-directional treatment relationship' and a 'reciprocal relationship', which usually prevails in self/mutual help initiatives.

Scarce, but growing evidence on the possible benefits of peer support include: reduced use and shortened stay in hospital beds; enhanced social support, functioning and quality of life, and increased self-esteem and positive outlook for people on the receiving end of peer support; improved quality of life with fewer hospitalizations for peer providers, and changes in attitudes of provider colleagues without a peer background, towards less stigmatization and less negativity (Peebles *et al.* 2007). With regard to documented chal-lenges such as role, relationship and confidentiality concerns, lack of resources, training, support and supervision for consumer providers, and disillusionments and stigmatization experiences of consumer providers, Peebles *et al.* (2007) suggest, with Mowbray *et al.* (1998), four ways to foster system transformation:

- Advance attention to structural matters, for example, definition of roles and responsi-bilities, recruitment and career advancement strategies;
- Improved supervision;
- Rethink of professional roles, credentialing, licensure;
- Communication of clear information about the role of peer providers for service users.

Certified Peer Specialists

Beginning in 1999 peer support was eligible for Medicaid funding and provided by Certified Peer Specialists, who had received training and certification by the Appalachian Consulting Group (ACG) in Georgia (www.trainingteams.org 10.8.08). More than 300 peers had been trained and certified in Georgia by 2007 and some $10 million annually are billed for peer support services (Peebles *et al.* 2007). The ACG under the directorate of Larry Fricks has since been active in assisting other states and initiatives with training and certification programmes (www.trainingteams .org/trainingteam3.0/PDF/SelfHelpNetwork/CPS_Appalachian_Consulting_Group_ Information_083107.pdf 20.8.08).

Ike Powell has designed the ACG national training programme, based on Pat Deegan's work (see pages 71), on three major sources of the disabling power of psychiatric health problems:

- symptoms;
- stigma;
- negative self-image.

and five stages or ways in which people relate to them

1. 'being overwhelmed by the symptoms;
2. giving in to the diagnosis, seeing no possibility for recovery, and becoming dependent on the system;
3. beginning to question how much their lives are really limited by the diagnosis and how much by their own belief system;
4. beginning to challenge what they had originally seen, or had been told, were limits;
5. beginning the process of moving outside or beyond the system for their supports. (Peebles *et al.* 2007)'

The Georgia/ACG national training programme 'helps peers understand and identify each stage, how people get "stuck" at one stage, and interventions that enable people to move on with their lives' (ibid., p 578).

Peebles *et al.* (2007) ascribe the successes of this and other pioneering work in Georgia – for example, the work initiatives of del Vecchio *et al.* (2000) – to a 'very well organized and outcome focused consumer movement' and look forward to the results of a randomized controlled study on Georgia's peer support services, which is currently underway. Some promising results have already been presented.

Peebles, Mabe, Davidson, Fricks, Buckley, Fenely (2007) conclude by saying that system transformations through recovery will change the relationships among administrators, practitioners and consumers of care into full partnerships. They suggest that empirical support for effectiveness and efficacy is necessary and highlight the importance of educational interventions for system transformation.

For information on peer support in mental health systems see also the website of the National Association of Peer Specialists (www.naops.org; 20.08.08), which also presents the Peer Specialist Compensation/Satisfaction 2007 Survey Report.

STEP UP

Dan Fisher (cf. pp 65) talks about the disappointments and risks of the above described approach and developments in an article in the *National Council Magazine* in 2007. (www.power2u.org/articles/fisher/consumers-step-up.html 20.8.08) In the article he deplores the severe changes to the concept of peer support and recovery through the institutionalization of peer support as a reimbursable service. One of the reasons for this is, he says, that supervision by traditionally trained clinicians with little understanding of peer support and recovery has led to a reinforcement of the medical model and a misunderstanding of recovery as 'just another term for remission'. As a member of the US President's New Freedom Commission (2003) and in line with its bold vision of 'a future when everyone with a mental illness would recover' he concludes that consumers/survivors/ex-patients 'will need to almost completely redesign it'. His question: 'What would a consumer-driven, transformed, recovery-based system look like?' is a renewed commitment to the expertise of people with a lived experience and their leadership for transformation:

S: Services and supports need to be consumer-driven;
T: Training needs to be consumer-driven;
E: Evaluation and research needs to be consumer-driven;
P: Policy and planning needs to be consumer driven.

The National Coalition of Mental Health Consumer/Survivor Organizations, which was funded in 2007 (www.ncmhcso.org 20.8.08), should unite the powers of the movement – United for Power- and **STEP UP**.

The Coalition's statement of purpose speaks about the authentic voice of the consumer/survivor movement leading transformation with a vision of recovery that 'goes far beyond treatment, because it is about *all* the elements that go into good lives – housing, education, jobs, social relationships, and full participation in the community' and which was echoed in the New Freedom Mental Health Commission Report, which sees a 'future when everyone with mental illness will recover'.

The Coalition of Mental Health Consumer/Survivor Organisations' policy priorities include funding for peer-run networks, services and alternatives, and social security reform to better enable people to return to work, as well as control of the influence of the pharmaceutical industry, protection of people's rights and facilitation of voting (www.ncmhcso.org; 20.8.08). The Coalition proposes a 'new consensus for the mental health field:

- **Recovery:** Recovery is real and possible for everyone. To recover, we need services and supports that treat us with dignity, respect our rights, allow us to make choices, and provide assistance with our real-life, self-defined needs. This range of services must include consumer-run and -operated programmes.
- **Self-determination:** Self-determination is essential for recovery to occur. We need to be in control of our own lives.
- **Holistic choices:** We need choices that meet our self-defined needs. We need a wide range of recovery-oriented services and supports to assist us in achieving our goals. These include assistance with housing, education, and career development, all of which can be consumer-run. We need these opportunities to achieve full integration into the community.
- **Voice:** We must have a voice in our recovery and in the policies facilitating our recovery. We are the most authentic voice in the mental health system, since mental health decisions affect every aspect of our lives. We bring our *lived experience*, therefore, we must be central in any dialogues and decisions about mental health issues at all levels. This is empowerment.
- **Personhood:** We are whole human beings and will campaign to remove stigma and discrimination. We have the same dreams as all members of the community and the ability to make our own decisions. A barrier-free community is one free from discrimination and stigma.' (www.ncmhcso.org 20.8.08)

The Coalition supports the SAMHSA consensus statement on recovery (page 13) and in times of evidence-based practice is committed to enriching the field with its 'full range of lived experiences', notably captured in their proposition 'We are the evidence!'

This bodes well for the emerging evidence-base for recovery-orientation as it includes an urgent call for a partnership approach which allows all experiences and all forms of evidence to be used at all levels. Co-operative and co-ordinated efforts with service users, carers, their spokespeople and public health advocates offer formidable chances to reduce stigma, discrimination and social exclusion, which are currently seriously limiting clinical and other efforts towards recovery. While the task appears huge, the combination of the wisdom and energy of the consumer movement and the current need of many clinicians – and academics – in psychiatry world-wide to overcome reductionistic and uninspired conceptual frameworks, might just work in favour of substantial changes now.

CHAPTER 8

The Significance of Discovering Recovery for the Authors

The importance of the narratives of personal experiences told by individuals with psychiatric diagnoses impressed us in a way that we, as authors, also wanted to accept the challenge to reveal some personal things about ourselves.

MICHAELA AMERING

Not only my colleagues, but many of my friends and family members are often surprised that I spend so much time with service users and pay so much attention to the user/survivor movement. I also wonder about this sometimes and try to understand my motives.

And many users/suvivors ask themselves: why are they attracted to psychiatrists? What kind of power-dynamics operate in such relationships?

Harald Hofer was one of the most important people in my life. When he was first confronted with psychiatry, he was a young man and the psychiatry of the 70s was doing its thing. Not unlike his childhood with an alcoholic father, a sadistic grandmother, and many years in foster care, Harald experienced psychiatry which offered and enforced 'help', as a dangerous assault. He placed his personal experiences in the service of the user movement. His commitment, fighting spirit, and his wisdom have put many things in motion in Austria. But it is still much too little, and his premature death has left us with a painful void.

During the years of our friendship we had many difficult confrontations – they were always about power. It took many years for Harald to be willing to see that the two of us were on the same level, and he did not spare either of us any of the steps or any of the necessary confrontation along the way to that conclusion. Both of us suffered often from the difficulties of our friendship: and always both of us profited from it. In 2004 I was able to accompany Harald as he was dying. Hospice care made it possible for him to live in a self-determined fashion until the very end. This was possible because he was so strong and wise in dealing with his pain, his fears, and the insanities of the situation. But also it would not have happened had I not dedicated myself to care for him as if I were next of kin and assumed responsibility for any kind of difficulties that might

Recovery in Mental Health: Reshaping scientific and clinical responsibilities Michaela Amering and Margit Schmolke
Copyright © 2009 John Wiley & Sons, Ltd

occur in connection with his diagnosis of schizophrenia. The staff of one hospice which rejected him outright, explained to me that the team could not tolerate the contradiction between their hospice ideology – to do nothing against the will of the patient – and psychiatry's task which they presumed was to treat people against their will. Harald had enough friends who were willing to help, an advance directive in place, and a male hospice nurse who became his accomplice and worked with him not just by providing nursing care, but also as a helper in his day-to-day life, along with all its craziness.

Ron Coleman recruited me for my work in Birmingham and thus gave me one of my most important experiences in psychiatry. When Laurie Ahern tells me 'What you say, is relevant for us. We can listen, when you speak about psychosis and about psychiatry, we like to hear what you have to say', she validates my work. When Wilma Boevink writes to me that she is impressed with the fact that I had formulated my dilemmas about psychiatric work so early, I can be proud about my doubts and my questions and my questioning. Christian Horvath and Crazy Industries go beyond letting me partake of their many wonderful ideas and initiatives, by giving me feedback about my work, which allows me to assess my strengths and weaknesses in an extremely accurate fashion.

I am a researcher. It is part of my work to read and to hear what the smartest people in psychiatric research have to say. I consider this a great privilege, and I relish it greatly.

Another privilege is being accepted in a user-oriented sub-culture. The experiences of people who are current or former service users and who are now speaking out for themselves and for others, are particularly valuable to me. Helen Glover, Jan Wallcraft, Diana Rose, Judi Chamberlin, Mary Nettle, Mary Maddock, Michaela Jägersberger, Stephanus Binder, Peter Lehmann, Hannelore Klafki, Antje Müller, Regina Bellion and their many colleagues in the limelight are extraordinary personalities, who have very special talents and have made exceptional contributions. What they all have in common is an ability to argue convincingly that their stories, their paths and their impressive developments are not so extraordinary after all, but that recovery is important and possible for everyone. I have come to the conclusion that they are right.

Every day I deal with people who occasionally lose their minds. I do not envy them. I am attracted to them and want to help. Sometimes I am able to do just that. Unfortunately, I still don't understand why some people become psychotic at certain times, but not at others. Or why some of us never have such experiences. I am quite hurt by this, since I feel I have a responsibility to understand, as a psychiatrist and as a human being. I hope never to become psychotic myself, and if it were to happen, I would like to be treated rather carefully. Maybe even with particular respect, since I do believe that a person in such a situation deserves that. Psychiatric illnesses are caused, in my opinion, by rather complicated combinations of factors. They are not self-determined and cannot be reduced to a single cause. I also agree with Gotthold Ephraim Lessing when he says: 'A person who does not lose her mind over certain things has no mind to lose'. I have come to grips with the fact that I am healthy – and as insensitive as an armadillo! I try to bear the misery, injustice and inconsistencies of the world mostly by forgetting about them, by not letting things get to me too much, or by looking the other way. And I am quite content that I can pull this off, more or less.

I do not believe that anyone takes something on on behalf of me by getting crazy. Nor do I believe that anything productive must be forthcoming when a person is flooded by psychotic anxiety and continues to be plagued by the same thoughts, voices, or impressions. But I have a great respect for people who sometimes experience such an intense exposure to the risks, profundities, secrets and ironies of human existence and who are able to survive this. I learn a lot from these survivors or heroes, as my friend Margit Schmolke calls them. The clarity and authenticity they demand from those who surround them, feels good to me. Their courage makes me hopeful. I want to be able to give something back. Recovery-concepts might be the right framework for this.

MARGIT SCHMOLKE

As a psychotherapist and researcher the concerns of the recovery movement have become increasingly important to me. The contributions of users about their work and in the form of their personal stories at many conferences has always moved and convinced me. I also found it curious that my research interest in the health and creative aspects of people with mental illnesses during the 90s coincided with the implementation and publication of several studies on recovery. Back then, I did not know too much about this subject, and find it exciting to see how the various threads from different directions are coming together around the recovery-concept. During my long-term work at the Dynamic-Psychiatric Hospital, Menterschwaige, in Munich I was fortunate to have several mentors, who opened my eyes and helped me find an emotional and intellectual approach to the profound suffering of the patients – and to their unique strengths and resources. This became possible through the joint exploration of their personal biographies. Often they were able to find creative ways to make use of their innermost resources to improve and enhance their lives. Sometimes this process took a long time, took many circuitous routes and required repeated hospital stays. During my work as a therapist at Bellevue Hospital in New York I encountered many people with severe psychiatric conditions. They too had hidden recovery-resources and it was difficult to stand by and watch as these lay fallow and were ignored by many staff members. I learned that the recovery-process takes its time and has its own dynamics, and that we clinicians should become partners in this process.

During a study I undertook for my doctoral thesis I evaluated interviews with people with a diagnosis of schizophrenia. When I discovered that these people were also healthy and had many coping-strategies and ways of dealing with problems, even in the midst of severe emotional distress and when psychiatric symptoms were present, it was a very uplifting experience for me (Schmolke 2001). Today I would certainly delete the adjective 'schizophrenic' and change title and text in accordance with 'person-first' language. I was very pleased to collaborate on this book with Michaela Amering, who has brought the idea of recovery home to me. I share with her an interest in the frequently unconventional and surprising twists and turns in the lives of people who have experienced severe personal crises. It has been a wonderful, enlightening and enriching collaboration!

References

Aderhold V, Stastny P (2007) Full disclosure: toward a participatory and risk-limiting approach to neuroleptic drugs. *Ethical Human Psychology and Psychiatry* **9/1**: 35–61.

Adewuya AO, Makanjuola ROA (2005) Social distance towards people with mental illness amongst Nigerian university students. *Social Psychiatry and Psychiatric Epidemiology* **40**: 865–8.

Alanen YO (1997) *Schizophrenia: its Origins and Need-adapted Treatment*. Karnac Books, London.

Albee GW, Gullotta TP (1997) Primary prevention's evolution. In: GW Albee, TP Gullotta (eds.). *Primary Prevention Works* (pp 3–22). Sage, Thousand Oaks, CA.

Allardyce J, Gaebel W, Zielasek J, van Os J (2007) Deconstructing Psychosis Conference February 2006. The validity of schizophrenia and alternative approaches to the classification of psychosis. *Schizophrenia Bulletin* **33/4**: 863–7.

American Psychiatric Association (2000) *Diagnostic and Statistical Manual of Mental Disorders* 4th Ed text revision. APA, Washington, DC.

American Psychological Association (2008) The road to resilience. www.apahelpcenter.org (25.07.08).

Amering M (2008) Recovery – why not? *Psychiatrische Praxis* **35**: 55–6.

Amering M, Schmolke M (2007) *Recovery. Das Ende der Unheilbarkeit*. Psychiatrie-Verlag, Bonn.

Amering M, Stastny P, Hopper K (2005) Psychiatric advance directives: qualitative study of informed deliberations by mental health service users. *British Journal of Psychiatry* **186**: 247–52.

Amering M, Sibitz I, Güssler R, Katschnig H (2002a) *Wissen-geniessen-besser leben. Ein Seminar für Menschen mit Psychoseerfahrung*. Psychiatrie-Verlag, Bonn.

Amering M, Hofer H, Rath I (2002b) The 'First Vienna Trialogue' – experiences with a new form of communication between users, relatives and mental health professionals. In: Lefley HP, Johnson DL (eds.). *Family Interventions in Mental Illness: International Perspectives*. Praeger, London, Westport, CT, pp 105–24.

Amering M, *et al.* (1999) Psychiatric wills of mental health professionals: a survey of opinions regarding advance directives. *Social Psychiatry and Psychiatric Epidemiology* **34**: 30–4.

Ammon G (1983) The principle of social energy in the holistic thought of Dynamic Psychiatry. *Dynamic Psychiatry* **16**: 169–84.

Anderson M, Jenkins R (2003) Mental health promotion and prevention. *Dynamic Psychiatry* **36**: 231–46.

Andreasen NC, *et al.* (2005) Remission in schizophrenia: proposed criteria and rationale for consensus. *American Journal of Psychiatry* **162**: 441–9.

Andresen R, Caputi P, Oades L (2006) Stages of recovery instrument: development of a measure of recovery from serious mental illness. *Australian and New Zealand Journal of Psychiatry* **40**: 972–80.

Andresen R, Oades L, Caputi P (2003) The experience of recovery from schizophrenia: towards an empirically-validated stage model. *Australian and New Zealand Journal of Psychiatry* **37**: 586–94.

Angermeyer MC, Matschinger H (2005) Causal beliefs and attitudes to people with schizophrenia. Trend analysis based on data from two population surveys in Germany. *British Journal of Psychiatry* **186**: 331–4.

Angermeyer MC, Beck M, Dietrich S, Holzinger A (2004) The stigma of mental illness: patients' anticipations and experiences. *International Journal of Social Psychiatry* **50/2**: 153–62.

Angermeyer MC, Buyantugs L, Kenzine DV, Matschinger H (2004) Effects of labelling on public attitudes towards people with schizophrenia: are there cultural differences? *Acta Psychiatrica Scandinavia* **109**: 420–5.

Angermeyer MC, Matschinger H (2004) Public attitudes to people with depression: have there been any changes over the last decade? *Journal of Affective Disorder* **83**: 177–82.

Angermeyer MC, Matschinger H (2003) Public beliefs about schizophrenia and depression: similarities and differences. *Social Psychiatry and Psychiatric Epidemiology* **38**: 526–34.

Angermeyer MC, Cooper B, Link BG (1998) Mental disorder and violence: results of epidemiological studies in the era of de-institutionalization. *Social Psychiatry and Psychiatric Epidemiology* **33**: 1–6.

Anthony W (2006) Personal accounts: what my MS has taught me about severe mental illnesses. *Psychiatric Services* **57**: 1081–2.

Anthony WA (2004) The principle of personhood: the field's transcendent principle. *Psychiatric Rehabilitation Journal* **27/3**: 205.

Anthony W, Rogers ES, Farkas M (2003) Research on evidence-based practices: future directions in an era of recovery. *Community Mental Health Journal* **39**: 101–14.

Anthony W (1993) Recovery from mental illness. The guiding vision of the mental health service system in the 1990s. *Psychosocial Rehabilitation Journal* **16**: 11–23.

Antonovsky A (1987) *Unraveling the Mystery of Health. How People Manage Stress and Stay Well*. Jossey-Bass, San Francisco.

Antonovsky A (1979) *Health, Stress and Coping*. Jossey-Bass, San Francisco.

APAL (2004) Guia Latinoamericana de diagnostico psiquiatrico (GLADP). Editorial de la Universidad de Guadalajara, Mexico.

APA – American Psychiatric Association (1994) *Diagnostic and Statistical Manual of Mental Disorders*. 4th Ed. American Psychiatric Association, Washington, DC.

Appelbaum PS (2003) Ambivalence codified: California's new outpatient commitment statute. *Psychiatric Services* **54**: 575–6.

Banzato CEM, Mezzich JE, Berganza CE (eds.) (2005) Philosophical and methodological foundations of psychiatric diagnosis. *Psychopathology* **38**: special issue, July/August 2005.

Bauer J (2004) *Das Gedächtnis des Körpers. Wie Beziehungen und Lebensstile unsere Gene steuern*. Piper, München.

Beck M, Dietrich S, Matschinger H, Angermeyer MC (2003) Alcoholism: low standing with the public? Attitudes towards spending financial resources on medical care and research on alcoholism. *Alcohol and Alcoholism* **38**: 602–5.

Becker T, Kilian R (2006) Psychiatric services for people with severe mental illness across Western Europe: what can be generalized from current knowledge about differences in provision, costs and outcomes of mental health care? *Acta Psychiatrica Scandinavica* **113** (Suppl 429): 9–16.

Becker T, Vazquez-Barquero JL (2001) The European perspective of psychiatric reform. *Acta Psychiatrica Scandinavica* **104** (Suppl 410): 8–14.

Bedregal LE, O'Connell MJ, Davidson L (2006) The Recovery Knowledge Inventory: assessment of mental health staff knowledge and attitudes about recovery. *Psychiatric Rehabilitation Journal* **30/2**: 96–103.

Bender D, Lösel F (1997) Protective and risk effects of peer relations and social support on antisocial behaviour in adolescents from multi-problem milieus. *Journal of Adolescence* **20/6**: 661–78.

Ben-Dor S (2001) Personal account. Schizophrenia. *Schizophrenia Bulletin* **27**: 329–32.

Bengel J, Strittmatter R, Willmann H (1999) *What keeps people healthy? The current state of discussion and the relevance of Antonovsky's salutogenic model of health*. Expert report commissioned by the Federal Centre for Health Education. Research and Practice of Health Promotion. Vol 4. Federal Centre for Health Education (FCHE), Cologne, Germany.

Bentall RP (2003) *Madness explained. Psychosis and Human Nature*. Penguin Books, London.

Berger H (2008) Health promotion – a change in the paradigms of psychiatry. www.hpps.net/document-01 Task Force on Health Promoting Psychiatric Services (10.08.08).

Berger H, Paul R, Heimsath E (2005) *Task Force on Health Promoting Psychiatric Services*. www.ec.europa.eu/health (30.08.08).

Berger H (1999) Health promotion – a change in the paradigms of psychiatry. In: Berger H, Krajic K, Paul R (eds.). *Health Promoting Hospitals in Practice: Developing Projects and Networks*. HPH Series Vol 3. Health Promotion Publications, Gamburg, pp 42–53.

Berkman LF (1995) The role of social relations in health promotion. *Psychosomatic Medicine* **57/3**: 245–54.

Bhui K, Rüdell K, Priebe S (2006) Assessing explanatory models for common mental disorders. *Journal of Clinical Psychiatry* **67**: 964–71.

Bleuler M (1978) *The Schizophrenic Disorders: Long-term Patient and Family Studies*. Yale University Press, New Haven.

Bleuler E (1950) *Dementia praecox or the group of schizophrenias*. International University Press, first published in 1911 (translated by J Zinkin).

Bock, T (2006a) *Lichtjahre, Psychosen ohne Psychiatrie*. Psychiatrie-Verlag, Bonn.

Bock T (2006b) *Eigensinn und Psychose. Non-Compliance als Chance*. Paranus-Verlag, Neumünster.

Bock T, Priebe S (2005) Psychosis seminars: an unconventional approach. *Psychiatric Services* **56/11**: 1441–3.

Bock T, Naber D (2003) 'Anti-stigma campaign from below' at schools – experience of the initiative Irre menschlich Hamburg e.V. *Psychiatrische Praxis*. **30/7**: 402–8.

Bock T (1992) Wieviel Krankheit braucht der Mensch? – Risiken der Prävention aus der Sicht der Psychiatrie. In: Paulus P (ed.). *Prävention und Gesundheitsfoerderung. Perspektiven für die psychosoziale Praxis*. GwG-Verlag, Kőln. pp 109–18.

Boevink W (ed.) (2006) *Stories of Recovery. Working Together towards Experiential Knowledge in Mental Health Care*. Trimbos-Institute, Utrecht.

Boevink W (2003) Recovery: Mitreden – mitmachen – selbst aktiv werden. Wie in den Niederlanden Psychiatrie-Erfahrene Partizipation neu definieren. *Psychosoziale Umschau* **18/3**: 37–9.

Boevink W (2002) Two sides of recovery. Paper presented at the 10th Triptych Congress, Roermond, the Netherlands, November. www.peter-lehmann-publishing.com/articles/boevink_recovery.htm (31.08.08).

Borg M, Davidson L (2008) The nature of recovery as lived in everyday experiences. *Journal of Mental Health* **17/2**: 129–40.

Borg M, Kristiansen K (2004) Recovery-oriented professionals: helping relationships in mental health services. *Journal of Mental Health* **13/5**: 493–505.

Borg M, Topor A (2003) *Virksomme relasjoner. Om bedringsprosesser ved alvorlige psykiske lidelser*. Kommuneforlaget, Oslo.

Borkin JR, *et al.* (2000) Recovery attitudes questionnaire: development and evaluation. *Psychiatric Rehabilitation Journal* **24**: 95–102.

Britten N, *et al.* (2004) The expression of aversion to medicines in general practice consultations. *Social Science and Medicine* **59**: 1495–1503.

Buckner JC, Mezzacappa E, Beardslee WR (2003) Characteristics of resilient youths living in poverty: the role of self-regulatory processes. *Developmental Psychopathology* **15/1**: 139–62.

Burns T, *et al.* (2008) The impact of supported employment and working on clinical and social functioning: results of an international study of individual placement and support. *Schizophrenia Bulletin* (Epub ahead of print).

Burns T, Firn M (2002) *Assertive Outreach in Mental Health: a Manual for Practitioners*. Oxford Medical Publications, Oxford University Press.

Campbell J (1997) How consumers/survivors are evaluating the quality of psychiatric care. *Evaluation Review* **21**: 357–63.

Campbell J, Schraiber R (1989) *The Well-being Project: Mental Health Clients Speak for Themselves*. California Department of Mental Health, Sacramento, CA.

Campbell-Orde T, Chamberlin J, Carpenter J, Leff HS (2005) Measuring the promise: a compendium of recovery measures, Vol II. http://www.power2u.org/downloads/pn-55.pdf (20.08.08)

Camus A (1983) *The Myth of Sisyphus and Other Essays*. Vintage Books, London (translated by J O'Brien).

Cicchetti D. Rogosch FA (1997) The role of self-organization in the promotion of resilience in maltreated children. *Development and Psychopathology* **9**: 797–815.

Chamberlin J (1978) *On Our Own: Patient-controlled Alternatives to the Mental Health System*. McGraw-Hill, New York.

Chinman M, *et al.* (2006) Toward the implementation of mental health consumer provider services. *Journal of Behavioral Health Services Research* **33/2**: 176–95.

Ciompi L, Hoffmann H (2004). Soteria Berne: an innovative milieu therapeutic approach to acute schizophrenia based on the concept of affect-logic. *World Psychiatry*: 140–6.

Ciompi L (1980) Catamnestic long-term study on the course of life and aging of schizophrenics. *Schizophrenia Bulletin* **6/4**: 606–18.

Coatsworth JD, Duncan L (2003) Fostering resilience. A strengths-based approach to mental health. A CASSP discussion paper. Pennsylvania CASSP Training and Technical Assistance Institute, Harrisburgh, PA.

Cohen LJ (1994) Psychiatric hospitalization as an experience of trauma. *Archives of Psychiatric Nursing* **VIII/2**: 78–81.

Coleman R (2006) *Recovery – an Alien Concept*. 2nd ed. P & P Press, UK.

Coleman R, Baker P, Taylor K (2006) *Working towards Recovery*. P & P Press, UK.

Coleman R, Smith M (2005) *Working With Voices*. P & P Press, UK.

Colombo A, Bendelow G, Fulford B, Williams S (2003) Evaluating the influence of implicit models of mental disorder on processes of shared decision making within community-based multi-disciplinary teams. *Social Science and Medicine* **56/7**: 1557–70.

Connor KM, Davidson JR (2003) Development of a new resilience scale: the Connor-Davidson Resilience Scale (CD-RISC). *Depression and Anxiety* **18/2**: 76–82.

Consumers in NHS Research (1999) *R & D in the NHS: How Can You Make a Difference?* NHS Executive, Leeds.

Consumers in NHS Research Support Unit (2001) *Involving consumers in research and development in the NHS: briefing notes for researchers*. Consumers in NHS Support Unit, London.

Copeland ME (2008). *Remembering Kate – a story of hope*. www.mentalhealthrecovery.com/art_kate.php (18.08.08).

Copeland ME (1997) *Wellness Recovery Action Plan*. Peach Press, Dummerston, VT.

Corrigan PW (2007) How clinical diagnosis might exacerbate the stigma of mental illness. *Social Work* **52**: 31–9.

Corrigan PW (2006) Recovery from schizophrenia and the role of evidence-based psychosocial interventions. *Expert Review of Neurotherapeutics* **6**: 993–1004.

Corrigan PW, *et al.* (2004) Examining the factor structure of the Recovery Assessment Scale. *Schizophrenia Bulletin* **30**: 1035–41.

Corrigan PW, Penn DL (1999) Lessons from social psychology on discrediting psychiatric stigma. *American Psychologist* **54**: 765–76.

Corrigan PW, *et al.* (1999) Recovery as a psychological construct. *Community Mental Health Journal* **35**: 231–9.

Cox J, Campbell A, Fulford KWM (2006) *Medicine of the Person*. Kingsley Publishers, London.

Crane-Ross D, Lutz WJ, Roth D (2006) Consumer and case manager perspectives of service empowerment: relationship to mental health recovery. *Journal of Behavioural Health Services Research* **33**: 142–55.

Crow T (2002) Should schizophrenia as a disease entity concept survive into the third millennium? In: (eds. Maj M, Sartorius N). *Schizophrenia. WPA Series Evidence and Experience in Psychiatry*, Vol 2, 2nd ed pp. 40–43. John Wiley, Chichester.

Crumlish N, *et al.* (2005) Early insight predicts depression and attempted suicide after 4 years in first-episode schizophrenia and schizophrenieform disorder. *Acta Psychiatrica Scandinavica* **112**: 449–55.

Davidson L. (in press) *The Roots of Recovery: What can be Learned from 300 Years of Efforts to Treat People with Mental Illnesses as People*. Wiley-Blackwell, Chichester.

Davidson L, *et al.* (2008) Using qualitative research to inform mental health policy. *The Canadian Journal of Psychiatry* **533**: 137–44.

Davidson L, Roe D (2007) Recovery from versus recovery in serious mental illness: one strategy for lessening confusion plaguing recovery. *Journal of Mental Health* **16/4**: 459–70.

Davidson L, *et al.* (2007) Creating a recovery-oriented system of behavioral health care: moving from concept to reality. *Psychiatric Rehabilitation Journal* **31**: 23–31.

Davidson L, *et al.* (2006a) The top ten concerns about recovery encountered in mental health system transformation. *Psychiatric Services* **57/5**: 640–5.

Davidson L, *et al.* (2006b) Play, pleasure, and other positive life events: 'non-specific' factors in recovery from mental illness? *Psychiatry* **69/2**: 151–63.

Davidson L, *et al.* (2006c) Peer support among adults with mental illness: a report from the field. *Schizophrenia Bulletin* **32**: 443–50.

Davidson L, *et al.* (2005a) Recovery in serious mental illness: paradigm shift or shibboleth? In: Davidson L, Harding C, Spaniol L (eds.) *Recovery from Mental Illness: Research Evidence and Implications for Practice*. Centre for Psychiatric Rehabilitation, Boston University. pp 5–26

Davidson L, Harding C, Spaniol L (eds.) (2005b) *Recovery from Mental Illness: Research Evidence and Implications for Practice*. Centre for Psychiatric Rehabilitation, Boston University.

Davidson L, *et al.* (2005c) Process of recovery in serious mental illness: findings from a multinational study. *American Journal of Psychiatric Rehabilitation* **8**: 177–201.

Davidson L (2003) *Living Outside Mental Illness: Qualitative Studies of Recovery in Schizophrenia*. NYU Press, New York.

Davidson L, *et al.* (1996) Hospital or community living? Examining consumer perspectives on deinstitutionalization. *Psychiatric Rehabilitation Journal* **19**: 49–58.

Davidson L, Strauss JS (1992) Sense of self in recovery from severe mental illness. *British Journal of Medical Psychology* **65**: 131–45.

Dawson J, Szmukler G (2006) Fusion of mental health and incapacity legislation. *British Journal of Psychiatry* **188**: 504–9.

Deegan PE, Rapp C, Holter M, Riefer M (2008) Best practices: a program to support shared decision-making in an outpatient psychiatric medication clinic. *Psychiatric Services* **59**: 603–5.

Deegan PE (2007) The lived experience of using psychiatric medication in the recovery process and a shared decision-making program to support it. *Psychiatric Rehabilitation Journal* **31/1**: 62–9.

Deegan PE, Drake RE (2006) Shared decision-making and medication management in the recovery-process. *Psychiatric Services* **57/11**: 1636–9.

Deegan P (2005a) Recovery as a journey of the heart. In: Davidson L, Harding C and Spaniol L (eds.) *Recovery from Severe Mental Illnesses: Research Evidence and Implications for Practice*. (pp 57–68) Vol 1. Center for Psychiatric Rehabilitation, Trustees of Boston University.

Deegan P (2005b) The importance of personal medicine: a qualitative study of resilience in people with psychiatric disabilities. *Scandinavian Journal of Public Health* **33** (Suppl 66) 29–35.

Deegan P (1996) Recovery and the conspiracy of hope. Paper, presented at the Sixth Annual Mental Health Services Conference of Australia and New Zealand, Brisbane, Australia. http://www.bu.edu/resilience/examples/deegan-recovery-hope.pdf (20.8.08)

Deegan P (1992) The independent living movement and people with psychiatric disabilities: taking back control over our own lives. *Psychosocial Rehabilitation Journal* **15**: 3–19.

Deegan P (1988) Recovery: the lived experience of rehabilitation. *Psychosocial Rehabilitation Journal* **11**: 11–19.

Del Vecchio P, Fricks L (2007) Guest editorial. Special issue on mental health recovery and system transformation. *Psychiatric Rehabilitation Journal* **31/1**: 7–8.

Del Vecchio P, Fricks L, Johnson JR (2000) Issues of daily living for persons with mental illness. *Psychiatric Rehabilitation Skills* **4**: 410–23.

Department of Health (2001) *Making it Happen – a Guide to Delivering Mental Health Promotion*. HMSO, London.

Department of Health (2000) *Working Partnerships. Consumers in Research. Third annual report*. Department of Health, London.

Department of Health (1999) *Patient and public involvement in the new NHS*. Department of Health, London.

Department of Health (1998) *Research – What's in it for Consumers? Report of the Standing Advisory Committee on Consumer Involvement in the NHS Research & Development Programme*. Department of Health, London.

De Sisto MJ, *et al.* The Maine and Vermont three-decade studies of serious mental illness. I and II. Matched comparison of cross-sectional outcome. *British Journal of Psychiatry* **167**: 331–8 and 338–42.

Detels R, McEwan J, Beaglehole R, Tanaka H (eds.) (2002) *Oxford Textbook of Public Health*. 4th ed. Oxford University Press.

Dietrich S, Matschinger H, Angermeyer M (2006) The relationship between biogenetic causal explanations and social distance toward people with mental disorders: results from a population survey in Germany. *International Journal of Social Psychiatry* **52**: 166–74.

Dinniss S, *et al.* (2007) Making DREEM come true. *Mental Health Today* **Jul-Aug**: 30–3.

Drake RE, *et al.* (2003) Fundamental principles of evidence-based medicine applied to mental health care. *Psychiatric Clinics of North America. Special issue: Evidence-based practices in mental health care* **26/4**: 811–20.

Drake RE, *et al.* (2000) Evidence-based treatment of schizophrenia. *Current Psychiatry Reports* **2**: 393–7.

Drayton M, Birchwood M, Trower P (1998) Early attachment experience and recovery from psychosis. *British Journal of Clinical Psychology* **37**: 269–84.

Dressing H, Salize HJ (2004) Compulsory admission of mentally ill patients in European Union Member States. *Social Psychiatry and Psychiatric Epidemiology* **39/10**: 797–803.

Dumont JM, *et al.* (2006) *Mental Health Recovery: What Helps and What Hinders? A National Research Project for the Development of Recovery Facilitating Performance Indicators. Phase II Technical Report: Development of the Recovery Oriented Systems Indicators (ROSI) Measures to Advance Mental Health Systems Transformation.* National Technical Assistance Center, National Association of State Mental Health Program Directors, Alexandria, VA.

Dumont J, Campbell J (1994) *A preliminary report for the Mental Health Reform Report Card Task Force of the MHSIP Ad Hoc Advisory Group.* Center for Mental Health Services, Rockville, MD.

Dunbar MM (1991) Shaking up the status quo: how AIDS activists have challenged drug development and approval procedures. *Food, Drug and Cosmetic Law Journal* **46**: 673–706.

Duyme M, Dumaret A-C, Tomkiewicz S (1999) How can we boost IQs of 'dull children'?: a late adoption study. *Proceedings of the National Academy of Sciences of the USA* **96**: 8790–4.

Edward K, Warelow P (2005) Resilience: when coping is emotionally intelligent. *Journal of the American Psychiatric Nurses Association* **11/2**: 101–2.

Engel GL (1977) The need for a new medical model: a challenge for biomedicine. *Science* **8**: 129–36.

Estroff SE (1989) Self, identity, and subjective experiences of schizophrenia: in search of the subject. *Schizophrenia Bulletin* **15/2**: 189–96.

European Commission (2005) Green Paper. *Improving the Mental Health of the Population: Towards a Strategy on Mental Health for the European Union.* Brussels. http://ec.europa.eu/health/ph_determinants/life_style/mental/green_paper/mental_gp_en.pdfmental_gp_en.pdf (10.08.08).

Farkas M (2007) The vision of recovery today: what it is and what it means for services. *World Psychiatry* **6/2**: 4–10.

Farkas M, Gagne C, Anthony W, Chamberlin J (2005) Implementing recovery-oriented evidence-based programs: identifying the critical dimensions. *Community Mental Health Journal* **41**: 141–58.

Faulkner A (2000) *Strategies for Living: a Report of User-led Research into People's Strategies for Living with Mental Distress.* Mental Health Foundation, London.

Faulkner A, Thomas P (2002) User-led research and evidence-based medicine. *British Journal of Psychiatry* **180**: 1–3.

Finzen A (2003) *Schizophrenie – die Krankheit behandeln.* Psychiatrie-Verlag, Bonn.

Finzen A (2001) *Psychose und Stigma. Stigmabewältigung – zum Umgang mit Vorurteilen und Schuldzuweisung.* Psychiatrie-Verlag, Bonn.

Fisher B, Neve H, Heritage Z (1999) Community development, user involvement, and primary health care. Editorial. *BMJ* **318**: 749–50.

Fleischhacker WW (2002) Pharmalogical treatment of schizophrenia. In: (eds. Maj M, Sartorius N). *Schizophrenia. WPA Series Evidence and Experience in Psychiatry*, Vol 2, ed. pp 75–113. John Wiley, Chichester.

Foster JR (1997) Successful coping, adaptation and resilience in the elderly: an interpretation of epidemiologic data. *Psychiatric Quarterly* **68/3**: 189–219.

Freidl M, Lang T, Scherer M (2003) How psychiatric patients perceive the public's stereotype of mental illness. *Social Psychiatry and Psychiatric Epidemiology* **38**: 269–75.

Freitas AL, Downey G (1998) Resilience: a dynamic perspective. *International Journal of Behavioral Development* **22/2**: 263–85.

Frese FJ, Stanley J, Kress K, Vogel-Scibilia S (2001) Integrating evidence-based practices and the recovery model. *Psychiatric Services* **52**: 1462–8.

Frey D, Rogner O, Schueller M, Koerte C, Havemann D (1985) Psychological determinants in the convalescence of accident patients. *Basic and Applied Social Psychology* **6/4**: 317–28.

Friborg O, Hjemdal O, Rosenvinge JH, Martinussen M (2003) A new rating scale for adult resilience: what are the central protective resources behind healthy adjustment? *International Journal of Methods in Psychiatric Research* **12**: 65–76.

Frueh BC, *et al.* (2000) Trauma within the psychiatric setting: conceptual framework, research directions, and policy implications. *Administration and Policy in Mental Health* **28/2**: 147–54.

Fuchs Ebaugh HR (1988) *Becoming an Ex. The Process of Role Exit*. The University of Chicago Press, Chicago.

Gaebel W, Baumann A, Witte AM, Zaeske H (2002) Public attitudes towards people with mental illness in six German cities: results of a public survey with a special consideration of schizophrenia. *European Archives of Psychiatry and Clinical Neuroscience* **252**: 278–87.

Gardner W, *et al.* (1999) Patients' revision of their beliefs about the need for hospitalization. *American Journal of Psychiatry* **156/9**: 1385–91.

Garmezy N (1991) Resiliency and vulnerability to adverse developmental outcomes associated with poverty. *American Behavioral Scientist* **34**: 416–30.

Garmezy N (1985) Competence and adaptation in adult schizophrenia patients and children at risk. In: Cancro R, Dean SR (eds.) *Research in the Schizophrenic Disorders: The Stanley R Dean Award Lectures*. Vol 2. Spectrum Publications, New York.

Garmezy N (1974) Children at risk: the search for the antecedents of schizophrenia. Part I: Conceptual models and research methods. *Schizophrenia Bulletin* **8**: 14–90.

Geanellos R (2005) Adversity as opportunity: living with schizophrenia and developing a resilient self. *International Journal of Mental Health Nursing* **14**: 7–15.

Glover H (2005) Recovery based service delivery: are we ready to transform the words into a paradigm shift? *Australian e-Journal for the Advancement of Mental Health (AeJAMH)* **4/3**: 1–4. http://www.auseinet.com/journal/vol4iss3/glovereditorial.pdf (28.08.08).

Glover H (2003) A series of thoughts on personal recovery. http://www.mentalhealth.org.uk (24.08.06).

Goldowsky M (2003) On confronting myself and the world. *Psychiatric Services* **54**: 823–4.

Goodare H, Lockward S (1999) Involving patients in clinical research. *BMJ* **319**: 724–5.

Giorgi A (1997) The theory, practice, and evaluation of the phenomenological method as a qualitative research procedure. *Journal of Phenomenological Psychology* **28**: 235–60.

Greenblat L (2000) First person account: understanding health as a continuum. *Schizophrenia Bulletin* **26**: 243–5.

Greve N (2007) Was lange währt ... wird nicht immer gut: Risiken der chronischen Betreuung. *Soziale Psychiatrie* **118**: 15–17.

Grusky O, Tierney K, Spanish MT (1989) Which community mental health services are most important? *Administration and Policy in Mental Health* **17/1**: 3–16.

Gullestad M (1989) *Kultur og hverdagsliv*. Det bla bibliotek. Universitetsforlaget, Oslo, Norway.

Gunkel S, Kruse G (eds.) (2004) Salutogenese und Resilienz – Gesundheitsförderung, nicht nur, aber auch durch Psychotherapie? In: Gunkel S, Kruse G (eds.) *Salutogenese, Resilienz und Psychotherapie. Was hält gesund? Was bewirkt Heilung?* (pp 5–68). Hannoversche Ärzte-Verlags-Union, Hannover.

Häfner H (2005) *Das Rätsel Schizophrenie. Eine Krankheit wird entschlüsselt*. C H Beck, München.

Hamann J, Leucht S, Kissling W (2003) Shared decision making in psychiatry. *Acta Psychiatrica Scandinavica* **107/6**: 403–9.

Hanson RF, *et al.* (2006) Relations among parental substance use, violence exposure and mental health: the national survey of adolescents. *Addictive Behaviors* **31/11**: 1988–2001.

Hansson L (2006) Determinants of quality of life in people with severe mental illness. *Acta Psychiatrica Scandinavica* **113** (Suppl 429): 46–50.

Harding C (2005) Recovery, resilience, and schizophrenia. Paper presented at the Section Symposium on Recovery, Hope and Schizophrenia. Chairs: M Amering, M Schmolke, World Congress of the World Psychiatric Association, September 10–15, 2005, Cairo.

Harding CM, *et al.* (1987a) The Vermont longitudinal study of persons with severe mental illness I: methodology, study sample, and overall status 32 years later. *American Journal of Psychiatry* **144/6**: 718–26.

Harding CM, *et al.* (1987b) The Vermont longitudinal study of persons with severe mental illness II: long-term outcome of subjects who retrospectively met DSM-III criteria for schizophrenia. *American Journal of Psychiatry* **144/6**: 727–35.

Harding CM, Zahniser JH (1994) Empirical correction of seven myths about schizophrenia with implications for treatment. *Acta Psychiatrica Scandinavica Suppl.* **384**: 140–6.

Hartmann CE (2002) Personal accounts: life as death: hope regained with ECT. *Psychiatric Services* **53**: 413–14.

Hasson-Ohayon I, *et al.* (2006) Insight into psychosis and quality of life. *Comprehensive Psychiatry* **47**: 265–9.

Hatfield AB, Lefley HP (1993) *Surviving Mental Illness. Stress, Coping and Adaptation*. Guilford Press, New York.

Hauser S, Allen J, Golden E (2006) *Out of the Woods: Tales of Resilient Teens*. Harvard University Press, Cambridge, MA.

Henderson C, *et al.* (2008) A typology of advance statements in mental health care. *Psychiatric Services* **59/1**: 63–71.

Henderson P, *et al.* (2007) Community development and community care. Reflections on practice and policy. *Journal of Community Work and Development* **9**: 35–45.

Henderson C, *et al.* (2004) Effect of joint crisis plans on use of compulsory treatment in psychiatry: single blind randomised controlled trial. *BMJ*, doi:10.1136/bmj.38155.585046.63.

Herman JL (1997) *Trauma and Recovery. From Domestic Abuse to Political Terror*. B & T.

Herrman H, Saxena S, Moodie R (eds.) (2005) *Promoting Mental Health: Concepts, Evidence and Practice*. A report of the World Health Organization, in collaboration with the Victorian Health Promotion Foundation and the University of Melbourne. WHO, Geneva.

Herrman H (2005) Public health perspectives on resilience and positive health. Paper presented at the symposium on Resilience in mental health promotion: interdisciplinary perspectives. Chairs: M Schmolke, O Ray. World Congress of the World Psychiatric Association (WPA), September 10–15, 2005, Cairo.

Herrman H, Moodie R, Walker L, Verins I (2003) International collaborations on mental health promotion: a Western Pacific initiative. *Dynamic Psychiatry* **36**: 272–89.

Herrman H (2001) The need for mental health promotion. *Australian and New Zealand Journal of Psychiatry* **35/6**: 709–15.

Hinterhuber H (1973) Catamnestic studies on schizophrenia. A clinical-statistical study of lifelong course. *Fortschritte der Neurologie Psychiatrie und ihrer Grenzgebiete* **41/10**: 527–58.

Hollnagel M, Malterud K (1995) Shifting attention from objective risk factors to patients' self-assessed health resources: a clinical model for general practice. *Family Practice* **12**: 423–9.

Holtz TH (1998) Refugee trauma versus torture trauma: a retrospective controlled cohort study of Tibetan refugees. *Journal of Nervous and Mental Disease* **186/1**: 24–34.

Holzinger A, Müller P, Priebe S, Angermeyer MC (2002) Die Prognose der Schizophrenie aus der Sicht der Patienten und ihrer Angehörigen. Eine explorative Studie. *Psychiatrische Praxis* **29**: 154–9.

Holzinger A, *et al.* (2003) Patients' and their relatives' causal explanations of schizophrenia. *Social Psychiatry and Psychiatric Epidemiology* **38**: 155–62.

Hopper K (2007) Rethinking social recovery in schizophrenia: what a capabilities approach might offer. *Social Science and Medicine* **65/5**: 868–79.

Hopper K, Harrison G, Janca A, Sartorius N (2007) *Recovery from Schizophrenia: an International Perspective: a Report from the WHO Collaborative Project, the International Study of Schizophrenia*. Oxford University Press.

House JS (2001) Social isolation kills, but how and why? Editorial comment. *Psychosomatic Medicine* **63**: 273–4.

Huber G, Gross G, Schüttler R (1975) A long-term follow-up study of schizophrenia: psychiatric course of illness and prognosis. *Acta Psychiatrica Scandinavica* **52/1**: 49–57.

Husserl E (1970) *The Crisis of European Sciences and Transcendental Phenomenology* (translated by Carr D). Northwestern University Press, Evanstown, IL.

Hutchinson DS, Henry A (2006) The health promotion of people with psychiatric disabilities. Introduction. *Psychiatric Rehabilitation Journal* **29/4**: 239–40.

Hutchinson DS, *et al.* (2006) A framework for health promotion services for people with psychiatric disabilities. *Psychiatric Rehabilitation Journal* **29/4**: 241–50.

International Early Psychosis Association Writing Group (2005) International clinical practice guidelines for early psychosis. *British Journal of Psychiatry* **187** (Suppl 48): s120–s4.

Iwaniec D, Larkin E, Higgins S (2006) Research review: risk and resilience in cases of emotional abuse. *Child and Family Social Work* **11/1**: 73–82.

Jacobson N, Greenley D (2001) What is recovery? A conceptual model and explication. *Psychiatric Services* **52**: 482–5.

Jamison KR (1997) *An Unquiet Mind*. Vintage Books.

Jerrell JM, Cousins VC, Roberts KM (2006) Psychometrics of the recovery process inventory. *Journal of Behavioral Health Services and Research* **33/4**: 464–73.

Kaltiala-Heino R, Laippala P, Salokangas RKR (1997) Impact of coercion on treatment outcome. *International Journal of Law and Psychiatry* **20/3**: 311–22.

Katsakou C, Priebe S (2006) Outcomes of involuntary hospital admission – a review. *Acta Psychiatrica Scandinavica* **114/4**: 232–41.

Katschnig H, Freeman H, Sartorius N (eds.) (2006) *Quality of Life in Mental Disorders*. 2nd ed. John Wiley, Chichester.

Kavanagh K, *et al.* (2003) Educating inpatients about their medications: is it worth it? *Journal of Mental Health* **12**: 71–80.

Kelly J, Murray RM (2002) A century of schizophrenia is enough. In: (eds.) Maj M, Sartorius N. *Schizophrenia. WPA Series Evidence and Experience in Psychiatry*, Vol 2, 2nd ed. pp 65–8. John Wiley, Chichester.

Kersting K (2003) Lessons in resilience. APA online. *Monitor on Psychology* **34/8**. www.apa.org/monitor/sep03/lessons.html (25.07.08).

Kickbusch I (2003) The contribution of the World Health Organization to a new public health and health promotion. *American Journal of Public Health* **93**: 383–8.

King G, Willoughby C, Specht JA, Brown E (2006) Social support processes and the adaptation of individuals with chronic disabilities. *Qualitative Health Research* **16/7**: 902–25.

Kjellin L, *et al.* (1997) Ethical benefits and costs of coercion in short-term inpatient psychiatric care. *Psychiatric Services* **48/12**: 1567–70.

Knuf A (2004) Vom demoralisierenden Pessimismus zum vernünftigen Optimismus. Eine Annäherung an das Recovery-Konzept. *Soziale Psychiatrie* **1**: 38–41.

Lam JN, Grossman FK (2006) Resiliency and adult adaptation in women with and without self-reported histories of childhood sexual abuse. *Journal of Traumatic Stress* **10/2**: 175–96.

Laub J, Sampson R (2003) *Shared Beginnings, Divergent Lives: Delinquent Boys to Age 70*. Harvard University Press, Cambridge, MA.

Lauber C, Nordt C, Braunschweig C, Rössler W (2006) Do mental health professionals stigmatize their patients? *Acta Psychiatrica Scandinavica* **113** (Suppl 429): 51–9.

Laugharne R, Priebe S (2006) Trust, choice and power in mental health: a literature review. *Social Psychiatry and Psychiatric Epidemiology* **41/11**: 843–52.

Lebel J, Goldstein R (2005) The economic cost of using restraint and the value added by restraint reduction or elimination. *Psychiatric Services* **56**: 1109–14.

Lecic-Tosevski D, *et al.* (2003) WPA Consensus statement on psychiatric prevention. *Dynamic Psychiatry* **36**: 307–15.

Lehtinen V (2002) The need for an integrated and need-adapted approach in treating schizophrenia. In: (eds.) Maj M, Sartorius N. *Schizophrenia. WPA Series: Evidence and Experience in Psychiatry*, Vol 2, 2nd ed. pp 235–7. John Wiley, Chichester.

Leppert K, Resilienzskala RS (2002) In: Brähler E, Schumacher J, Strauss B (eds.) *Diagnostische Verfahren in der Psychotherapie. Band 1. Diagnostik für Klinik und Praxis* (pp 295–8). Hogrefe, Göttingen.

Lester H, Gask L (2006) Delivering medical care for patients with serious mental illness or promoting a collaborative model of recovery? *British Journal of Psychiatry* **188**: 401–2.

Leucht S, Heres S (2006) Epidemiology, clinical consequences, and psychosocial treatment of nonadherence in schizophrenia. *Journal of Clinical Psychiatry* **67** (Suppl 5): 3–8.

Liberman RP, Kopelowicz A (2005) Recovery from schizophrenia: a concept in search of research. *Psychiatric Services* **56/6**: 735–42.

Link BG, Phelan JC (2001) Conceptualizing stigma. *Annual Review of Sociology* **27**: 363–85.

Link BG, *et al.* A modified labelling theory approach in the area of mental disorders: an empirical assessment. *American Sociological Review* **54**: 400–23.

Lobnig H, Krajic K, Pelikan JM (1999) The international WHO-network on health promoting hospitals: state of development of concepts and projects. In: Berger H, Krajic K, Paul R (eds.) *Health Promoting Hospitals in Practice: Developing Projects and Networks*. HPH Series Vol 3. Health Promotion Publications, Gamburg.

Lösel F (1994) Resilience in childhood and adolescence. *Children Worldwide* **21**: 8–11.

Lovell AM, Cook J, Velpry L (2008) Violence towards people with severe mental disorders: a review of the literature and of related concepts. *Revue d'Épidémiologie et de Santé Publique* **56/3**: 197–207.

Ludwig AM, Farrelly F (1966) The code of chronicity. *Archives of General Psychiatry* **15**: 562–8.

Luthar SS, Cicchetti D, Becker B (2000) The construct of resilience: a critical evaluation and guidelines for future work. *Child Development* **71/3**: 543–62.

Lutz R, Mark N (1995) Zur Gesundheit von Kranken. In: Lutz R, Mark N (eds.) *Wie gesund sind Kranke? Zur seelischen Gesundheit psychisch Kranker*. (pp 11–24) Verlag für Angewandte Psychology, Göttingen.

Lyssy R (2001) *Swiss Paradise*. Rüffer and Rub, Zürich.

Maj M, Sartorius N (eds.) (2002) Schizophrenia. WPA Series, *Evidence and Experience in Psychiatry*, Vol 2, 2nd ed. John Wiley, Chichester.

Malterud K, Hollnagel H (2004) Positive self-assessed general health in patients with medical problems – a qualitative study from general practice. *Scandinavian Journal of Primary Health Care* **22**: 11–15.

Malterud K, Hollnagel M (1999) Encouraging the strengths of women patients: a case study from general practice on empowering dialogues. *Scandinavian Journal of Public Health* **27**: 254–9.

Masten AS, Reed MG (2002) Resilience in Development. In: Snyder CR, Lopez SJ (eds.) *Handbook of Positive Psychology*. Oxford University Press, New York.

Masten AS (2001) Ordinary magic: resilience processes in development. *American Psychologist* **56**: 227–38.

Matschinger H, Angermeyer MC, Link BG (1991) Variation of response structures in relation to degree of personal involvement – a methodological study exemplified by the 'Discrimination Devaluation Scale'. *PPmP Psychotherapie, Psychosomatic, medizinische Psychologie*. **41**: 278–83.

McCabe R, Priebe S (2004) Explanatory models of illness in schizophrenia: comparison of four ethnic groups. *British Journal of Psychiatry* **185**: 25–30.

McGorry PD (1992) The concept of recovery and secondary prevention in psychotic disorders. *Australian and New Zealand Journal of Psychiatry* **26**: 3–17.

McNaught M, Caputi P, Oades LG, Deane FP (2007) Testing the validity of the Recovery Assessment Scale using an Australian sample. *Australian and New Zealand Journal of Psychiatry* **41/5**: 450–7.

Mead S, Copeland ME (2005) What recovery means to us: consumers' perspectives. In: Davidson L, Harding C, Spaniol L (eds.) *Recovery from Mental Illness: Research Evidence and Implications for Practice*. (pp 69–81) Centre for Psychiatric Rehabilitation, Boston University.

Meehan TJ, King RJ, Beavis PH, Robinson JD (2007) Recovery-based practice: do we know what we mean or mean what we know? *Australian and New Zealand Journal of Psychiatry* **42**: 177–82.

Meise U, *et al.* (2000) '. . . . not dangerous, but nevertheless frightening': A program against stigmatization of schizophrenia in schools. '. . . nicht gefährlich, aber doch furchterregend'. Ein Programm gegen Stigmatisierung von Schizophrenie in Schulen. *Psychiatrische Praxis* **27**: 340–6.

Mezzich JE (2007a) Psychiatry for the Person: articulating medicine's science and humanism. *World Psychiatry* **6/2**: 1–3.

Mezzich JE (2007b) The dialogal basis of our profession: Psychiatry *with* the Person. *World Psychiatry* **6/3**: 129–30.

Mezzich JE, Salloum IM (2007) On person-centered integrative diagnosis. *Die Psychiatrie* **4/4**: 262–5.

Mezzich JE (2005a) Positive health: conceptual place, dimensions and implications. *Psychopathology* **38/4**: 177–9.

Mezzich JE. (2005b) Proposal for a WPA Institutional Program on Psychiatry for the Person: From Clinical Care to Public Health. Paper presented and endorsed at the WPA General Assembly, World Congress of the World Psychiatric Association, Cairo, September 12, 2005.

Mezzich JE (2003) Comprehensive diagnosis as formulation and process towards health promotion. *Dynamic Psychiatry* **36**: 221–319.

Mezzich JE, Üstün TB (2002) International Classification and Diagnosis: critical experience and future directions. *Psychopathology* **35** Special issue.

Modestin J, *et al.* (2003) Long-term course of schizophrenic illness: Bleuler's study reconsidered. *American Journal of Psychiatry* **160/12**: 2202–8.

Monahan J, *et al.* (1996) Coercion to inpatient treatment: initial results and implications for assertive treatment in the community. In: Dennis DL, Monahan J (eds.) *Coercion and Aggressive Community Treatment*. Plenum Press, New York.

Mookadam F, Arthur HM (2004) Social support and its relationship to morbidity and mortality after acute myocardial infarction: systematic overview. *Archives of Internal Medicine* **164/14**: 1514–18.

Mowbray CT, Moxley DP, Collins ME (1998) Consumers as mental health providers: first-person accounts of benefits and limitations. *Journal of Behavioral Health Services and Research* **25/4**: 397–411.

Mullen KD (1986) Wellness: the missing concept in health promotion programming for adults. *Health Values* **10/3**: 34–7.

National Institute for Mental Health in England (NIMHE). *Emerging Best Practice in Mental Health Recovery*, UK Version 1, NIMHE, 2004 http://www.psychminded.co.uk/news/news2005/feb05/Emergingbestpractices.pdf

Newmann R (2005) APA's resilience initiative. *Professional Psychology: Research and Practice* **36/3**: 227–9.

New York City Department of Health and Mental Hygiene (2003) There is no health without mental health. NYC Vital Signs **2/3**: 1–4. http://www.nyc.gov/health/survey.

National Institute for Mental Health in England (2004) Emerging best practices in mental health recovery. NHS. http://www.nimhe.csip.org.uk (24.06.08).

Noordsy DL, *et al.* (2000) Recovery-oriented psychopharmacology: redefining the goals of antipsychotic treatment. *Journal of Clinical Psychiatry* **61** (Suppl 3): 22–9.

Oades L, *et al.* (2005). Collaborative recovery: an integrative model for working with individuals who experience chronic and recurring mental illness. *Australasian Psychiatry* **13**: 279–84.

O'Connell MJ, *et al.* (2005) From rhetoric to routine: assessing recovery-oriented practices in a state mental health and addiction system. *Psychiatric Rehabilitation Journal* **28/4**: 378–86.

Ogawa K, *et al.* (1987) A long-term follow-up study of schizophrenia in Japan – with special reference to the course of social adjustment. *British Journal of Psychiatry* **151**: 758–65.

Olds D, Hill P, Mihalic S, O'Brien R (1998) *Blueprints for Violence Prevention. Book Seven: Prenatal and Infancy Home Visitation by Nurses*. Center for the Study and Prevention of Violence, Boulder, CO.

Onken SJ, *et al.* (2007) An analysis of the definitions and elements of recovery: a review of the literature. *Psychiatric Rehabilitation Journal* **31/1**: 9–22.

Onken SJ, *et al.* (2002) *Mental Health Recovery: What Helps and What Hinders?* A National Research Project for the Development of Recovery Facilitating Performance Indicators. Phase I Research Report: a National Study of Consumer Perspectives. National Technical Assistance Center, National Association of State Mental Health Program Directors, Alexandria (VA).

Opp G, Fingerle M, Freytag A (eds.) (1999) *Was Kinder stärkt. Erziehung zwischen Risiko und Resilienz*. Ernst Reinhardt, München.

Orley J (1998) Application of promotion principles. In: Jenkins R, Üstün TB (eds.) *Preventing Mental Illness: Mental Health Promotion in Primary Care* (pp 469–77). John Wiley, Chichester.

Oshio A, Kaneko H, Nagamine S, Nakaya M (2003) Construct validity of the Adolescent Resilience Scale. *Psychological Reports* **93**: 1217–22.

Othaganont P, Sinthuvorakan C, Jensupakarn P (2002) Daily living practice of the life-satisfied Thai elderly. *Transcultural Nursing* **13/1**: 24–9.

Parker C (2001) First person account: landing a Mars lander. *Schizophrenia Bulletin* **27**: 717–18.

Parnas J (2002) On defining schizophrenia. In: (eds. Maj M, N Sartorius N). *Schizophrenia. WPA Series Evidence and Experience in Psychiatry*, Vol 2, 2nd ed.), pp 43–5. John Wiley, Chichester.

Peebles SA, *et al.* (2007) Recovery and systems transformation for schizophrenia. *Psychiatric Clinics of North America* **30**: 567–83.

Perkins L (2003) Personal accounts: mental illness, motherhood, and me. *Psychiatric Services* **54**: 157–8.

Pescosolido B, Gardner CB, Lubell KM (1998) How people get into mental health services: stories of choice, coercion and 'muddling through'. *Social Science and Medicine* **46**: 275–86.

Phelan JC (2002) The stigma of mental illness: some empirical findings. In: (eds.) Maj M, Sartorius N. *Schizophrenia. WPA Series Evidence and Experience in Psychiatry* Vol 2, 2nd ed. pp 287–9. John Wiley, Chichester.

Phelan JC, Link BG (1998) The growing belief that people with mental illnesses are violent: the role of the dangerousness criterion for civil commitment. *Social Psychiatry and Psychiatric Epidemiology* **33**: 7–12.

Pollard JA, Hawkins JD, Arthur MW (1999) Risk and protection: are both necessary to understand diverse behavioural outcomes in adolescence? *Social Work Research* **23**: 145–58.

Priebe S, McCabe R (2006) The therapeutic relationship in psychiatric settings. *Acta Psychiatrica Scandinavica* **113** (Suppl 429): 69–72.

Priebe S (2003) The future of psychiatric care – dreams and nightmares. *Psychiatrische Praxis* **30** (Suppl) S48–S53.

Priebe S, Broker M, Gunkel S (1998) Involuntary admission and posttraumatic stress disorder symptoms in schizophrenia patients. *Comprehensive Psychiatry* **39/4**: 220–4.

Pull CB (2002) The diagnosis of schizophrenia: a review. In: (eds. Maj M, Sartorius N). *Schizophrenia. WPA Series Evidence and Experience in Psychiatry*, Vol 2, 2nd ed (pp 1–37) John Wiley, Chichester.

Puschner B, *et al.* (2005). Compliance-Interventionen in der medikamentösen Behandlung Schizophrenieerkrankter. Befunde aktueller Übersichtsarbeiten. *Psychiatrische Praxis* **32**: 62–7.

Rabinowitz J, Levine SZ, Haim R, Häfner H (2007) The course of schizophrenia: progressive deterioration, amelioration or both? *Schizophrenia Research* **91**: 254–8.

Raeburn J, Rootman I (1998) *People-centred Health Promotion*. John Wiley, Chichester.

Ralph RO (2004) Verbal and visual definitions of recovery: focus on Recovery Advisory Group recovery model. In: Ralph RO, Corrigan PW (eds.) *Recovery in Mental Illness: Broadening our Understanding of Wellness*. American Psychological Association, Washington, DC.

Ralph RO, Corrigan PW (2004) *Recovery in Mental Illness: Broadening our Understanding of Wellness*. American Psychological Association, Washington, DC.

Ralph RO, Kidder K (2000) *What is Recovery? A Compendium of Recovery and Recovery Related instruments*. Human Services Research Institute, Cambridge, MA.

Ralph RO, Kidder K, Phillips D (2000) *Can we measure Recovery?* www.ccamhr.ca/resources/A_Compendium_of_Recovery_Measures1.pdf (31.08.08).

Ralph RO (2000a) Introduction. Consumer contributions to mental health: a report of the Surgeon General. *Psychiatric Rehabilitation Skills* **4/3**: 379–82.

Ralph RO (2000b) *Review of recovery literature: a synthesis of a sample of recovery literature* 2000. http://www.nasmhpd.org/general_files/publications/ntac_pubs/reports/ralphrecovweb.pdf (31.08.08)

Ralph RO, *et al.* (1999) *Recovery advisory group recovery model, a work in progress*. Presentation at the National Mental Health Statistics Conference, Washington, DC, June 1999. www.mhsip.org/recovery (31.08.08).

Ramon S, Healy B, Renouf N (2007) Recovery from mental illness as an emerging concept and practice in Australia and the UK. *International Journal of Social Psychiatry* **53/2**: 108–22.

Raphael B, Schmolke M, Wooding S (2005) Interrelationships between mental and physical health and illness. In: Herrman H, Saxena S, Moodie R (eds.) *Promoting Mental Health: Concepts, Evidence and Practice. A report of the World Health Organization, in collaboration with the Victorian Health Promotion Foundation and the University of Melbourne*. WHO, Geneva.

Rapp CA (1998) *The Strengths Model*. Oxford University Press, New York.

Rapp CA, Wintersteen R (1989) The strengths model of case management: results from twelve demonstrations. *Psychosocial Rehabilitation Journal* **13/1**: 23–32.

Rappaport J (1981) In praise of paradox: a social policy of empowerment over prevention. *American Journal of Community Psychology* **9/1**: 1–25.

Ray O (2005) Psycho-neuro-endocrino-immunology perspectives on resilience. Paper presented at the symposium on Resilience in mental health promotion: interdisciplinary perspectives. Chairs: M Schmolke, O Ray. World Congress of the World Psychiatric Association September 10–15, 2005, Cairo.

Read J, Perry BD, Moskowitz A, Connolly J (2001) The contribution of early traumatic events to schizophrenia in some patients: a traumagenic neurodevelopmental model. *Psychiatry* **64/4**: 319–45.

Repper J, Perkins R (2003) *Social Inclusion and Recovery: a Model for Mental Health Practice*. Elsevier Health Sciences, London.

Rettenbacher MA, Burns T, Kemmler G, Fleischhacker WW (2004) Schizophrenia: attitudes of patients and professional carers towards the illness and antipsychotic medication. *Pharmacopsychiatry* **37**: 103–9.

Resnick SG, Fontana A, Lehman AF, Rosenheck RA (2005) An empirical conceptualization of the recovery orientation. *Schizophrenia Research* **75**: 119–28.

Riba M (2005) The value of resilience in psycho-oncology. Paper presented at the symposium on Resilience in mental health promotion: interdisciplinary perspectives. Chairs: M Schmolke, O Ray. World Congress of the World Psychiatric Association, September 10–15, 2005, Cairo.

Richardson CR (2005) Integrating physical activity into mental health services for persons with serious mental illness. *Psychiatric Services* **56/3**: 324–31.

Richardson G (2002) Mental health promotion through resilience and resiliency education. *International Journal of Emergency Mental Health* **4/1**: 65–76.

Ridgeway P, *et al.* (2002) *Pathways to Recovery: a Strengths Recovery Self-help Workbook*. University of Kansas School of Social Work, Office of Mental Health Research and Training, Lawrence, KS.

Riecher-Rössler A, *et al.* (2006) Early detection and treatment of schizophrenia: how early? *Acta Psychiatrica Scandinavica* **113** (Suppl 429): 73–80.

Riecher-Rössler A, Rössler W (1993) Compulsory admission of psychiatric patients – an international comparison. *Acta Psychiatrica Scandinavica* **87**: 231–6.

Riecher A, Rössler W, Löffler W, Fatkenheuer B (1991) Factors influencing compulsory admission of psychiatric patients. *Psychology and Medicine* **21/1**: 197–208.

Riedel-Heller SG, Matschinger H, Angermeyer MC (2005) Mental disorders – who and what might help? Help-seeking and treatment preferences of the lay public. *Social Psychiatry and Epidemiology* **40**: 167–74.

Ritsher JB, Otilingam PG, Grajales M (2003) Internalized stigma of mental illness: psychometric properties of a new measure. *Psychiatry Research* **121**: 31–49.

Ritsher JB, Phelan JC (2004) Internalized stigma predicts erosion of morale among psychiatric outpatients. *Psychiatry Research* **129**: 257–65.

Roberts G, Hollins S (2007) Recovery: our common purpose? *Advances in Psychiatric Treatment* **13**: 397–9.

Robins CS, *et al.* (2005) Consumers' perceptions of negative experiences and 'sanctuary harm' in psychiatric settings. *Psychiatric Services* **56**: 1134–8.

Roe D, Chopra M, Rudnick A (2004) Persons with psychosis as active agents interacting with their disorder. *Psychiatric Rehabilitation Journal* **28**: 122–8.

Rogers A, *et al.* (1998) The meaning and management of neuroleptic medication: a study of patients with a diagnosis of schizophrenia. *Social Science and Medicine* **47**: 1313–23.

Romme M, Escher S (1993) *Accepting Voices*. MIND, London.

Rose D, Thornicroft G, Slade M (2006) Who decides what evidence is? Developing a multiple perspectives paradigm in mental health. *Acta Psychiatrica Scandinavica* **113** (Suppl 429) 109–14.

Rose D (2003a) Having a diagnosis is a qualification for the job. *BMJ* **326**: 1331.

Rose D (2003b) Collaborative research between users and professionals: peaks and pitfalls. *Psychiatric Bulletin* **27**: 404–6.

Rose D, *et al.* (2003) Patients' perspectives on electroconvulsive therapy: systematic review. *BMJ* **326**: 1363.

Rose D (2001) *Users' Voices: the Perspective of Mental Health Service Users on Community and Hospital Care*. London, Sainsbury Centre for Mental Health.

Roessler W, *et al.* (1999) Does the place of treatment influence the quality of life of schizophrenics? *Acta Psychiatrica Scandinavica* **100**: 142–8.

Royal College of Psychiatrists (1995) *Fact sheet on ECT*. RCP, London.

Royle J, Oliver S (2001) Consumers are helping to prioritize research. *BMJ* **253**: 48–9.

Rüsch N, Angermeyer MC, Corrigan PW (2005a) Mental illness stigma: concepts, consequences, and initiatives to reduce stigma. *European Psychiatry* **20**: 529–39.

Rüsch N, Angermeyer MC, Corrigan PW (2005b) Das Stigma psychischer Erkrankung: Konzepte, Formen und Folgen. *Psychiatrische Praxis* **32**: 221–32.

Rutter D, *et al.* (2004) Patients or partners? Case studies of user involvement in the planning and delivery of adult mental health services in London. *Social Science and Medicine* **58**: 1973–84.

Rutter M (2006) Implications of resilience concepts for scientific understanding. *Annals of the New York Academy of Sciences* **1094**: 1–12.

Rutter M (2005) The promotion of resilience in the face of adversity. Paper given at the conference on Resilience – Development in Spite of Adversities, organised by the Training Institute of Systemic Therapy and Counselling, Zürich, February 9–12, 2005. Available on CD by Auditorium Verlag, Schwarzach/M., duenninger@t-online.de

Rutter M (1999) Resilience concepts and findings: implications for family therapy. *Journal of Family Therapy* **21/2**: 119–44.

Rutter M (1995) Psychosocial adversity: risk, resilience and recovery. *Southern African Journal of Child and Adolescent Mental Health* **7/2**: 75–88.

Rutter M (1985) Resilience in the face of adversity. Protective factors and resistance to psychiatric disorder. *British Journal of Psychiatry* **147**: 598–611.

Sadler JZ, Fulford B (2004) Should patients and their families contribute to the DSM-V process? *Psychiatric Services* **55/2**: 133–8.

Salyers MP, Tsai J, Stultz TA (2007) Measuring recovery orientation in a hospital setting. *Psychiatric Rehabilitation Journal* **31/2**: 131–7.

Sartorius N (2002) Iatrogenic stigma of mental illness. *BMJ* **324**: 1470–1.

Saxena S, Thornicroft G, Knapp M, Whiteford H (2007) Resources for mental health: scarcity, inequity, and inefficiency. *The Lancet* **370**: 878–89.

Sayce L (2000) *From Psychiatric Patient to Citizen. Overcoming Discrimination and Social Exclusion*. Macmillan Press, London.

Scheier MF, Carver CS, Bridges MW (1994) Distinguishing optimism from neuroticism (and trait anxiety, self mastery, and self-esteem): a re-evaluation of the Life Orientation Test. *Journal of Personality and Social Psychology* **67/6**: 1063–78.

Scherman MH, Lowhagen O (2004) Drug compliance and identity: reasons for non-compliance – experiences of medication from persons with asthma/allergy. *Patient Education and Counseling* **54**: 3–9.

Schmolke M (2005) The concept of resilience in psychological research. Paper presented at the symposium on Resilience in mental health promotion: interdisciplinary perspectives. Chairs: M Schmolke, O Ray. World Congress of the World Psychiatric Association, September 10–15, 2005, Cairo.

Schmolke M, Lecic-Tosevski D (eds.) (2003a) Health promotion – an integral component of effective clinical care. Special Issue. *Dynamic Psychiatry* 36: 221–319.

Schmolke M, Lecic-Tosevski D (eds.) (2003b) Editorial. Health promotion – an integral component of effective clinical care. *Dynamic Psychiatry* 36: 221–230.

Schmolke M (2001) *Gesundheitsressourcen im Lebensalltag schizophrener Menschen. Eine empirische Untersuchung*. Psychiatrie-Verlag, Bonn.

Schore A (2001) Effects of a secure attachment relationship on right brain development, affect regulation, and infant mental health. *Infant Mental Health Journal* **22/1–2**: 7–66.

Schrank B, Stanghellini G, Slade M (2008) Hope in psychiatry: a review of the literature. *Acta Psychiatrica Scandinavica* **118/6**: 421–33.

Schrank B, *et al.* (2006) Schizophrenia and psychosis on the Internet. Schizophrenie und Psychose im Internet. *Psychiatrische Praxis* **33**: 277–81.

Schürmann I (1997) Beziehungsformen zwischen Langzeitnutzern und Professionellen im Kontext der Moderne. In: Zaumseil M, Leferink K (eds.) *Schizophrenie in der Moderne - Modernisierung der Schizophrenie*.(239–79) Edition Das Narrenschiff im Psychiatrie Verlag, Bonn.

Seedhouse D (2002) *Total Mental Health Promotion: Mental Health, Rational Fields and the Quest for Autonomy*. John Wiley, Chichester.

Seikkula J, *et al.* (2006) Five year experience of first episode non-affective psychosis in open dialogue approach: treatment principles, follow-up outcomes and two case studies. *Psychotherapy Research* **16/2**: 214–28.

Seikkula J, Trimble D (2005) Healing elements of therapeutic conversation: dialogue as an embodiment of love. *Family Process* **44/4**: 461–75.

Seikkula J, Olson ME (2003) The open dialogue approach to acute psychosis: its poetics and micropolitics. *Family Process* **42/3**: 403–18.

Seligman M, Peterson C (2003) Positive clinical psychology. In: Aspinwall LG, Staudinger UM (eds.) *A Psychology of Human Strengths. Fundamental Questions and Future Directions for a Positive Psychology.* (pp 305–17) American Psychological Association, Washington, DC.

Seligman, MEP (1975) *Helplessness: on Depression, Development and Death.* Freeman, San Francisco.

Shaw K, McFarlane A, Bookless C (1997) The phenomenology of traumatic reactions to psychotic illness. *Journal of Nervous and Mental Disease* **185/7**: 434–41.

Shih M (2004) Positive stigma: examining resilience and empowerment in overcoming stigma. *Annals of The American Academy of Political and Social Science* **591**: 175–85.

Shin S, Lukens EP (2002) Effects of psycho-education for Korean Americans with chronic mental illness. *Psychiatric Services* **53**: 1125–31.

Sibitz I, Katschnig H, Goessler R, Amering M (2006) 'knowing – enjoying – better living' – a seminar for persons with psychosis to improve their quality of life and reduce their vulnerability. *Psychiatrische Praxis* **33/4**: 170–6.

Sibitz I, *et al.* (2005) 'Pharmacophilia' and 'pharmacophobia' – determinants of patients' attitudes towards antipsychotic medication. *Pharmacopsychiatry* **38/3**: 107–12.

Sibitz I, Amering M (2003) Wissen – Geniessen – Besser leben: Ein Seminar für Menschen mit Psychoseerfahrung. Pro mente sana aktuell zum Themenschwerpunkt 'NutzerInnen-Orientierung: Ein Konzept wird konkret'. *Heft* **3**: 30–1.

Smith GM, *et al.* (2005) Pennsylvania State Hospital system's seclusion and restraint reduction program. *Psychiatric Services* **56**: 1115–22.

Silverstein SM, Bellack AS (2008) A scientific agenda for the concept of recovery as it applies to schizophrenia. *Clinical Psychology Review*, doi: 10.1016/j.cpr.2008.03.004

Slade M, Amering M, Oades L (2008) Recovery. An international perspective. *Epidemiologia e Psichiatria Sociale* **17/2**: 128–37.

Slade M, Hayward M (2007) Recovery, psychosis and psychiatry: research is better than rhetoric. *Acta Psychiatrica Scandinavia* **116**: 81–3.

Solomon P (2004) Peer support/peer provided services underlying processes, benefits, and critical ingredients. *Psychiatric Rehabilitation Journal* **27/4**: 392–401.

Sowers W (2007) Recovery: an opportunity to transcend our differences. *Psychiatric Services* **58/1**: 5.

Sowers W/Quality Management Committee of the American Association of Community Psychiatrists (2005) Transforming systems of care: the American Association of Community Psychiatrists' guidelines for recovery oriented services. *Community Mental Health Journal* **41/6**: 757–74.

Spagnolo AB, Murphy AA, Librera LA (2008) Reducing stigma by meeting and learning from people with mental illness. *Psychiatric Rehabilitation Journal* **31/3**: 186–93.

Stastny P, Lehmann P (2007) (eds.) *Alternatives Beyond Psychiatry.* Peter Lehmann Publishing, Shrewsbury UK, Eugene, OR, USA.

Stastny P, Amering M (2006) Consumer-interests and the quality of life concept – common ground or parallel universes? In: (eds.) Katschnig H, Freeman H, Sartorius N. *Quality of Life in Mental disorders* pp 175–83. 2nd ed, John Wiley, Chichester.

Stastny P (2004) Strukturelle Etablierung von Empowerment-Projekten. Chancen und Grenzen am Beispiel der USA. In: (hrsg.) A Knuf, U Seibert. *Selbstbefähigung fördern. Empowerment und psychiatrische Arbeit.* Psychiatrie-Verlag, Bonn.

Strauss JS (2008) Prognosis in schizophrenia and the role of subjectivity. *Schizophrenia Bulletin* **34/2**: 201–3.

Strauss JS (1989) Subjective experiences of schizophrenia: toward a new dynamic psychiatry – II. *Schizophrenia Bulletin* **15/2**: 179–87.

Strauss JS, Harding CM, Hafez H, Liberman P (1987) The role of the patient in recovery from psychosis. In: (eds.) Strauss JS, Böker W, Brenner H. *Psychosocial Treatment of Schizophrenia* (pp 160–6). Hans Huber, Toronto.

Strauss JS, *et al.* (1985) The course of psychiatric disorders. III: longitudinal principles. *British Journal of Psychiatry* **155**: 128–32.

Svanberg POG (1998) Attachment, resilience and prevention. *Journal of Mental Health* **7/6**: 543–78.

Swartz MS, *et al.* (2001) Effects of involuntary outpatient commitment and depot antipsychotics on treatment adherence in persons with severe mental illness. *Journal of Nervous and Mental Disease* **189/9**: 583–92.

Tait L, Lester H (2005) Encouraging user involvement in mental health services. *Advances in Psychiatric Treatment* **11**: 168–75.

Tammet D (2007) *Born on a Blue Day*. Schuster and Schuster, New York. http://www. mtholyoke.edu/acad/misc/profile/names/ghornste.shtml *Bibliography of First-Person Narratives of Madness*, 3rd ed.

Telford R, Faulkner A (2004) Learning about service user involvement in mental health research. *Journal of Mental Health* **13/6**: 549–59.

Thornicroft G (2006) *SHUNNED: Discrimination against People with Mental Illness*. Oxford University Press, Oxford.

Thornicroft G, Tansella M (2005) Growing recognition of the importance of service user involvement in mental health service planning and evaluation. *Epidemiologie Psychiatria Sociale* **14/1**: 1–3.

Thornton H (2002) Patient perspectives on involvement in cancer research in the UK. *European Journal of Cancer Care* **11**: 205–9.

Tondora J, Davidson L (2006) Practice Guidelines for Recovery Oriented Behavioral Health care. Department of Mental Health and Addiction Services, Hartford, CT. http://www.ct.gov/dmhas/LIB/dmhas/publications/practiceguidelines.pdf (20.08.08).

Tones K, Tilford S (2003) An empowerment model of health promotion. In: Sidell M I *et al.* (eds.) *Debates and Dilemmas in Promoting Health. A Reader*. 2nd ed. Palgrave, McMillan/OPU, Basingstoke.

Topor A (2001) *Managing the contradictions. Recovery from Severe Mental Disorders*. Stockholm Studies of Social Work 18. Akademitryck AB, Edsbruk, Sweden.

Townsend W, *et al.* (1999) Emerging best practices in mental health recovery. Ohio Department of Mental Health. http://www.tacinc.org/Docs/HS/MHRecovery.pdf (24.06.08).

Trivedi P, Wykes T (2002) From passive subjects to equal partners. Qualitative review of user involvement in research. *British Journal of Psychiatry* **181**: 468–72.

Turner-Crowson J, Wallcraft J (2002) The recovery vision for mental health services and research: a British perspective. *Psychiatric Rehabilitation Journal* **25/3**: 245–54.

Tyreman S (2005) The expert patient: outline of UK government paper. *Medicine, Health Care and Philosophy* **8**: 149–51.

Tyrer P (2002) Commentary: Research into mental health services needs a new approach. *Psychiatric Bulletin* **26**: 406–7.

US Department of Health and Human Services (1999) *Mental Health: A Report of the Surgeon General – Executive Summary*. US Department of Health and Human Services, Substance Abuse and Mental Health Services Administration (SAMHSA), Center for Mental Health Services, National Institute of Health, National Institute of Mental Health, Rockeville, MD.

US Department of Health and Human Services (2003) President's New Freedom Commission on Mental Health. http://www.mentalhealthcommission.gov/reports/FinalReport/downloads/FinalReport.pdf.page 1 (30.08.08).

Van Os J, *et al.* (2006) Standardized remission criteria in schizophrenia. *Acta Psychiatrica Scandinavica* **113**: 91–5.

Vieta E (2005) Improving treatment adherence in bipolar disorder through psychoeducation. *Journal of Clinical Psychiatry* **66** Suppl 1: 24–9.

Vogelsanger V (1999) Gesünder durch Selbsthilfegruppen. *Pro Mente Sana Aktuell* **2**: 14–15.

Wahl OF (1999) Mental health consumers' experience of stigma. *Schizophrenia Bulletin* **25**: 467–78.

Wagnild GM, Young HM (1993) Development and psychometric evaluation of the Resilience Scale. *Journal of Nursing Measurement* **1/2**: 165–178.

Walker L, Rowling R (2002) Debates, confusion, collaboration and emerging practice. In: Rowling L, Martin G, Walker L (eds.) *Mental Health Promotion and Young People: Concepts and Practice* (pp 1–9). McGraw Hill, Sydney.

Wallcraft J, Schrank B, Amering M. (in press) *Handbook of Service User Involvement in Mental Health Research*. Wiley-Blackwell, Chichester.

Walsh F (1998) *Strengthening Family Resilience*. Guilford Press, New York.

Ware NC, *et al.* (2008) A theory of social integration as quality of life. *Psychiatric Services* **59/1**: 27–33.

Ware NC, *et al.* (2007) Connectedness and citizenship: redefining social integration. *Psychiatric Services* **58**: 469–74.

Warner R (2007) Review of Recovery from Schizophrenia: an International Perspective. A Report from the WHO Collaborative Project, the International Study of Schizophrenia. *American Journal of Psychiatry* **164**: 1444–5.

Warner R (2004) *Recovery from Schizophrenia. Psychiatry and Political Economy* (3rd ed). Brunner-Routledge, New York.

Warner R (2002) Reducing the stigma associated with schizophrenia. In: (eds.) Maj M, Sartorius N. *Schizophrenia. WPA Series Evidence and Experience in Psychiatry* Vol 2, 2nd ed pp 290–2. John Wiley, Chichester. http://www.mhsip.org/2003%20presentations/Plenary/RidgewayPlenary.pdf

Warner R (1999) The emics and etics of quality of life assessment. *Social Psychiatry and Psychiatric Epidemiology* **34/3**: 117–21.

Warner R, Taylor D, Powers M, Hyman J (1989) Acceptance of the mental illness label by psychotic patients: effects on functioning. *American Journal of Orthopsychiatry* **59**: 398–409.

Welter-Enderlin R, Hildenbrand B (eds.) (2006) *Resilienz – Gedeihen trotz widriger Umstände*. Carl Auer, Heidelberg.

Werner EE, Smith RS (2001) *Journeys from Childhood to Midlife: Risk, Resilience, and Recovery*. Cornell University Press, Ithaca, NY.

Werner EE (1993) Risk, resilience and recovery: perspectives from the Kauai longitudinal study. *Development and Psychopathology* **5**: 503–15.

WHO European Ministerial Conference on Mental Health. (2005a) Mental Health Action Plan for Europe: Facing the Challenges, Building Solutions. Helsinki, Finland, 12–15 January 2005. EUR/04/5047810/7.

WHO (2005b) Mental Health Declaration for Europe: Facing the Challenges, Building Solutions. http://www.euro.who.int/document/mnh/edoc06.pdf. (08.03.08)

WHO (2001) *Strengthening mental health promotion*. Fact Sheet no 220. World Health Organization, Geneva.

WHO, UNESCO, UNICEF (1992) Comprehensive school health promotion. Suggested guidelines for action. *Hygie* **11/3**: 8–15.

WHO (1992) *The ICD-10 Classification of Mental and Behavioural Disorders: Clinical Descriptions and Diagnostic Guidelines*. WHO, Geneva.

WHO (1986) *Ottawa Charter of Health Promotion*. WHO, Geneva.

Wiersma D (2006) Needs of people with severe mental illness. *Acta Psychiatrica Scandinavica* **113** (Suppl 429): 115–19.

Williams B, Healy D (2001) Perceptions of illness causation among new referrals to a community mental health team: 'explanatory models' or 'exploratory map'? *Social Science and Medicine* **53**: 465–76.

Williams L (1998) A 'classic' case of borderline personality disorder. *Psychiatric Services* **49**: 173–4.

Wisdom JP, *et al.* (2008): 'Stealing me from myself': identity and recovery in personal accounts of mental illness. *Australian and New Zealand Journal of Psychiatry* **42**: 489–95.

Wolff S (1995) The concept of resilience. *Australia and New Zealand Journal of Psychiatry* **29/4**: 565–74.

Woodbridge K, Fulford B (2004) *Whose Values? A Work-book for Value-based Practice in Mental Health Care*. The Sainsbury Centre for Mental Health, London

WPA (2003) Essentials of the World Psychiatric Association's International Guidelines for Diagnostic Assessment (IGDA). *British Journal of Psychiatry* **182** (Suppl 45): 37–66.

Wustmann C (2004) Resilienz. Widerstandsfähigkeit von Kindern in Tageseinrichtungen foerdern. Beltz, Weinheim.

Wüstner K (2001) Subjective theories of illness as objective for genetic counselling – the Wiedemann-Beckwith-syndrome as example. *Psychotherapy Psychosomatic Medicine and Psychology* **51/8**: 308–19.

Young SL, Ensing DS (1999) Exploring recovery from the perspective of people with psychiatric disabilities. *Psychiatric Rehabilitation Journal* **22**: 219–31.

Zygmunt A, Olfson M, Boyer CA, Mechanic D (2002) Interventions to improve medication adherence in schizophrenia. *American Journal of Psychiatry* **159**: 1653–64.

Index